BASIC
ENVIRONMENTAL
HEALTH

BASIC ENVIRONMENTAL HEALTH

Annalee Yassi
Tord Kjellström
Theo de Kok
Tee L. Guidotti

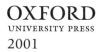

OXFORD
UNIVERSITY PRESS
2001

OXFORD
UNIVERSITY PRESS

Oxford   New York

Athens   Auckland   Bangkok   Bogotá   Buenos Aires   Calcutta
Cape Town   Chennai   Dar es Salaam   Delhi   Florence   Hong Kong   Istanbul
Karachi   Kuala Lumpur   Madrid   Melbourne   Mexico City   Mumbai
Nairobi   Paris   São Paulo   Shanghai   Singapore   Taipei   Tokyo   Toronto   Warsaw

and associated companies in
Berlin   Ibadan

Copyright © 2001 by the World Health Organization

Published by Oxford University Press, Inc.,
198 Madison Avenue, New York, New York, 10016
http://www.oup-usa.org

Oxford is a registered trademark of Oxford University Press.

Library of Congress Cataloging-in-Publication Data
Basic environmental health / Annalee Yassi . . . [et al.].
p. cm.   Includes bibliographical references and index.
ISBN 0-19-513558-X
1. Environmental health.
I. Yassi, Annalee.
RA565.B376 2001   615.9′02—dc21   00-032400

9 8 7 6 5

Printed in the United States of America
on acid-free paper

PREFACE

This book is intended to be used as a textbook at the university level. It is basic and interdisciplinary in its approach, in recognition of the wide variety of professional groups for whom training in environmental health is desirable. The text is only one component of a "teaching kit" in environmental health; a Teacher's Guide, with a variety of interactive exercises, and a chart book of tables and graphs, ready for transparency projection, supplement the text (available from EHG, WHO, 1211 Geneva, Switzerland, Fax: +41-22-7914123, email:pfistera@ who.ch; www.who.int/[search the Environment program]).

The target groups for the book include university students in public health, medicine, nursing, other health professions, engineering, environmental science, management, and others needing a basic introduction to environmental health (including students interested in environmental law, geography, urban planning and social work). The book and the teaching kit can be used in courses to form a component of a traditional program at university level, or in stand-alone courses for in-service training of government agency staff, industry professionals and managers, and interested people in non-governmental organizations or community groups.

The textbook is divided into 12 chapters, each with defined objectives. The first section, Chapters 1–4, introduces the concepts and methods applied in environmental health. Chapter 1 is an overview of the macro-level influences on health, touching on various social science disciplines. Chapter 2 describes the nature of environmental health hazards, introducing toxicology, microbiology, health physics, injury analysis, and psychosocial concepts. Chapter 3 lays out the basic approach to risk assessment and includes a discussion of epidemiological methods. Chapter 4 outlines the principles of risk management. The second section organizes the discussion by route of exposure. Chapter 5 addresses air quality; Chapter 6 water and sanitation; and Chapter 7 food and agricultural issues. The third section is sustainable development: Chapter 8—settlements and urbanisation, Chapter 9–energy, Chapter 10–industry, and Chapter 11–global concerns. Chapter 12 ties the course together focusing on ethical issues and the concrete application of the course material.

Thus the book can form the basis of a full semester course or its equivalent. While it is meant to be a "primer," extensive referencing to other publications should allow as comprehensive a coverage of any topic as the educational setting requires.

The problem solving exercises in the Teacher's Guide can be used to adjust the level of complexity of the course for individual students or the class as a whole. In interdisciplinary classes, for example, the teacher may require more in-depth research from students in the areas of their own disciplines compared to others in different disciplines, who would in turn focus on areas of their own expertise. This permits each student to achieve a maximum learning experience while contributing optimally to the group. It also simulates the real world scenario in which professionals in different disciplines are expected to understand each other, while depending on each other for the more complex details.

The text and teaching kit are part of a sustained effort by WHO, UNEP, UNESCO, and CRE to promote strengthened teaching in environmental health for a wide variety of students at university level.

Winnipeg, Manitoba, Canada   A.Y.
Auckland, New Zealand   T.K.

ACKNOWLEDGMENTS

This text was developed with the assistance of the United Nations Environment Programme (UNEP), Conference of European University Rectors (CRE), and the United Nations Educational Scientific and Cultural Organisation (UNESCO), and under the overall auspices of the Office of Global and Integrated Environmental Health of the World Health Organisation (WHO). It was tested at workshops in Visby, Sweden; Budapest, Hungary; Cape Town, South Africa; and Amman, Jordan where valuable comments were provided by the participants. Comments received in meetings of reviewers held in Geneva in June 1994 and November 1995, and by many others were also incorporated.

Dr. Theo de Kok (University Maastricht, The Netherlands), the third author of the book, has been developing distance learning materials, in conjunction with this text. Merri Weinger (education specialist, WHO) is the primary author of the Teacher's Guide.

There are many people who have made valuable contributions to this text to date; these and others will hopefully continue to contribute by supplying case studies from which others could learn. Among the many contributors, several stand out for specific mention.

Dr. Jerry Spiegel (formerly of Manitoba Environment, Winnipeg, Canada and now with the Liu Centre for the study of Global Issues at the University of British Columbia, Vancouver, Canada) served as the major editor of the book and contributed substantially to the chapter on risk management. He also wrote a large section of the industry chapter and extensively rewrote other parts of the text.

Dr. Alan Pinter (Johan Béla National Institute of Health [NIH], Budapest, Hungary), and Dr. Evert Nieboer (McMaster University, Hamilton, Canada) both had substantial input to the book, particularly to the toxicology sections, and Dr. Avrum Regenstreif had major input to the chapter on settlements and urban development. The following individuals (listed in alphabetical order) also served as reviewers and contributed valuable comments and materials:

Dr. Pedro Más Bermejo, Director, National Institute of Hygiene Epidemiology and Microbiology, La Habana, Cuba

Dr. Helen Dolk, London School of Hygiene and Tropical Medicine, London, UK

Professor Hunay Evliya, Cukurova University, Turkey

Professor Maria Alvim Ferraz, University of Oporto, Portugal

Professor H.N.B. Gopalan, UNEP, Nairobi, Kenya

Dr. Steve Hrudey, University of Alberta, Canada

Dr. Steven Markowitz, Mount Sinai School of Medicine, New York, USA

Dr. S. Miyagawa, Division of Food and Nutrition, WHO, Geneva

Dr. Monica Nordberg, Karolinska Institute, Stockholm, Sweden

Dr. Peter Orris, Cook County Hospital, Chicago, USA

Dr. Peri Pamir, CRE, Geneva

Dr. David Rapport, University Guelph, Canada

Dr. Yasmin von Schirnding, Environmental Health, Johannesburg, South Africa

Dr. Colin Soskolne, University of Alberta, Canada

Dr. Carl-Einar Stalvant, Stockholm University, Sweden

Ms. Adrienne Taylor, Auckland, New Zealand

Professor Dr. Henk van de Plas, Copernicus Steering Committee, The Netherlands

Dr. Susan van de Vynckt, UNESCO, Paris

and others.

In addition, valuable assistance in assembling the material was provided by Sandrine Chorro (France), and Elissa Neville and Ingra Schellenberg (Canada). The enormous help provided by Simone Beaudet, Lisa Springer, Mavis Puchlik, Dr. Sande Harlos, and Dr. Anthony Morham at the University of Manitoba (Canada) was invaluable; as was the editing assistance provided by Donne Flanigan and Jennifer Dundas. The skillful proofreading and editing conducted by Myrna McGill was especially appreciated.

The support of the Occupational and Environmental Health Unit in the Department of Community Health Sciences at the University of Manitoba, where this book was drafted, rewritten, edited and assembled, deserves special recognition. This project was partially funded through a Programme Development Grant from this University.

The Occupational Health Program of the University of Alberta (Canada) contributed to the production of this work and managed final preparation of the figures. The artwork was drawn, adapted, or enhanced for this book by Ms. Sam Motyka, Health Sciences Media Services, University of Alberta Hospitals, Capital Health Authority, Edmonton, Alberta (Canada). Funding for the preparation of some figures came from the Tripartite Fund for Occupational Health at the University of Alberta.

The final review and editing was coordinated by Dr. Tord Kjellström at the University of Auckland with the assistance of Suzanne Jackson and Adrienne Taylor.

CONTENTS

BASIC
ENVIRONMENTAL
HEALTH

1

INTRODUCTION

LEARNING OBJECTIVES

After studying this chapter you will be able to do the following:

- explain the basic relationship between environmental factors and health, and how the interrelationship between economic development, the environment, and health can be seen in an ecosystem framework
- interpret environmental health in historical context with respect to changes in technology, economic development, and social organization
- describe the basic requirements for a healthy environment
- discuss the importance of the workplace to environmental health
- explain the basic issues and concerns with respect to methods of measuring environmental quality, exposure, and health effects
- describe the larger socioeconomic issues affecting environmental health

BIRTH, LIFE, DEATH, AND THE ENVIRONMENT

When human beings first appeared in the world, their maximum life expectancy is believed to have been around 30 or 40 years. Due to the hostile environment in which they lived, they had a short life expectancy compared to that which characterizes most societies today. Still, it was long enough for them to have children and to establish themselves as the species most capable of modifying their environment for better or worse.

To survive, the first humans had to cope with the following:

- the constant search for sufficient food and drinking water while avoiding plants that contained natural toxins (like poisonous toadstools) or rancid infected meat
- infections and parasites that spread from person to person or animal to person, often through food, drinking water, or insect vectors
- injuries from falls, fires, and animal attacks
- cold and hot temperatures, rain, snow, natural disasters, and other adverse conditions.

These health hazards all occurred in the natural environment. In some societies the "traditional hazards" listed above still dominate environmental health concerns. However, as human beings brought these hazards under control in some regions, "modern hazards" caused by technological and industrial development took over as the primary threat to health and well-being.

Over the last few decades, life expectancy has increased significantly in most countries, as examples of survival curves show (Fig. 1.1). Some investigators say that this is largely due to improvements made in the living environment. Others say that improvements in nutrition are an essential reason for longer lives. Still others say that the changes could not have happened without improved medical diagnosis and treatment of illnesses. All of these statements are probably correct. Progress in health has gone hand in hand with improvements in environmental quality, nutrition, and medical care. People who are sick now are more likely to survive because of improved medical care, and the much greater number who are healthy at any given time are likely to stay healthy and fit because of improved nutrition and control of environmental health hazards. Pro-

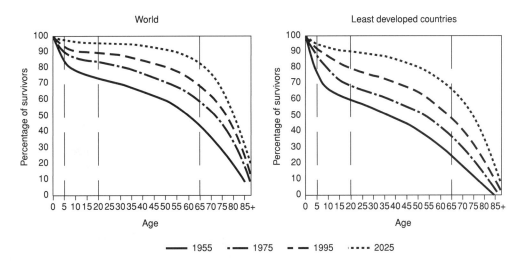

Figure 1.1 Survival curves, 1955–2025. From WHO, 1998a, with permission.

jections of survival and world population through to year 2025 indicate a continual improvement of life expectancy (Fig. 1.1).

Environmental health science is essentially about two things: hazards in the environment, their effects on health, and the variations in sensitivity to exposures within populations; and the development of effective means to protect against hazards in the environment. This book will describe the major environmental hazards that can affect health, show how these hazards can be assessed, and demonstrate how the resulting adverse health effects can be reduced or avoided. The roles of various professionals in protecting health will be explored and the fundamental principles that all environmental health professionals need to understand, regardless of where they work, will be described.

HEALTH AND THE ENVIRONMENT

An Ecosystem Perspective

The term *ecosystem*, coined in the 1930s, can be defined as a system of dynamic interdependent relationships among living organisms and their physical environment. It is a bounded entity that has acquired self-stabilizing mechanisms and an internal balance that has been evolving over the course of centuries. Within a stable ecosystem one species does not eliminate another; otherwise the food supply of the predator species would disappear. Stable and balanced ecosystems will survive longest. An ecosystem cannot sustain massive amounts of materials and energy being consumed by one species without depriving other species and eventually endangering the viability of the entire ecosystem. Similarly, an ecosystem's capacity to absorb wastes and to replenish soil and fresh water is not limitless. At some point an external load can overwhelm the ecosystem's balance, resulting in rapid change or a collapse of the ecosystem. Just as the concept of homeostasis (the body system's capability to function in a coordinated way to ensure the constancy of its internal environment) is now generally understood

The Gaia Hypothesis

James Lovelock, a British atmospheric scientist, advanced the hypothesis that the earth and all its components (including the geosphere and the water, gas, nutrients, energy cycles, and all living organisms) constitute a global homeostatic mechanism that ensures constancy of the environment. This hypothesis is known as the *Gaia hypothesis*, as the word *Gaia* comes from the Greek goddess Mother Earth. Lovelock contends that the global biosphere acts in a self-regulating manner, using feedback mechanisms to counter externally imposed disturbances. For example, the heat output of the sun has increased by about 30% since our planet was formed. Yet the earth has maintained a relatively constant temperature. This is believed to be due to the increased solar energy stimulating an increase in photosynthesis, which reduces carbon dioxide levels in the atmosphere. This in turn reduces the "greenhouse" capacity of the atmosphere, causing it to cool and thereby compensate for more heat from the sun. Similarly, the Gaia hypothesis suggests that oxygen has accumulated in the atmosphere to a level that is optimal for biological life on Earth, reflecting the balance of positive and negative feedback from the variety of interdependent living organisms. These changes have taken place very slowly over thousands or millions of years, while the currently debated increase in greenhouse gases has taken place in a few decades.

The controversy surrounding the Gaia hypothesis is due in part to the fact that it cannot be scientifically tested. Additionally, the hypothesis is seen by some investigators to imply that nature acts in a purposeful manner, a concept that does not fit comfortably with the mechanistic view of the world that prevails in contemporary Western civilization. Nonetheless, the Gaia hypothesis has stimulated awareness of the interdependencies within ecosystems and the balance of nature, which, within limits, serve to sustain the planet's life support systems. It has also provided a powerful vision or analogy for treating the Earth with the same respect one would show a mother.

Source: Lovelock, 1988; see also McMichael, 1993.

and accepted, these complex, compensating mechanisms seem to apply to ecosystems as well (see Box 1.1).

Definitions of Health and Environment

In the Constitution of the World Health Organization, *health* is defined as "a state of complete physical, mental and social well-being and not merely the absence of disease or infirmity" (WHO, 1948). This is the most commonly quoted modern definition of health. The concepts of disease, disability, and death tend to be much easier for health professionals to address than this idealistic concept of health. As a result, health sciences have largely been disease sciences since they focus on treating illness or injury rather than enhancing health. In some languages (e.g., Swedish) distinct terms for sick care and health care are in common usage, but unfortunately, this difference is not articulated in the English language.

Similarly inclusive definitions of environment in the context of health have been proposed. Last (1995) defined *environment* as "[All] that which is external to the individual human host. [It] can be divided into physical, biological, social, cultural, any or all of which can influence health status in populations." This definition is based on the notion that a person's health is basically determined by genetics and the environment. From the parents of an individual come genetic factors (genes), consisting of the DNA in each body cell. The genes existed when the embryo was first formed and do not generally change during the course of one's life. If a gene does change (as in the case of a mutation), it may lead to loss of function, cell death, and occasionally to cancer, as a result of very specific mutations. Some studies have suggested that genes provide a built in "clock of self-destruction," as the body can only function properly for a limited time. The limit for most individuals is within the range of 70 to 100 years. An individual's genetic material is one of the major factors that determines how he or she is affected by environmental exposure. While everybody will have problems if subjected to high enough exposures to an environmental hazard, some people are affected at lower exposures because they have preexisting or concomitant risk factors or conditions, and some people are affected at quite low exposures because of an inherited susceptibility (Jedrychowski and Krzyzanowski, 1995).

Poverty, poor living and working conditions, and lack of education have been repeatedly identified as major impediments to health. Over the years it has become clear that substantial improvements in health cannot be achieved without improvements in social and economic conditions. Providing relevant health services in the context of these conditions is addressed in the Health for All policy of the World Health Organization (WHO), established at a conference in Alma Ata in 1978. The final declaration stated that a goal of governments, international organizations, and the world community should be "the attainment by all people of the world by the year 2000 of a level of health that will permit them to lead a socially and economically productive life." It was explicitly noted that this could be attained only through a fuller and better use of the world's resources: "Health is only possible where resources are available to meet human needs and where the living and working environment is protected from life-threatening and health-threatening pollutants, pathogens and physical hazards" (WHO, 1992a).

Environmental pollution and degradation have a huge impact on people's lives. Every year hundreds of millions of people suffer from respiratory and other diseases associated with indoor and outdoor air pollution. Hundreds of millions of people are exposed to unnecessary physical and chemical hazards in the workplace and living environment. Half a million die as a result of road accidents. Four million infants and children die every year from diarrheal diseases, largely as a result of contaminated food or water. Hundreds of millions of people suffer from debilitating intestinal parasites. Two million people die from malaria every year while 267 million are ill with it at any given time. Three million people die each year from tuberculosis and 20 million are actively ill with it. Hundreds of millions suffer from poor nutrition. Almost all of these health problems could be prevented (WHO 1992a).

As noted in the book *Our Planet, Our Health* (WHO, 1992a), the responsibility for protecting and promoting good health extends to all groups in society. No longer is good health the responsibility of only traditional health care professionals, such as doctors, nurses, sanitary engineers, and safety officers, who seek to cure disease, care for the sick, remove pathogens, and reduce injuries. Human well-being is now clearly the responsibility of planners, architects, teachers, employers, industrial managers, and all others who influence the physical or social environment. That is why this book is geared for teaching people in many professions. Naturally, health professionals have a special role in environmental health, but they need to work with all groups in society to promote good health. The ability to work in teams and adopt a transdisciplinary approach is key to being able to solve environmental health problems (Somervile and Rapport, 2000).

Human Interaction with the Environment

Human health ultimately depends on a society's capacity to manage the interaction between human activities and the physical, chemical, and biological environments (Fig. 1.2). It must do this in ways that safeguard and promote human health, while at the same time protecting the integrity of the natural systems on which a healthy environment depends. The physical and biological environments include everything from the immediate home and work environments to regional, national, and global environments. This includes maintaining a stable climate and continued availability of safe environmental resources (soil, fresh water, clean air). It also includes continued functioning of the natural systems that receive the waste produced by human societies without exposing people to pathogens and toxic substances and without compromising the well-being of future generations.

The idea of an inextricable link between human health and the environment has long been recognized. Over 100 years ago, Chief Seattle, an indigenous leader

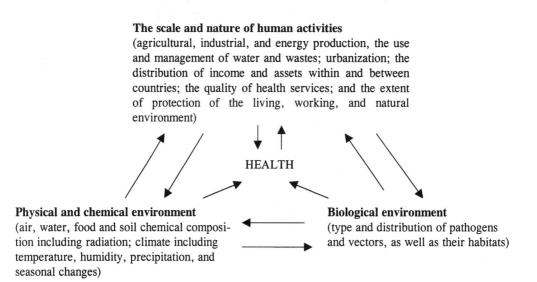

Figure 1.2 Interaction between human activities and the physical, chemical, and biological environments. Adapted from WHO, 1992a, with permission.

in Washington Territory during the western expansion of the United States, spoke movingly of our relationship to earth in a much-quoted speech: "We are a part of the web of life and whatever we do to the web we do to ourselves." Thus, when we think of health as a state of complete physical, mental, and social well-being, we must recognize that this also implies a context of ecological well-being.

The concept of sustainable development requires that a modern economy not harm the environment to the extent that it closes off opportunities for future generations. Thus, the World Commission on Environment and Development (WCED), in the report, *Our Common Future*, defined "sustainable development" as "[d]evelopment that meets the needs of the present without compromising the ability of future generations to meet their own needs" (WCED, 1987). To promote health, which implies the full development of human potential, an adequately prosperous economy, a viable environment, and a convivial community are needed (Dean and Hancock, 1992). These qualities should be reflected in a society's economic activity, which must not destroy the human and social capital or the resources of society. The benefits of economic activity need to be equitably distributed both within and among nations, societies, and communities (Hertzman et al., 1994). Because of the need for this kind of distribution, equity is an integral part of sustainable development. Agenda 21, the United Nations Program of Action for Environment and Development, agreed upon at Rio de Janeiro in 1992, reiterated this relationship, stating that "[h]uman beings are at the centre of concerns for sustainable development. They are entitled to a healthy and productive life in harmony with nature" (UN, 1993). While virtually every aspect of human health is closely linked to the physical and social environment, we will focus here on the interaction between health and the environment according to the factors described in Figure 1.2: *biological pathogens* and their vectors and reservoirs; physical and chemical agents in an environment that are *independent of human activities* and can impair human health by either their presence (e.g., naturally occurring radionuclides, ultraviolet light) or their absence (e.g., iodine, iron); and noxious physical and chemical agents *added* to the environment *by human activities* (e.g., nitrogen oxides, polycyclic aromatic hydrocarbons, particulates arising from fossil fuel combustion, waste produced by industry, biomedical waste, and radioactive waste).

Socioeconomic factors control how resources are used. Whether a person is hungry, adequately fed, or overfed, depends not only on the state of his or her natural resources but also on the socioeconomic factors that influence such things as how agricultural practices result in use or misuse of those resources and whether safe, nutritious, and affordable food is available. Health also depends on how people feel about their society—including how much trust and social cohesion exists in their community (Putnam, 1993; Kawachi et al., 1999). The following definition of *environmental health* is thus applicable: "Environmental health comprises those aspects of human health, including quality of life, that are determined by physical, biological, social, and psychosocial factors in the environment. It also refers to the theory and practice of assessing, correcting, controlling, and preventing those factors in the environment that can potentially affect adversely the health of present and future generations" (WHO, 1993a).

Sometimes there is an ethical dilemma between promoting human health and protecting the environment. One extreme position is that any control limiting the exploitation of resources may inhibit an individual's or a community's attempts to enhance their standard of living, therefore infringing on their rights and freedoms as well as decreasing their ability to maintain health. At the other extreme is the position that any action to protect the environment and maintain the integrity of the ecosystem is justified regardless of the impact on human activity and health. The United Nations has stated that ensuring human survival should be taken as a first-order principle, one that takes precedence over all others. The first order assigned to meeting human survival is consistent with the United Nations Universal Declaration of Human Rights (UN, 1948), which states that "all people have the right to a standard of living adequate for the health and well-being of themselves and their family, including food, clothing, housing, health care, and the necessary social services." Respect for nature and control of environmental degradation is a "second-order" principle, which should guide all human activities, except when these activities conflict with the first principle. In reality, most such conflicts are more apparent than real and arise from a faulty understanding of the human-environment interaction, or a dysfunctional social and economic system.

Sustainable development implies that everyone eventually must have access to the environmental resources that meet their needs. This must also be done with a continuous commitment to improve general understanding of how the environment and health are linked. It must be done without overwhelming the finite absorptive capacities of the global ecosystem.

Human Ability to Adapt

Human beings, like all living things, depend on their environments to meet their health needs, including their needs for food, water, shelter, and security. Deficiencies may happen because of inadequate resources, waste or an inequitable distribution of these resources. When people are exposed to hostile or unsafe environments, microorganisms, toxins, excessive radiation, or armed enemies, their health invariably suffers. Compared with most other species, however, humans have extraordinary abilities to adapt to and influence their environment to meet their needs. For example, people have learned to produce and gather food and to limit their exposure to parasites and extreme weather conditions. They take collective measures to protect themselves against hostile beings and adverse conditions. They have also acquired practices (e.g., ethics, cultures) and structures (e.g., cities, highways, dams) that enable them to better cope with the natural environment.

While there are many ways to make the environment healthier, more often than not, environmental health hazards are beyond the control of the affected individual. This may be the case with the following conditions:

- industrial pollution
- poor services of drinking water and sanitation
- poor housing and town planning
- lax control over eating establishments or food industry

BOX 1.2

The Concept of Supportive Environments for Health

In the concept of supportive environments, determinants of the health of entire populations are addressed, including the following:

- the role of local environmental factors in the healthy development of the community
- an approach that enables and promotes health, as well as protects from environmental hazards
- creation of equity in health within a community
- the importance of sustainable development as a health issue
- people's understanding of environment in a broad sense
- people's sense of involvement and personal interest in restoring or creating a healthy environment.

Source: Haglund et al., 1992.

- poor quality roads
- poor conditions in the workplace.

Adaptation and change to improve a community's environment then require decisions and actions by leaders of industry, government, and institutions. To achieve this, decision makers may have to feel some community pressure, decision makers and their technical advisers may need better training, and resources for environmental and health protection may have to be reallocated. The environmental health professional is likely to be one person to whom the community looks for advice on how to find solutions to their concerns, and to help empower them with increased capacity to understand the issues, consider the options, and formulate action plans.

Supportive Environments for Health

Supportive environments are the conditions that countries or communities try to create to achieve their health targets (see Box 1.2). The focus is on how good environments enhance health rather than on the health impact of bad environments. This effort involves such practices as building healthy housing, promoting healthy lifestyles, cleaning up industrial pollution, reducing traffic hazards, reducing tobacco smoking, and changing dietary habits. In poor communities the most important issues may be basic sanitation and water supply, improved maternal and child health care, and the control of communicable diseases.

The concept of empowering communities to take control over the determinants of their health is indeed the key feature of health promotion. The WHO, in the now much quoted Ottawa Charter (WHO, 1986) defined health promotion as "the process of enabling people to increase control over, and to improve, their health."

Economic and Industrial Development and Environmental Health

While it is well known that biological agents and naturally occurring chemical and physical hazards have existed throughout human history, there is also a long history of environmental pollution from anthropogenic sources (human activities). Even in ancient times, sites of production and manufacturing were contaminated with pollution. A good example is lead contamination in the area around smelters centuries ago and the horrible odor and water pollution associated with tanneries. By modern standards, the scale of most of these enterprises was very small, however. The technology was that of the individual artisan using traditional work practices that had not substantially changed for centuries. The resulting pollution was usually restricted to the immediate area. Pollution from human waste was considered more of a problem, as it effectively limited the size of cities. As great a problem as pollution was occupational health and safety, as workers were subjected to intense exposure to a variety of hazards at the workplace.

The Industrial Revolution marked a dramatic turning point in the interaction between economic activity and the environment. Industrial pollution was first identified as an obvious and serious issue in the early 1800s, when it became obvious that production on an industrial scale, using the breakthrough technology of the time, resulted in pollution on a scale never before seen. This pollution was largely the result of the energy requirements of a technology based on iron and steel, which led to more widespread air pollution as well as local concentrations of pollution near the factory site.

The United Kingdom, home of the Industrial Revolution, was the first country to suffer from industrial pollution on a massive scale. It became particularly obvious during the later years of the reign of Queen Victoria (the Victorian era). Mass production led to the recruitment of hundreds of thousands of new workers into a wage-earning class. These workers soon became consumers themselves. Production soared and the profits created a pool of capital that was then reinvested in further industrial expansion. The new industrial cities became infamous. A well-studied example was the city of Manchester, but the export of new technology created many other examples in the British Isles, Europe, and elsewhere. At that time much of what is now the developing world was under colonialism. It would be many years before these areas would suffer similar problems in the course of their own economic development. The colonial system restricted most manufacturing to the colonizing country, which sold manufactured goods in the colonies and bought raw materials and food from them.

Industrial pollution may have been a serious problem in the Victorian era, but it was not high on the list of social priorities of the day. Considered much more important at that time were social issues, such as child labor, class-based poverty, alcohol and drug abuse (mostly gin and opium), welfare services (or the absence thereof), corruption, and prostitution. All of these issues were related to the urbanization that accompanied the recruitment of an industrial work force. The principal health concerns of the day were communicable diseases, which were out of control in the squalid, densely populated cities. These problems became a national crisis in England and Scotland and it soon became obvious that one reason for the crisis was that there was no effective local governmental responsibility for these problems.

The First Environmental Crisis

The first wave of sustained and broad-based environmental concern appeared in Europe in the nineteenth century in response to serious public health problems associated with adulterated food and water contamination. The primary threats at the time were agents of infectious disease for the general public and disabling and often fatal injury in the workplace. This increase in awareness, which led to political action, came at a time of great social unrest and eventually reform. Child labor, prostitution, alcohol and drug abuse, exploitative employment practices, crime, and land ownership, which was concentrated in the hands of a few, often absent landowners, were all part of the emerging big picture in Europe at the time, particularly in economically developed countries such as England, Scotland, France, the German states, and the Austro-Hungarian Empire. A reform movement in the middle of the century tackled all of these problems with legislation that was generally piecemeal and not always entirely effective. Together, these reforms greatly reduced the magnitude of the problems but did not solve them.

In 1848 the British parliament passed the first broad-based public health law. This was a significant event in the midst of a reform movement that reached all sectors of urban life. Industrial pollution, however, was largely ignored at the time. In part because the government saw its role as protecting the rights of factory owners, The Public Health Act concentrated on environmental problems of a different type, namely clean water and health hazards related to infectious diseases. The prevailing economic theory was that unconstrained economic growth would benefit all levels of society and that maximal profits were needed to attract investment. Another reason for neglecting the environment was that other pressing social issues were so obvious and so severe that pollution seemed much less important as an issue. At the time, there was essentially no public health science that addressed chemical pollution, even though scientific understanding of the health effects of toxic chemical exposures was relatively sophisticated. The history of environmental pollution concerns and actions (see Box 1.3) is largely a story of the issue of industrial pollution catching up with other public health issues on the public agenda after first being neglected.

The intrinsic inefficiencies of Victorian technology ensured that pollution would remain a problem until the early twentieth century, which was characterized more by technological refinement than innovation. Applied chemistry and chemical engineering expanded spectacularly in the late 1700s and early 1800s. This led to the introduction of many processes that generated pollution, particularly in the production of sulphuric acid, soap, bleach, and soda ash (sodium carbonate). Organic chemistry developed later and introduced many new synthetic chemicals. However, in this era most of these chemicals were biodegradable—i.e., eventually they could be broken down by natural processes in the environment. Chemicals that persisted for longer in the environment mostly came later, except for metals such as lead.

Just before and during World War II, major advances in engineering and chemistry substantially changed the face of industry, especially in the chemical sector. Synthetic rubbers, solvents, plastics, and pesticides became available and were often more effective and cheaper to produce than the older products. Many of these new synthetic chemicals were based on chlorine chemistry. A large number of them turned out to be difficult to break down by natural processes and, as a result, persisted in the environment. Changes in technology and a greater demand from consumers in North America, Japan, and Europe also led to huge increases in the volume of hazardous materials. In the postwar years, production expanded massively, along with a well-documented increase in industrial pollution that led to a public outcry in the 1960s and '70s in many countries.

The Second Wave of Environmental Concern

The second wave of public environmental concern, which came in the mid- to late twentieth century, was dominated by two broad movements that came together into what was called the *environmental* or *ecology movement*. In the first movement, which had its roots in the nineteenth century, conservation of natural resources and preservation of special sites of natural or historic significance were important priorities. Until the mid-twentieth century its major achievement was the designation in various countries of certain areas as parks, wilderness areas, and other protected lands. The second movement focused on substances that could be toxic to humans or damaging to the environment. It grew in part out of concerns at the turn of the century with food and drug adulteration; its greatest achievement was food and drug safety laws, mostly in the early twentieth century. The pure food and drug movement adopted environmental pollutants as a central issue following the massive increase in production following World War II. The new "toxics movement" was particularly inspired by the 1962 publication of the highly influential book *Silent Spring* by Rachel Carson. Toxic exposures that took place in the workplace were often much more intense than those caused by emissions and effluents leaving the plant site. Unfortunately, during this era, the environmental movement did very little directly toward improving workers' health, as the two problems were not obviously linked at the time. The issue of workers' health advanced more slowly, as part of the movement to improve workers' rights.

These public movements, and the UN Conference on the Human Environment in 1972, persuaded many national governments to introduce legislation that curbed industrial pollution, mostly by requiring companies to limit emissions or effluents of pollution. This environmental movement peaked in the early 1970s, but it left a lasting framework of regulations, new technology, and policies aimed at preventing chemical pollution, particularly in the developed world. Although not completely effective, these actions did substantially reduce the total amount of industrial pollution for a time and resulted in many examples of successful environmental improvement. It would be an exaggeration to say that the developed world solved the problem of industrial pollution or even reduced it to acceptable levels, but the scale of the problem was significantly reduced.

The focus during this era was almost entirely on particular chemicals that were relatively toxic. Omitted from the concern of the 1970s were carbon dioxide and relatively nontoxic chemicals such as the chlorofluorocarbons. These were not generally understood to be serious environmental hazards until the late

1980s, even though scientists had given warnings about their toxic effects much
earlier (see Box 1.3). These chemicals have since become a major environmental concern.

The Third Wave of Environmental Concern

In the 1980s and into the 1990s, the accelerated rate of economic development,
combined with a substantial increase in world population, introduced a critical
new factor into the environmental equation. Until the 1980s the levels of production in the developing world were relatively low compared to those in the
developed countries. As a consequence, industrial pollution in developing countries tended to be confined to local areas, as it had been in Europe and America
in earlier times. Recently, however, production levels in these countries have increased very rapidly along with the demand for goods and the capacity for di-

rect trading among countries because of the globalization of trade. Much of the production in this new sector is relatively undercapitalized and therefore it is often based on expedient, cheaper technologies. There are usually few controls over effluents and emissions, and the result is increases in industrial pollution.

Since 1987 and the publication of the seminal report *Our Common Future* (WCED, 1987), environmental planning and economic development have become oriented toward "sustainable development," the level of production and activity that can be undertaken in one generation without compromising environmental integrity or depleting the resources to support the next generation. This concept, which is roughly equivalent to the idea in biology of living within the carrying capacity of the ecosystem for a society, has entered the mainstream of economic thought and environmental management. It represents a way of thinking about development that takes into account resource management, pollution, social development, and human health.

New environmental concerns continue to emerge. Some toxicologists are focusing on chemicals that disrupt the endocrine system and are persistent in the environment (see Chapter 2). Certainly the concerns about global environmental change (see Chapter 11) have generated renewed interest in the environment that will likely persist for decades to come.

BASIC REQUIREMENTS FOR A HEALTHY ENVIRONMENT

Clean Air

Air is essential for life itself; without it we could survive only a few minutes. Air pollution is one of the most serious environmental problems in societies at all levels of economic development. As many as 500 million people are exposed daily to high levels of indoor air pollution in the form of smoke from open fires or poorly designed stoves. More than 1500 million people live in urban areas with dangerously high levels of air pollution (WHO, 1992a). Industrial development has been associated with the emission of large quantities of gaseous and particulate substances from both industrial production and from burning fossil fuels for energy and transportation. When technology was introduced to control air pollution by reducing emissions of particles, it was found that the gaseous emissions continued and caused problems of their own. Although current efforts to control both particulate and gaseous emissions have been partially successful in much of the developed world, there is recent evidence that air pollution is a health risk even under these relatively favorable conditions (WHO/NILU, 1996).

In rapidly developing societies, sufficient resources may not be initially invested in air pollution control because of other economic and social priorities. The rapid expansion of industry in these countries has occurred at the same time as automobile and truck traffic has increased, demands for power for the home have grown, and populations have concentrated in large urban areas, or megacities. The result is some of the worst air pollution problems in the world.

In many traditional societies and in societies where household energy sources considered to be clean are not yet widely available, air pollution is a serious problem because inefficient and smoky fuels are used to heat buildings and to cook, causing air pollution both outdoors and indoors. The result can be acute irritation of mucous membranes, respiratory infections, lung disease, eye problems, and increased risk of cancer. Women and children in poor communities in developing countries are particularly exposed to air pollution.

The quality of air indoors is also a problem in many developed countries because buildings have been built to be airtight and energy efficient. Chemicals produced by heating and cooling systems, smoking, and evaporation from building materials accumulate indoors and create a pollution problem.

Safe and Sufficient Water

Water is essential to life. We need to drink a minimum of 1 to 2 liters per day. After about 4 days without water, a person will die. Water is also essential for plants, animals, and agriculture, so throughout history, people have clustered along the shores of lakes and rivers to get water for households and agriculture. Water also provides natural transportation, is used for disposal of wastes, and plays an essential role in the farming, fishing, and industrial sectors. Although fresh water is considered a renewable resource, there is a limited supply. Moreover, it is unequally distributed among the countries and people of the world. In many regions, shortages of fresh water are the main obstacle to agricultural and industrial production. In some cases this has led to difficult conflicts (e.g., the difficulties of sharing water resources among the countries of the Middle East). These shortages lead to poverty and soil degradation; many cities and agricultural regions are drawing water from underground aquifers faster than these sources are able to replenish themselves.

The quality of fresh water is of great importance to maintaining good health. A high proportion of life- and health-threatening infections are transmitted through contaminated water or food; as much as 80% of all sickness and disease in some developing countries has been attributed to the lack of safe water and appropriate means to dispose of excrement (WHO, 1992a). Nearly half the world's population suffers from diseases associated with insufficient or contaminated water, which affect mostly the poor in virtually all developing countries. Two thousand million people are at risk of waterborne and foodborne diarrheal diseases, which are the main cause of nearly four million child deaths each year. Cholera epidemics, which are also frequently transmitted by unsafe drinking water, are increasing in frequency. Schistosomiasis (200 million people infected) and dracunculiasis (10 million people infected) are two of the most serious water-based diseases. Insect vectors breeding in water transmit other life-threatening diseases such as malaria (267 million infected), filariasis (90 million infected), onchocerciasis (18 million infected), and dengue fever (30 to 60 million infected) (WHO, 1992a).

Water shortages usually lead to problems of water quality, since sewage, industrial effluent, and agricultural and urban runoff overload the capacity of water bodies to break down biodegradable waste and to dilute nonbiodegradable waste. Water pollution is most serious in cities where controls on industrial emissions are not enforced and sewers, drains, and sewage treatment plants are often lacking.

Food provides the energy for our bodies to function. The equivalent of about 1000 to 2000 calories is required each day for a person to stay alive, depending on a person's body weight and level of physical activity. Without food, most people would die after about 4 weeks. Food also provides essential vitamins and trace elements, without which people develop deficiency diseases.

The output of the world's food-producing systems has matched the population growth over the last few decades (Fig. 1.3). There is no global shortage of food or lack of capacity to produce it at this time. Nonetheless, the success in global agriculture has not been shared equally. Asia and Latin America have substantially increased their per-capita food production, while Africa's food production has not kept pace with population growth, and the countries of the former Soviet Union have had a dramatic decrease in food production. For a large part of the world's population, undernutrition and the infections associated with it remain a major cause of ill health and premature death. Foodborne pathogens cause millions of cases of diarrheal disease each year, including thousands in the developed world. Poor food distribution and its utilization are the main culprits in this situation. Rapid degradation of land and water resources also pose an important threat to future food production. To make matters worse, because of economic pressures to develop exports of agricultural products, increasingly, the best land is not being used for local food production. In many situations, food intake is the most important route of exposure for chemical environmental contaminants.

There are many health effects, other than foodborne diseases, that result from an inadequate diet, including starvation under disaster conditions, excess numbers of premature and underweight births, and nutrition so marginal as to weaken immune systems and deny millions of children proper growth and development. Food contaminated by toxins from plants and molds or those present in fish and shellfish can also be a serious problem, as is food contaminated directly by agri-

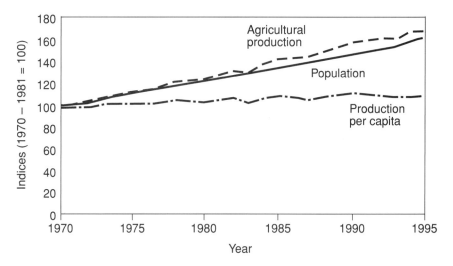

Figure 1.3 Trends in world food production and food production per capita. From WHO, 1997, with permission.

cultural chemical residues or indirectly through pollution of the soil by toxic metals and solvents.

Safe and Peaceful Settlements

A safe and peaceful place in which to live is also necessary for good health. Inadequate housing and community infrastructure other structures adversely affect the health of urban residents. Low income, uncertain employment, insecure residential tenure, and poor health go hand in hand with inadequate, overcrowded shelter lacking space and sanitation and with minimal health protection. Residents are exposed to disease pathogens, pollutants, violence, and injury hazards, often in conditions that breed alienation and psychosocial dysfunction. Drug abuse, family break-up, urban violence and suicide are believed to be associated with overcrowded housing and inadequate community support. Overcrowding enables the spread of acute respiratory infections, tuberculosis, meningitis, and intestinal parasites; infants, children, and the elderly are at particular risk as a result of less developed or reduced resistance. Injuries from burns or scalds are also associated with overcrowding, as it is more difficult to safely store hazardous household substances such as bleach or kerosene.

In urban areas of developing countries, a high proportion of housing is concentrated in informal settlements made of flammable materials and often built on dangerous sites. Disasters such as mudslides, floods, and hurricanes are particularly destructive in these crowded, inadequately prepared communities. Fear of eviction is also a constant worry for most tenants and inhabitants of these settlements. As these settlements usually have only rudimentary water supply systems and no sewers or drains, risk of infection associated with excreta is always high. An estimated 30% to 50% of the solid wastes generated in urban areas of developing countries is left uncollected (WHO, 1992c).

War and civil violence are also major factors in disrupting housing and threatening well-being, as, demonstrated in Somalia, Rwanda, and Bosnia Herzegovina.

Stable Global Environment

Human health and ecosystem health are inextricably linked. The long-range transport of air pollutants, the transboundary movement of hazardous products and wastes, stratospheric ozone depletion, climate change, and loss of biodiversity are among the global problems threatening the health of many communities (WHO, 1997). For example, when sulphur and nitrogen oxides are emitted from fossil fuel power plants, they are transported over long distances, often across national boundaries, and are converted to acids that eventually fall to the ground as acid rain or snow. Individuals' health may be affected by acidified water used and treated in water supplies, since it contains higher water concentrations of metals (e.g., copper and lead from pipes, or aluminium and mercury from soil and sediments). Also, the stratosphere's ozone layer is being damaged by various chemicals, including chlorofluorocarbons used in refrigeration. Damage of the ozone layer leads to increased ultraviolet radiation exposure to large populations, which in turn may cause eye cataracts, skin cancer, and other problems. Finally, the greenhouse effect, emissions of carbon dioxide and other greenhouse gases, and eventual global warming (McMichael et al., 1996) may also threaten a stable global environment that protects health.

The United Nations Environmental Programme (UNEP) launched the Global Environmental Project in 1995, a participatory process involving experts from over 100 countries. Its recent publication, *GEO-2000* (UNEP, 2000) noted that global emissions of CO_2 continue to rise, with an annual increase over the past decade of 1.3%, with the level in 1996 being almost four the 1950 total. GEO-2000 urges that alternative policies be swiftly implemented to avoid major environmental disasters.

MEASURING ENVIRONMENTAL QUALITY, HUMAN EXPOSURE, AND HEALTH IMPACT

Measuring Environmental Quality

The measurement of environmental hazards, levels of human exposure to these environmental hazards, and the resulting health impact are clearly interrelated. Specifically, the investigation of environmentally induced health effects always requires consideration of the nature of the hazard and levels of exposure. Even though it is pertinent to evaluate the extent of environmental change within the discipline of environmental health, however, the main purpose of this book is to focus on evaluating human exposure and health impact.

In many countries, measurements of pollutants in air, water, food, and sometimes soil have become routine. Most of the common measurements are made because of health concerns, but some relate to the agricultural or industrial use of the air, water, or soil. Examples of common measurements are sulphur dioxide (SO_2) and total suspended particulates (TSP) in air, which indicate the extent of pollution from coal use, diesel oil use, and specific industries (e.g., cement factories). Another common measurement is the concentration of *Escherichia coli* (*E. coli*) bacteria in water. This gives a good indication of the fecal contamination of the water and the extent to which the water can be used for drinking, bathing, or food processing. In certain dry areas of the world, well water can have very high natural concentrations of toxic metals, e.g., arsenic, and routine monitoring is necessary.

There is an important distinction between environmental quality monitoring and human exposure monitoring. The latter takes into account whether the polluted air has actually been inhaled, the polluted water has been drunk, and the polluted food has been eaten. In addition, human exposure monitoring takes into account the length of time a person spends in the polluted area and the amounts of pollutant that are consumed. In many countries, an occupational health inspector periodically monitors the quality of the workplace environment. During such surveys, hazardous exposures as well as safety and ergonomic aspects are taken into account.

Measuring Human Exposure to Environmental Hazards

The measurement or estimation of levels of exposure to an environmental pollutant or hazard is called *exposure assessment*. Human exposure can occur through several routes—most importantly, inhalation, ingestion, and skin contact. Assessment can be undertaken by a direct approach, an indirect approach, or a combination of the two. With the direct approach, pollutant concentrations taken in by an individual through food, water, air, or skin contact are measured directly. Field studies using personal monitors, questionnaires, and diaries provide the exposure data. Survey sampling techniques are used to select a sample of people that statistically represents the population of interest. Also, several reliable marker methods have been developed to estimate environmental exposures, e.g., blood lead levels can be used to estimate exposure to from all sources.

The indirect approach uses a mathematical model to estimate exposure. Information about how much time people spend in different environments (such as in their homes, workplaces, motor vehicles) is combined with data on pollutant concentrations in these microenvironments to estimate human exposure to airborne contaminants. Similarly, keeping diaries of food and beverage consumption can be invaluable when combined with data on contaminant levels and food and beverage products to estimate ingestion exposures.

Determining Health Effects and Risks in Human Populations

A *health effect* is the specific damage to health that an environmental hazard can cause in an individual person. Often the same hazard can cause a range of different effects of different severity. Traditional diagnostic tools can determine effects in the individual. The science of carrying out such health measurements in populations is called *epidemiology*, which is defined as "the study of the distribution and determinants of health-related states or events in specified populations, and the application of this study to the control of health problems" (Last, 1995). This definition highlights the fact that epidemiologists are concerned not only with death and disease but also with more positive health states and with the means to improve health.

The initial step in any epidemiological investigation involves the description of the problem at hand. A clear case definition, or definition of the health effect of concern (e.g., respiratory disease in children living in an area with air pollution), has to be established so as not to confuse investigators. Similarly, if the study is triggered by a pollution or exposure situation, the exposure type needs to be clearly defined. Describing case distributions by time, place, and person is usually an extremely useful first step in providing clues for the cause of the disease and any environmental factors involved (Beaglehole et al., 1993). There are two approaches to quantifying the number of cases occurring: measures of new cases (*incidence*) or of existing cases (*prevalence*). Incidence can only be measured within a defined time period (for acute infectious disease, incidence is often measured in days or weeks, whereas for chronic diseases it is often measured in years). Prevalence can only be measured at a specific point in time or over a relatively short defined period (called *period prevalence*).

Once a case definition has been established, it is important to define the population at risk of exposure and of developing the outcome of interest, to avoid counting people not at risk and thereby diluting the evaluation. The population at risk may be defined by factors such as age, gender, area, workplace, occupation, or ethnic group. Definitions of populations at risk become more difficult in situations where the illness of interest is chronic in nature, is indistinguishable from normally endemic illnesses, or involves long latency periods. In such settings, disease rates may need to be studied in relatively large population units (countries, provinces) over extended periods of time. After defining the cases and the population at risk, the number of cases and persons at risk can be used to calculate rates of disease occurrence (either as incidence rates or prevalence rates). The observed incidence (or prevalence) of the disease must be compared with disease occurrence in some reference (or control) population, with appropriate adjustments so that rates are compared using equivalent populations distributed by age, gender, and other similar aspects and according to similar case definitions. In this manner, investigators can determine whether there is indeed an increase in the health effects of concern and can gather information to isolate what might have caused it.

Environmental Health Monitoring

To quantify health effects by monitoring the health of populations, appropriate health indicators must be selected, monitoring methods must be developed, and data quality needs to be evaluated. Through standardization of health indicators and harmonization of sampling and measurement techniques, it is possible to compare data between jurisdictions. Health-monitoring strategies involve the application of different methods to get results in the most cost-effective way (see Table 1.1).

Monitoring strategies are dependent on available health care infrastructure. Use of records from hospital and medical services is more feasible in countries with national medical care services and centralized administrations than in countries where most services are provided by independent health care agencies and

TABLE 1.1

CHARACTERISTICS OF SELECTED APPROACHES TO HEALTH MONITORING

	Sample Population	Data Providers	Potential for Quantification of Environmental Impact
National registers	Entire population of country	Health care personnel Hospital records Laboratory records	Large, provided that health data are linked with good exposure data; confounding needs to be avoided
Local registries	Entire population of smaller administrative entities	Health care personnel Hospital records Laboratory records	Large, provided that health data are linked with good exposure data; conclusions can be generalized only if the population studied is representative
Sentinel networks	Population covered by data providers	Selected practitioners, laboratories, hospitals	Only if relevant exposure data are concurrently collected and the population studied is representative
Periodic health surveys	Ideally randomly drawn from population	Specifically trained survey team	Only if relevant exposure data are concurrently collected or are available from other sources

TABLE 1.2
USEFUL HEALTH INDICATORS

Physical Health	*Psychosocial Well-being*
PUBLIC	
Respiratory effects	Changes in the quality of life
Injuries	Changes in cultural/social patterns
Communicable diseases	Rates of crime
Cancer	Rates of drug and substance abuse
Effects on fertility and development (e.g., congenital anomalies)	Stress-related conditions
WORKERS	
Injuries	Changes in the quality of life
Days off work	Relocation
Long term activity limitations	Stress-related conditions
Respiratory effects	
Noise effects	
Dermatitis	
Effects on fertility and development	
Cancer	

private organizations. Surveys in which representative sampling strategies are used may provide a more realistic alternative in some situations. Each country has to develop its own strategy for health monitoring. Priority should be given to monitoring health and environmental variables that have (*a*) the greatest impact on the health of the population, and (*b*) the highest potential for prevention. Also to be considered is whether there is a strong commitment to intervene with preventive measures.

The types of information and indicators that may be used to assess the potential impacts of environmental exposures on physical and psychosocial health in both the general public and the workforce are listed in Table 1.2. These indicators of occupational or public health can be combined with those for biological monitoring (see Chapter 3) and environmental monitoring to describe the environmental health status of a population. Environmental health indicators are being incorporated into many environmental programs. Guidelines for the use of these indicators are provided in *Linkage Methods for Environmental Health Analysis* (Briggs et al., 1996), and are discussed further in *World Resources 1998–99: A Guide to the Global Environment* (WRI, 1998) a joint publication by the WRI, the United Nations Environment Programme (UNEP), the United Nations Development Programme (UNDP) and the World Bank.

PATTERNS OF ILLNESS THROUGHOUT THE WORLD

Demographic and Epidemiological Transitions

Over the last two centuries, a major shift in the health situation of most countries has taken place. In Europe, high mortality and high birth rates with people suffering from a variety of communicable diseases, have given way to a low-mortality, low–birth rate situation in which few cases of communicable diseases have occurred. This shift, which started in the last century and has continued to the present time, has been called the *demographic transition* (see Fig. 1.4), as it relates mainly to the crude birth rate and death rate. When both rates were high, the populations stayed stable. In those countries where they are now both low, the populations have again stayed stable, as in the Scandinavian countries. During the transition from high to low rates there is a period when death rates lower while the birth rate stays high; during this period the population will grow. The more the death rates decrease while birth rates remain stable, the more rapid is the growth of the population, a phenomenon that can be found in most developing countries. Many developed countries have more or less completed their demographic transition. The death rate in such countries now principally reflects diseases associated with aging.

The high pretransition death rates are very much linked to a high level of communicable disease, so the transition in death and birth rates is accompanied by a change in the pattern of the causes of death—less communicable disease and more chronic noncommunicable disease. This change in disease pattern over time has been called the *epidemiological transition*. Figure 1.5 shows how the mortality patterns changed in the United States in the twentieth century.

This pattern of change has been shown in all countries to follow economic development, as improvements in housing, sanitation, and community infrastructure reduce the risk of communicable disease. It is not just the improving economy itself that protects citizens' health but the improvements to water supply, shelter, and nutrition, which are part of the development of community services. As these improvements take place, chronic noncommunicable diseases become a more important factor, largely because of the longer life expectancy and increasing proportion of old people in communities.

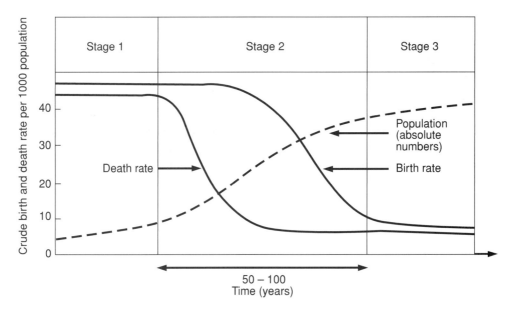

Figure 1.4 The demographic transition. From Kjellström and Rosenstock, 1990, with permission.

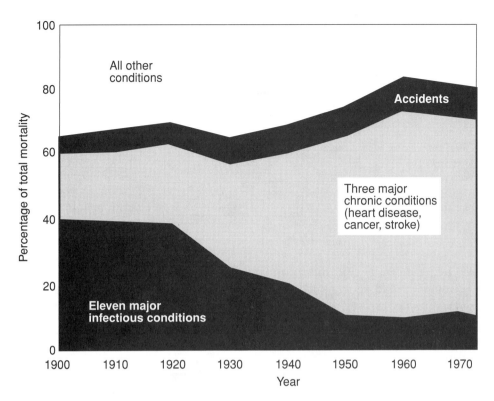

Figure 1.5 The epidemiological transition as it has occurred in the United States. From Beaglehole et al., 1993, with permission.

Mortality Trends

In many developing countries crude death rates are declining while in developed regions they remain steady. The data on life expectancy, which are a better measure of trends, as it takes into consideration differences in age structure, show that improvements in levels of health have been made throughout the world, although life expectancies are still much lower in developing countries than in developed regions.

Age-standardized mortality figures are generally not available for developing countries. Table 1.3 provides estimates of the proportion of deaths from various causes as a percentage of the total number of deaths. Although this gives a profile of what people in each country are dying of, it does not indicate which groups are dying at what age or at what rate. The differences between the two patterns shown in Table 1.3 reflect in part a different age composition in the two groups of countries. But this difference does not go far to explain the 10-fold disparity in mortality from infectious diseases in general or the 20-fold difference in mortality from tuberculosis. Such statistics are dramatic evidence of the pretransition state of the developing world.

As an unambiguous event, death is a good indicator for statistical comparisons of health situations in countries. Mortality rates, nonetheless have their limitations. They tell us little about suffering and loss of productivity related to morbidity; direct information on the incidence and prevalence of diseases would

TABLE 1.3

CAUSES OF DEATH IN DEVELOPED AND DEVELOPING COUNTRIES, 1993

	Deaths from all Causes (%)	
Cause of Death	Developed Countries	Developing Countries
Infectious and parasitic diseases	1.2	41.5
Chronic lower respiratory diseases	7.8	5.0
Malignant neoplasms	21.6	8.9
Diseases of the circulatory system	46.7	10.7
Maternal causes	0	1.3
Perinatal and neonatal conditions	0.7	7.9
External causes of mortality	7.5	7.9
Other and unknown causes	14.5	16.8

Source: WHO, 1995a.

be a better indicator. But this information is only available from surveys of limited temporal and geographic scope. Systems for registering cases of important communicable diseases, such as AIDS, yellow fever, leprosy, and cholera, exist in most countries. Annual data on cancer incidence are reported to the International Agency for Research on Cancer (IARC) from participating countries' registries.

At an individual level, the risk (%) of dying between the ages of 15 and 60 years from noncommunicable disease does not increase during the epidemiologic transition, it decreases (see Fig. 1.6). These transitions are also accompanied by a change in the types of environmental hazards to which people are exposed. In the pretransition stage, the dominant hazards are what we know to be the traditional hazards of poverty: unsafe drinking water, lack of sanitation, poor shelter, indoor air pollution from stoves and fireplaces, and injury hazards from poorly constructed buildings. As economic development and the epidemiologic transi-

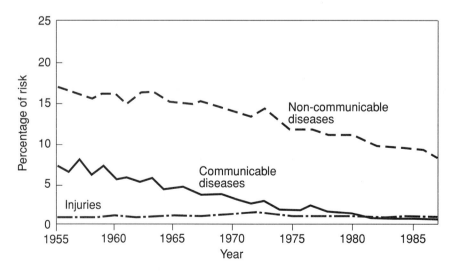

Figure 1.6 The epidemiological transition as it has occurred in Chile. From Murray et al., 1992, with permission.

tion progress, the hazards of the modern age start to dominate: air pollution from power stations, industry, and cars; water pollution from industry; and agricultural chemical exposures. The term *health hazard transition* has been coined to describe this change in types of environmental hazards (Kjellström and Rosenstock, 1990). All of these concepts are useful in describing the change that occurs in conjunction with economic and community development.

Murray and Lopez (1996), using different estimates of the world's largest killers from those used by the WHO, concluded that noncommunicable diseases, rather than infectious diseases, are the world's top killers, accounting for 56% of all deaths; infectious diseases account for 34% and injuries for 10%. While stressing that there is a lot of error in estimates, their assessment suggests that developing countries are further along in the transition than previously expected.

Burden of Disease

Many conditions that do not lead to people's deaths are still responsible for a high prevalence of illness or disability. *Burden of disease* measures the impact of ill health on communities (World Bank, 1993; Murray and Lopez, 1996; the term *public health impact* was used previously). Included in this concept is the impact of both morbidity and mortality on normal life and work capacity. Often the unit of calculation is in terms of life years lost, which statistically converts the duration and timing of illness and disability into a comparable scale, equivalent to the years that might have been lost from a fatal disease. Insurance companies apply the same approach when calculating compensation for permanent injury, e.g., 25% of death compensation for the loss of a limb, 50% compensation for blindness, etc.

Attempts have been made to express the burden of disease in a single number, namely the overall life-years-lost equivalent. This number has been given different names, such as *quality-adjusted life years* (QALYs) or *disability-adjusted life years* (DALYs). Each is based on a number of very uncertain assumptions and judgments about how a disease or disability period should be translated into number of disease free or disability free years lost prior to death. Thus, the final numbers need to be interpreted with caution. Although it is convenient to have a single number for burden of disease, it may be misleading, particularly when comparing disease patterns over time or between geographic regions, for which the impact of disease on well-being and productivity is not constant. For example, improved rehabilitation, technologies for mobility, and access policies have made physical disabilities much less of a handicap in some countries than they used to be. To assume that a particular type of disability is equivalent to a particular number of life-years-lost in every country at any time may seriously bias the interpretation of what these calculations mean.

The burden of disease can also be described as a series (or matrix) of numbers of mortality, morbidity, and disability. Although this description is more complex than using just one number, it offers the opportunity to highlight specific aspects of the burden, such as the impact on the use of health services. A "burden of disease matrix" would also make it possible to better identify the contributions to this burden of disease from specific environmental hazards, without the need to translate ill health into death. For instance, it has been estimated in Sweden that about 400,000 people are disturbed in their homes by traffic noise

BOX 1.4

The Disability-Adjusted Life Year Concept

To show how the calculations have been made for one specific example of burden of disease measurement, the DALY concept will be described here. The WHO and the World Bank undertook a joint exercise to attempt to quantify the extent of "healthy life" lost due to various diseases and conditions. Diseases were classified into 109 categories on the basis of the international classification of diseases (ninth revision). Using the recorded cause of death where available and expert judgment when records were not available, the study assigned all deaths in 1990 to these categories by age, gender, and demographic region. For each death, the number of years of life lost was defined as a difference between the actual age at death and the expectation of life at that age in a low-mortality population. The disability, and the incidence of cases by age, gender, and geographic region were estimated on the basis of community surveys or expert opinion. The number of years of healthy life lost was then obtained by multiplying the expected duration of the condition by a severity weight that measured the severity of the disability in comparison with loss of life. Diseases were grouped into six classes of severity or disability. The death and disability losses were then combined. As shown in Figure 1.7, the value of each year of life lost, shown on the left, rises steeply from 0 at birth to a peak at age 25 and then declines gradually with increasing age. The age weights reflected a consensus judgment, but other patterns could be used. Through using the combination of discounting (reducing by 3% so that future use of healthy life is valued at progressively lower levels) and age weights (e.g., using uniform age weight, with each year of life having the same value, therefore increasing the relative importance of childhood diseases), a pattern of DALYs lost by death at each age could be seen. As shown on the right, the death of a newborn girl represents a loss of 32.5 DALYs; a female death at age 30 means the loss of 29 DALYs; and a female death at age 60 represents 12 lost DALYs.

Source: World Bank, 1993.

and about 100 people die from lung cancer due to residential radon exposure in their homes. Is it possible to make a comparison of the health impact of noise disturbance and death with a common measurement unit? Would that be needed to guide decisions about financial input into prevention of different health risks? The methods for the measurement of the burden of disease (discussed further in Box 1.4) will need further development to produce useful information for decision making and priority setting for environmental hazards control. Two of the key issues are whether deaths in the future should be discounted using an economic analysis approach, and whether deaths at different ages should be given different values (Fig. 1.7). Considerable work is now being done to attempt to quantify the value of reducing health risks (Tengs et al. 1995) using economic methods such as contingent valuation, and comparing the results using various techniques (Spiegel, 2000). This type of analysis may be very useful for decision-makers.

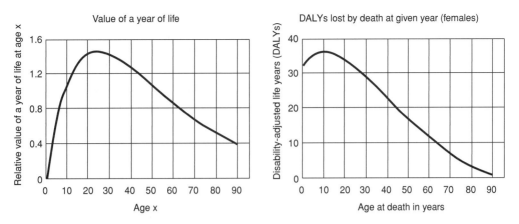

Figure 1.7 Age patterns of age value weights and disability adjusted life years (DALY) lost. From World Bank, 1993, with permission.

The sum of disease across all ages, conditions, and regions is referred to as the *global burden of disease* (GBD). Table 1.4 shows the GBD by cause and regional burden of disease in four of the eight World Bank regions.

Vulnerable Groups

By far the greatest risk factor for poor health is poverty. Particularly vulnerable groups include children, women, elderly people, racial minorities, disabled people, and indigenous peoples, all of whom are often vulnerable because they are not empowered to change their physical environments. Smaller body size, pre-existing diseases, pregnancy, and nutritional deficiencies are several factors that may also increase their vulnerability. Often we do not know how specific hazards affect subgroups of the population. The effects of the hazard on groups in populations that are in a minority or underrepresented in detailed studies may not be identified. There may also be subgroups that are more vulnerable because of where they live or work, because of personal illness (e.g., asthma), or because of biological factors of susceptibility as described below. (As noted in Chapter 3, levels of safe exposure to a contaminant for the general population are often adjusted to account for these vulnerable groups.)

Children As much as two-thirds of all preventable diseases due to environmental conditions occurs in children (WHO, 1997). Children are physically more vulnerable to environmental hazards than adults for several reasons. The metabolic processes of children are different from those of adults (Bearer, 1995). Children under the age of 5 are particularly susceptible because the liver's detoxification potential and kidney's filtration potential is not fully developed (WRI, 2000). Also, their bodies are still developing and the effect of an environmental insult can interfere with that development. The investigation of how toxins may affect fetal and child development is called *developmental toxicology*. Lead, for example, causes damage to the growing central nervous system in children. The metabolic rate per kilogram of body weight of children is much higher than that of an adult, in part because children are still developing and they are smaller. This means that their

TABLE 1.4

GLOBAL DISTRIBUTION OF DALY-LOSS BY DISEASE, 1990[a]

Cause	World	Sub-Saharan Africa	Latin America and the Caribbean	Formerly Socialist Economies of Europe	Established Market Economies
Population (millions)	5267	510	444	346	796
COMMUNICABLE) DISEASES (%	45.8	71.3	42.2	8.6	9.7
Tuberculosis	3.4	4.7	2.5	0.6	0.2
STDs and HIV	3.8	8.8	1.2	1.2	3.4
Diarrhoea	7.3	10.4	5.7	0.4	0.3
Vaccine preventable infections	5.0	9.6	1.6	0.1	0.1
Malaria	2.6	10.8	0.4	<0.05	<0.05
Respiratory infections	9.0	10.8	6.2	2.6	2.6
Maternal causes	2.2	2.7	1.7	0.8	0.6
Perinatal causes	7.3	7.1	9.1	2.4	2.2
Other	5.3	6.4	8.3	0.6	0.5
NONCOMMUNICABLE DISEASES (%)	42.2	19.4	42.8	74.8	78.4
Cancer	5.8	1.5	5.2	14.8	19.1
Nutritional deficiencies	3.9	2.8	4.6	1.4	1.7
Neuropsychiatric disease	6.8	3.3	8.0	11.1	15.0
Cerebrovascular disease	3.2	1.5	2.6	8.9	5.3
Ischemic heart disease	3.1	0.4	2.7	13.7	10.0
Other	19.3	9.9	19.8	25.0	27.3
INJURIES (%)	11.9	9.3	15.0	16.6	11.9
Motor vehicle	2.3	1.3	5.7	3.7	3.5
Intentional	3.7	4.2	4.3	4.8	4.0
Other	5.9	3.9	5.0	8.1	4.3
TOTAL (%)	100.0	100.0	100.0	100.0	100.0
Millions of DALYs	1362	293	103	58	94
DALYs per 1000 population	259	575	233	168	117

[a]Examples are of four of the eight World Bank regions. HIV, human immunodeficiency virus; STDs, sexually transmitted disease.
Source: World Bank, 1993.

respiratory rate, for example, is proportionately greater and they breathe in much more air pollution in relation to their body weight than an adult in similar circumstances. Children also have a greater chance of experiencing chronic effects of exposure to environmental hazards than adults, because when they are exposed to a carcinogen, the chances are much higher that they will live beyond the latency period (the years that it takes for a cancer to develop after exposure).

The physical environment of children is different from those of adults, even in the same home. Newborns remain in cribs and are not able to remove themselves from environmental hazards such as direct sunlight. They must count on adults to recognize and deal with dangerous environments. Toddlers live close to the ground and thus may be exposed to contaminants in soil and dust. They are constantly putting things in their mouths, as young children go through a phase of intense oral exploratory behavior, and they may be prone to pica, the practice of eating dirt.

Children are also vulnerable in a social sense. When families are not strong and poverty is severe, children are often exploited and deprived of their rights. Children are less able to protect themselves by making informed choices, protesting working conditions, or refusing to be exposed to hazards. In some countries, children are forced to work in hazardous environments to earn money to support themselves and their families. Under such conditions, which can amount to slavery, children have no protection and may be severely abused. When they are injured, there may be no one to support them or to replace their lost income. In extreme situations, children have been forced into prostitution where they experience a high risk of becoming infected with human immunodeficiency virus (HIV). It is estimated that there are over 20 million "street children" in Latin America alone. Child abuse and parental neglect contribute to childhood injuries and poisoning by drugs and other chemicals.

A child's environment also plays a significant role in the propagation of infectious diseases. Despite successes in tackling vaccine-preventable diseases, each year 2.8 million children die from them and a further 3 million suffer ill health as a result of these diseases (WHO, 1993b). Certain diseases are more prevalent in children (for example, asthma), and high concentrations of toxicant (for example, air pollution) will affect children before they affect adults. Many children are born prematurely, grow up in poverty, or do not have adequate nutrition. These conditions in turn decrease their ability to cope with an environmental hazard. One-third of children in developing countries weigh less than 2.5 kg at birth, and almost half the children in Africa show signs of malnutrition. There are numerous biological, chemical, and physical agents that, at low doses, have little effect on a mother but have profound effects, such as congenital and developmental problems, on the fetus. Listeria, methyl mercury, and radiation are prime examples of such agents.

Recognizing the vulnerability of children, the Ministers of Environment of the seven highly developed countries and Russia published the *1997 Declaration of the Environment Leaders of the Fight on Children's Environmental Health* (USEPA, 1997). The declaration highlights the problems of specific hazards, such as polluted water, air quality, lead, endocrine-disrupting chemicals, and environmental tobacco smoke, along with the general problem of appropriate risk assessment and standard setting, which must take into account the special situations of children.

Women The rapid increase in problems arising from the destruction of natural resources, rapid industrialization and urbanization, pollution and population pressures has a special impact on women (Sims, 1994). Women have less privileged status in society and less access to resources, although they are often obliged to fulfil multiple roles and function as producers, reproducers, and home managers. Of the 1.3 billion people living in poverty, 70% are women (UNDP, 1995).

Women may be at a disadvantage from birth onward because of inadequate nutrition, lack of education, heavy workloads, early marriage, and early and frequent pregnancies. In some countries, women who have no partners are at particularly high risk of poor health and are forced into poverty or prostitution because of insufficient opportunities to earn a living by themselves. Prostitution has grown to immense proportions in some developing countries (this applies to girls and boys as well as women). In addition, women suffer discrimination at the workplace and are often subjected to the worst working conditions. In rural areas, women have particularly heavy workloads, as they are responsible for gathering fuel, collecting water, and foraging.

Women's vulnerability during pregnancy and childbirth is evident from the very high levels of maternal mortality in most developing countries. In many low-income communities, there is a significantly higher incidence of certain diseases among women, because they spend more time in its contaminated environments. Women suffer more from diseases associated with inadequate water and sanitation and from respiratory problems associated with smoke in living environments where cooking or heating is on open fires or poorly designed stoves using coal or wood. An anthology entitled *Women, Health and the Environment* (Sims, 1994), published by the WHO, provides further examples and details in this area. The role of women in sustainable development has received increasing attention. In many societies, women have greater influence than men on rates of population growth, infant mortality, and various aspects of health and environmental degradation. Thus any socioeconomic pressures that are detrimental to women are detrimental to society as a whole and the global ecosystem.

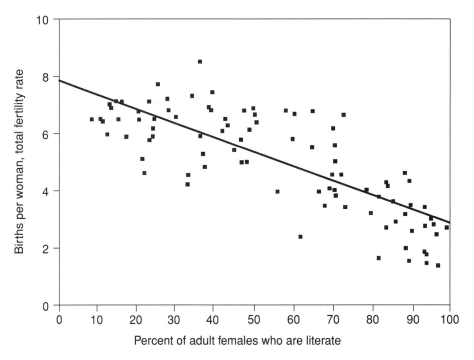

Figure 1.8 Fertility rate by female literacy, 1990. From WRI, 1994, with permission.

Women spend more time than men doing both paid and unpaid work in almost all developing and developed countries. Although more women are working outside the household than ever before, their wages still lag behind those of men. Many women work in low-paying jobs in the service sector and in the informal sector, for example, in food vending and trading in household goods, tailoring, domestic service, and artisanship. Women also contribute significantly to agricultural production and they traditionally harvest forest products, such as firewood, in many countries. Women usually bear primary responsibility for collecting, supplying, and managing water. In addition, women deliver basic health care in many parts of the world. Even so, in many societies, cultural and religious attitudes have resulted in discriminatory laws and/or practices that have prevented women from becoming equal partners in society. In almost all areas of the world, the literacy rate for women is lower than that for men.

Women's poverty, limited education, and economic opportunities and discrimination contribute to high fertility rates, which in turn lead to various problems, including strained resources and endangered health for women and children. The World Bank has shown that for every year of schooling a woman receives, her fertility rate is reduced by 10% and for every 1–3 years of schooling, child mortality rates are reduced by 15% (World Bank, 1993). The relationship between female literacy and fertility is shown in Figure 1.8; Figure 1.9 shows the relationship between child mortality and female literacy.

Education and training program for women have become a high priority in efforts to move toward sustainable development. These programs must, of course,

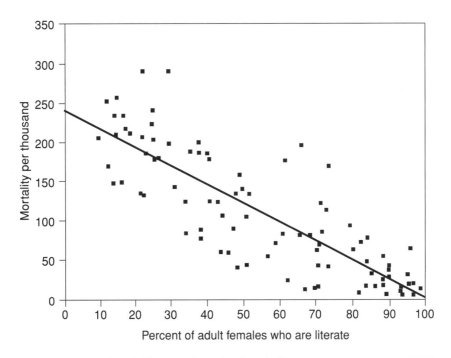

Figure 1.9 Mortality rate for children under 5 by female literacy, 1990–91. From WRI, 1994, with permission.

be combined with basic health services, expanded economic opportunities, and enforced civil rights. Many multilateral organizations, including many United Nations agencies, have been working together to recommend national and international actions toward these ends. One publication by the United Nations Population Fund, published as part of *Investing in Women: The Focus of the '90's* (Nafis, 1990), urges governments and international nongovernmental organisations to do the following:

- document and publicize women's vital contribution to development
- increase women's productivity and remove barriers to productive resources
- provide family planning and improve the health of women
- expand education
- establish equality of opportunity.

Elderly People The world is aging. This simple fact has immense implications for the provision of shelter, health care, and social support. Elderly persons are at an increased risk of having diseases. They are more likely to be malnourished than younger adults, for a variety of social, economic, and physiological reasons (including early dementia), and are therefore more vulnerable to many diseases. Especially important are diseases that decrease the body's ability to cope with hazardous exposures. Examples of such disabling conditions that are common in the elderly include emphysema, kidney disease, congestive heart failure, dementia, and diabetes. As with children, elderly persons with respiratory diseases are not able to tolerate air pollution. The elderly are more likely to have had a long exposure to a given toxin simply because they have been living longer. An older body also has less mass, and often metabolizes toxins at a slower rate. As in children, therefore, smaller doses of a given substance will have a greater effect on the elderly than on younger adults.

Recent rapid changes in lifestyles in many societies has led to changes in cultures that once had more respect for elders. As a result, the elderly are often impoverished without the social support of extended families, and are subject to some of the same patterns of vulnerabilities as children.

Disabled People It is estimated that there are 500 million disabled people in the world today, and this number is expected to double in the early part of the twenty-first century. Four out of five disabled people live in developing countries, and one third of them are children. Few countries are able to provide meaningful assistance, support, rehabilitation, and protection, thus many disabled people are particularly impoverished and subject to exploitation and chronic illness. Chronic psychiatric conditions, including addictions to alcohol or drugs, may also lead to malnutrition, self-mutilation, and depression. These conditions may decrease the body's ability to cope with environmental hazards.

Disabled people often have difficulty finding meaningful jobs that pay them an adequate living. They are often forced to take unwanted and dangerous jobs or face unemployment and poverty. The disabled, therefore, are sometimes at increased risk from environmental hazards because of their cultural milieu, in addition to their vulnerability as a result of their disability.

Indigenous Peoples In general, throughout the twentieth century the state of health of aboriginal peoples has remained far worse than that in populations of non-aboriginal origin in the same countries. For instance, infant mortality rates remain at a persistently higher level in aboriginal people in Canada (Fig. 1.10). In the early 1990s the infant mortality rate among registered Canadian Indians was still about twice as high as the national rate (Fig. 1.11), despite the gains made during the post–World War II years, particularly among Northwest Territories Inuit. The success of immunization programs in Canada substantially reduced the impact of such diseases as measles, rubella, mumps, poliomyelitis, tetanus, and diphtheria in aboriginal communities. Similarly, the availability of effective anti-tuberculosis therapy and the large scale control efforts of the 1950s resulted in a steep decline in tuberculosis mortality. Despite such improvements, the disparity between aboriginal and nonaboriginal Canadians remains great, with the former having an incidence of tuberculosis as much as ten times higher.

Within Inuit of one region of the Northwest Territories, the incidence of meningitis was 20 times higher among 5-year-olds, and 33 times higher among infants, compared to nonaboriginal communities (Hammond et al., 1988). While diarrheal diseases are less severe in Canadian aboriginal communities than in many developing countries, isolated outbreaks continue to be reported, highlighting the similarity between conditions experienced by Canada's aboriginal communities and that of many developing countries. Similarly, infections of the

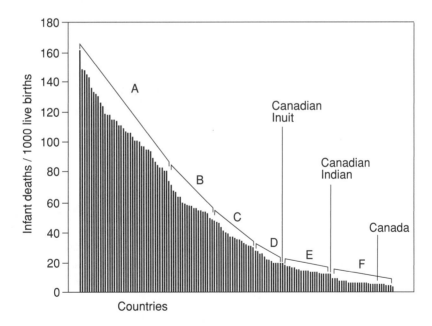

Figure 1.10 Infant mortality rates in different countries and among aboriginal populations in Canada. A, most sub-Saharan African countries, Afghanistan, Bangladesh, Haiti; B, some North African countries, India, Central America, Brazil; C, Venezuela, Argentina, China, some Asian and Middle Eastern countries; D, Korea, Malaysia, Chile, Panama, Uruguay, Romania, former USSR; E, Costa Rica, Cuba, Jamaica, Greece, Portugal, Eastern Europe; F, Western Europe, North America, Australiasia, Israel, Japan, Hong Kong. From Waldram et al., 1995, with permission.

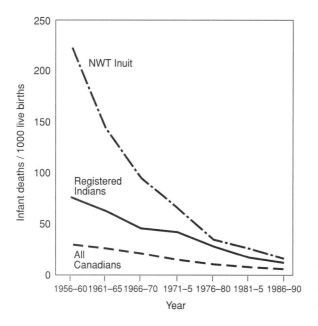

Figure 1.11 Infant mortality rate among Canadian registered Indians, Northwest Territories Inuit, and all Canadians. From Waldram et al., 1995, with permission.

respiratory tract are more common among aboriginal communities. Various housing surveys have documented the high proportion of aboriginal dwellings characterized by overcrowding, inadequate heating, and poor ventilation (Clatworthy and Stevens, 1987). These factors contribute to the high risk of respiratory infections.

Of particular concern is the increase in chronic diseases and the high prevalence of obesity in many aboriginal groups. Among the most serious health problems now affecting aboriginal peoples are injuries sustained as a result of accidents and violence. The high level of morbidity and mortality from such injuries has been attributed to the prevailing economic conditions and social stress that aboriginal peoples experience. For example, in Canadian aboriginal communities a high number of residential fires have occurred, which have been linked to personal behaviors such as smoking, drinking, leaving children unattended, and having suicidal intent. Contributing social environmental factors that are largely attributable to poverty include disconnection of electricity because the utility bill hasn't been paid, alcoholism, lack of fire protection in the community, nonadherence to building codes, lack of child care, and mental health problems. Moreover, acts of violence are intimately related to the mental health of individuals and the social health of a community. Suicide, which is particularly high among young adult males, is indicative of the alienation and despair occurring in these communities.

Many aboriginal people recognize that these problems must be resolved through a healing process undertaken by the communities themselves. The reestablishment of individual and community self-esteem has been actively pursued through the enhancement of positive traditional values and customs. A landmark conference entitled "Healing Our Spirit Worldwide" in Edmonton, Canada in 1992 brought together aboriginal groups from around the world who shared their experience in healing the wounds of violence and substance abuse. Such efforts, combined with the general move toward self-government, promise encouraging results. There is great benefit to be gained when environmental health professionals work with traditional healers who know the community and are often highly trusted so they can be effective agents of change.

IMPACT OF ENVIRONMENTAL FACTORS ON HEALTH

It is clear that the environment in which people live has a huge influence on their health. A safe water supply, food that is nutritionally sufficient, and interruption of the fecal–oral chain of disease transmission are essential to reducing the incidence of gastrointestinal diseases. Because of such simple measures, these diseases had already declined significantly in most of Europe and North America well before the introduction of therapeutic drugs and oral rehydration therapy. Likewise, immunization and the use of modern drugs have contributed to the dramatic decrease in mortality from infectious respiratory diseases. Reductions in overcrowding and overall improvements in housing and the working environment have also played a major role. Whereas noncommunicable disease risks have decreased through reduced air pollution in large cities of developed countries, the effect of other exposures, such as tobacco smoking, continue to pose major health risks.

The sharp increase in the incidence of lung cancer and the steady decrease in stomach cancer stand out as the most significant changes in cancer trends, the former being due mostly to past trends in tobacco smoking, the latter possibly to changes in the preservation of food and the amount of fruit and vegetables in the diet. It is not possible to accurately assess the burden of cancer attributed to environmental factors except for that related to occupational exposure to carcinogens (e.g., to asbestos, vinyl chloride, or benzene), urinary schistosomiasis, (related to stagnant water from dams, for example) which carries a high risk of bladder cancer, or hepatitis B virus (e.g., from improperly disposed needles), which is associated with a high incidence of liver cancer. The most significant cancer risk factors for the general population are tobacco smoking, alcohol consumption, dietary composition, and sexual behavior. The role of ionizing radiation in inducing cancers is also well established but forms only a small percentage of total incidence. Exposure to the ultraviolet component of sunlight is responsible for a significant number of skin cancers—much more so than ionizing radiation. Perhaps 5% of all cancers in the general population is due to exposure to environmental chemicals. The variety of chemicals produced, used in daily life, and released to the environment is rising, and exposure to them is of increasing concern.

Table 1.5 shows an estimate of the GBD from selected environmental threats in 1990 and potential worldwide reductions through environmental interventions (World Bank, 1993). It is estimated that 36 million DALYs, or 3% of the GBD, are preventable with currently available and feasible interventions in the workplace environment. Additional interventions are likely to become available in the future. These losses are caused by injuries and deaths in high-risk occupations and by chronic illness stemming from exposure to toxic chemicals, noise, stress, and physically disabling work patterns. If by removing urban air pollution

TABLE 1.5

ESTIMATED GLOBAL BURDEN OF DISEASE FROM SELECTED ENVIRONMENTAL
THREATS, 1990, AND POTENTIAL WORLDWIDE REDUCTIONS THROUGH
INTERVENTION IN THE WORKPLACE AND AMBIENT ENVIRONMENT

Type of Environment and Principal Related Diseases[a]	Burden from These Diseases (millions of DALYs/year)	Reduction Achievable Through Feasible Interventions[b] (%)	Burden Averted by Feasible Interventions (millions of DALYs/year)	Burden Averted per 1000 Population (DALYs/year)
OCCUPATIONAL	318	—	36	7.1
Cancers	79	5	4	0.8
Neuropsychiatric	93	5	5	0.9
Chronic respiratory	47	5	2	0.5
Musculoskeletal	18	50	9	1.8
Unintentional injury	81[c]	20	16	3.1
URBAN OUTDOOR AIR				
Acute respiratory infections	123	5	6	1.2
Chronic respiratory diseases	47	5	2	0.5
ROAD TRANSPORT				
(motor vehicle injuries)	32	20	6	1.2
All the above	473[d]	—	50	10.0

[a]The diseases shown are those for which there is substantial evidence of a relationship with the environment.
[b]Estimates are derived from the product of the efficacy of the interventions and the proportion of the global burden of disease that occurs among the exposed.
[c]Computed by subtracting motor vehicle injuries (32 million DALYs) from all unintentional injuries (113 million DALYs)
[d]Adjusted for double counting. However, this is based on current allocation of economic resources; much more could be achieved with a different prioritization for resource use.
Source: World Bank, 1993.

5% of all acute respiratory infectious and chronic respiratory diseases could be prevented, this would result in a decrease in a burden by 8 million DALYs each year, or 0.6% of the GBD (Table 1.5).

Local environmental impacts on especially vulnerable groups may be much greater. For example, airborne lead concentrations have been high in polluted urban environments where lead has come mainly from the exhaust of vehicles burning leaded gasoline. Elevated lead levels in children have been associated with impaired neuropsychological development, poor intellectual performance, and behavioral difficulties.

Diseases related to poor sanitation and inadequate water supply, inadequate garbage disposal and drainage, heavy indoor air pollution, and crowding probably account for nearly 30% of the total burden of disease (see Table 1.6). Modest improvements in household environments would avert almost one-quarter of this burden, mostly as a result of reductions in diarrhea and respiratory infections.

TABLE 1.6

ESTIMATED BURDEN OF DISEASE FROM POOR HOUSEHOLD ENVIRONMENTS
IN DEVELOPING COUNTRIES, 1990, AND POTENTIAL REDUCTION THROUGH
INTERVENTIONS

Principal Diseases Related to Poor Household Environments[a]	Relevant Environmental Problem	Burden from These Diseases in Developing Countries (millions of DALYs/year)	Reduction Achievable Through Feasible Interventions (%)[b]	Burden Averted by Feasible Interventions (millions of DALYs/year)	Burden Averted per 1000 Population (DALYs/year)
Tuberculosis	Crowding	46	10	5	1.2
Diarrhea[c]	Sanitation, water supply, hygiene	99	40	40	9.7
Trachoma	Water supply, hygiene	3	30	2	0.3
Tropical cluster[d]	Sanitation, garbage disposal, vector breeding around the home	8	30	2	0.5
Intestinal worms	Sanitation, water supply, hygiene	18	40	7	1.7
Respiratory infections	Indoor air pollution, crowding	119	15	18	4.4
Chronic respiratory diseases	Indoor air pollution	41	15	6	1.5
Respiratory tract cancers	Indoor air pollution	4	10	[e]	0.1
All of the above		338	—	79	19.4

Note: The demographically developing group consists of the demographic regions Sub-Saharan Africa, India, China, other Asian countries, Latin America, the Caribbean, and the Middle Eastern crescent.

[a]The diseases listed are those for which there is substantial evidence of a relationship with the household. (Examples of excluded conditions are violence related to crowding and guinea worm infection related to poor water supply.)

[b]Estimates are derived from the products of the efficacy of the interventions and the proportion of the burden of disease that occurs among the exposed.

[c]Includes diarrhoea, dysentery, cholera, and typhoid.

[d]Diseases within the tropical cluster most affected by the domestic environment are schistosomiasis, South American trypanosomiasis, and Bancroftian filariasis.

[e]Less than one.

Source: World Bank, 1993.

In a review of the links between development, environment, and health (WHO, 1997), the "environmental fraction" of the global DALY's for major disease and injury groups ranged between 10% and 90% (Table 1.7). The resulting approximate estimate of the environmental contribution to the global burden of disease and injury was 23% (WHO, 1997).

TABLE 1.7

PROPORTION OF GLOBAL DALYS ASSOCIATED WITH ENVIRONMENTAL
EXPOSURES, 1990

	Global DALYs (thousands)	Environmental fraction (%)	Environmental DALYs (thousands)	% of all DALYs	
				All Age Groups	Age 0–14 Years
Acute respiratory infections	116,696	60	70,017	5.0	4.50
Diarrheal diseases	99,633	90	89,670	6.5	6.10
Vaccine-preventable infections	71,173	10	7117	0.5	0.49
Tuberculosis	38,426	10	3843	0.3	0.04
Malaria	31,706	90	28,535	2.1	1.80
Unintentional injuries	152,188	30	45,656	3.3	1.60
Intentional injuries	56,459	NE	NE		
Mental health	144,950	10	14,495	1.1	0.08
Cardiovascular diseases	133,236	10	13,324	1.0	0.12
Cancer	70,513	25	17,628	1.3	0.11
Chronic respiratory diseases	60,370	50	30,185	2.2	0.57
Total these diseases	975,350	33	320,470	23.0	15.40
Other diseases	403,888	NE	NE		
Total all diseases	1,379,238	(23)	(320,470)		

NE, not estimated.
Source: WHO, 1997; DALY data from Murray and Lopez, 1996.

LINKS BETWEEN ENVIRONMENTAL AND OCCUPATIONAL HEALTH

Importance of the Workforce

The workforce of a country is the backbone of its development. A healthy, well-trained, and motivated workforce increases productivity and generates wealth that is necessary for the good health of the community at large. Injured and sick workers, quite apart from being a major source of morbidity to themselves and their families, affect the economy as a whole, as do lost workdays due to illness and injury. The environment in the workplace generally involves levels of higher human exposure to environmental hazards and more injuries than in the residential environment. Every year approximately 100 million work injuries and 200,000 occupational deaths are reported in addition to the millions of cases of illnesses due to chronic exposure to noise, infectious agents, biomechanical hazards, and toxic chemicals. The workforce therefore requires particular health protection to maintain productivity, social equity, and personal security. The *Encyclopaedia of Occupational Health and Safety* (ILO, 1998) is a good source of information about workers' health.

Linked Environmental and Occupational Health Hazards

The main reason for linking the occupational and general environments when addressing health concerns is that the source of the hazard is often the same. A common approach may work effectively in varied settings, particularly when it comes to the choice of chemical technologies for production. One example is the use of water-based paints instead of paints containing potentially toxic organic solvents. Another example is choosing nonchemical over chemical pest control methods.

Substituting one substance for another that is less acutely toxic may make good occupational health sense. However, if the new substance is not biodegradable or if it damages the stratospheric ozone layer, it is not an appropriate exposure control solution; it only moves the problem elsewhere. Chlorofluorocarbons (CFCs), widely used as refrigerant instead of the more acutely dangerous substance, ammonia, is the classic example of what is now known to have been an environmentally inappropriate substitution, for CFCs are the main cause of damage to the stratospheric ozone layer (see Chapter 11, Ozone Depletion and Ultraviolet Radiation).

Common Approaches and Human Resources

The scientific knowledge and training required to assess and control environmental health hazards are generally the same skills and knowledge required to address health hazards within the workplace. Toxicology, epidemiology, occupational hygiene, ergonomics, and safety engineering are basic sciences that underlie assessment in these two fields. It thus may make good sense for the same professions to monitor both areas, especially in countries with scarce resources (see Role of the Environmental Health Professionals, below).

The Workplace as a Sentinel for Environmental Hazards

Environmental health hazards have often been first identified from observations of adverse health effects in workers. The workplace is where the impact of industrial exposures is best understood. To conduct an epidemiological study it is necessary to define the exposed population, the nature and level of the exposure, and the specific health effect. It is generally easier to define the members of a workforce than it is to determine the membership of a community, particularly in a community that is transient. As well, the outcome of high levels of exposure typical of the workforce are almost always easier to delineate than more subtle changes attributable to low-level exposure.

Information on occupational health effects of many toxic exposures (including metals such as lead, mercury, arsenic, and nickel, as well as known carcinogens such as asbestos) has been used to calculate the health risk to the wider community. For example, as early as 1942, reports began to appear of cases of osteomalacia with multiple fractures among workers exposed to cadmium in a French factory producing alkaline batteries. During the 1950s and 1960s, cadmium intoxication was considered to be strictly an occupational disease. However, from the knowledge gained about the workplace came the recognition that the osteomalacia and kidney disease that was occurring in Japan at this time, "Itai itai" disease, was due to cadmium contamination of rice from irrigation water containing cadmium from a mine and metal refinery. Research in occupational epidemiology made a substantive contribution to the understanding and recognition of the environmental health effects.

The Total Exposure Concept

It is not enough to assess the exposure to a hazard from just one source. The sum of all exposures needs to be measured to assess health impacts and establish dose–response relationships. Pesticide exposure is a classic example where occupational exposure may be supplemented by substantive environmental exposure. This may come through food and water source contamination and through nonoccupational airborne exposure. In Central America, for example, some cotton growers using pesticides not only have little access to protective clothing but live very close to the cotton fields; many live in temporary housing with no walls for protection from aerial pesticide spraying. Workers also wash in irrigation channels containing pesticide residues, resulting in increased exposure (Michaels et al., 1985). Thus to understand the relationship between their pesticide exposure and the health effects that may be reported, all sources of exposure to pesticide should be taken into consideration. Other examples of exposure that may occur at the workplace as well as in the ambient environment are exposure to particulate matter from engine emissions (from industrial machines or traffic), benzene (as a solvent or from cigarette smoke), and polycyclic aromatic hydrocarbons (from products containing tar or from diet).

Consistency in Setting Standards

Environmental health standards are usually much stricter than occupational health standards, as shown, for example, by the guideline values recommended by the WHO for selected chemicals for each exposure situation given in Table 1.8. The rationale for the difference is that the community includes many subgroups that are relatively sensitive, including the very old, the ill, young children, and pregnant women, whereas the workforce is at least healthy enough to work. Also, it is often argued that risk is more "acceptable" to a work force, as these people are benefiting by having a job and are therefore more willing to accept the risk. Many ethical and scientific debates rage around the question of standards and their degree of protection and for whom. Linking occupational and environmental health can be a positive contribution to sorting out these controversies. In this regard, tightening the connection between occupational and environmental health may facilitate greater consistency in setting standards.

TABLE 1.8

COMPARISON BETWEEN WHO HEALTH-BASED GUIDELINES FOR AIR IN THE WORKPLACE AND IN THE GENERAL ENVIRONMENT (WHO AIR QUALITY GUIDELINES)

Chemical	Workplace Guideline $\mu g/m^3$ (8-hr mean)	General Environment Guideline $\mu g/m^3$ (annual mean)
Lead	30–60	0.5–1.0
Cadmium	10	0.01–0.02
Manganese	300	1
Mercury	50	1
Formaldehyde	500	100 (24 hours)
Nitrogen dioxide	900	150 (24 hours)
Sulfur dioxide	1300	50

Source: WHO, 1987a and several Technical Report Series issues.

Incentives for Prevention

Although the workplace is usually the site of more intense exposures, the impact of these hazards on the general public has often been a major force in stimulating cleanup efforts, both inside the workplace and in the surrounding community. For example, the discovery of high levels of lead in workers' blood by an industrial hygienist in a lead foundry in Bahia, Brazil led to investigations of lead in the blood of children in nearby residential areas (Nogueira, 1987). The finding that the children had high lead levels was a major impetus in the company to take action to reduce occupational exposures as well as lead emissions from the factory, although workers in the foundry are still exposed to substantially higher exposures than would be tolerated by the general community. For more about the relationship between occupational and environmental health, see the section by Yassi and Kjellström in the *Encyclopaedia of Occupational Health and Safety* (ILO, 1998).

OBSTACLES TO AND OPPORTUNITIES FOR RESOLVING ENVIRONMENTAL HEALTH PROBLEMS

Demographic Issues

The impact of people on the environment is related to the size of the population and to the level of consumption. Both expand independently and both lead to increasing pressure on the environment as both a supplier of resources and a repository of waste. Limited resources have made development in the poorest countries of the world difficult, with increasing demand for water, food, and energy for domestic use being in direct proportion to the number of users. Meanwhile, more people are moving to urban areas where the infrastructures are rarely able to keep up with the influx of new citizens. In temperate and sub-Arctic countries, energy needs may be greater than in other parts of the world because of the climate. Countries in these areas are generally highly developed, and the high level of consumption accompanying their affluence (which until recently, in many countries, was not accompanied by much genuine concern for the environment or the need for conservation of resources) has magnified global problems.

Different areas of the world have different rates of population growth. The global annual increase is thought to have stabilized, with an increase of about 81 million people added each year for 1990–95 (WRI, 2000). Nevertheless, the world population, which was 5.3 billion in 1990, and more 5.9 billion in 1999 is expected to be between 7.7 and 11.2 billion by the year 2050 (WRI, 2000). Because of the differences in rates of increase, the proportion of the world's population in North America and Europe has been shrinking while in other parts of the world it has been expanding or has remained stable (see Fig. 1.12). These projections are based on expected trends in birth and death rates, and adjustments to the projections will be necessary as new information becomes available. Improvements in the provision of health care may alter the pattern of mortality, and the AIDS pandemic will have a major influence on population growth, especially in Africa, where children and young adults are most affected. Changes

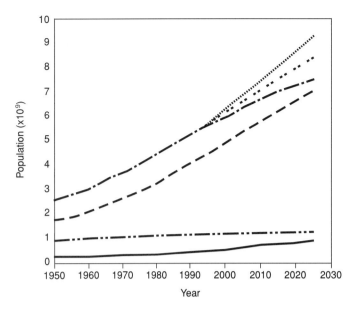

Figure 1.12 World population trends and projections. ———— least developed countries, medium variant; – – – developing countries, medium variant; — - - — developed countries, medium variant; — - — - world population, low variant; ·········· World population, high variant; - - -- - - world population, medium variant. From WHO, 1992a, with permission.

in lifestyle, such as in reproductive and dietary habits, age at marriage, or tobacco, alcohol, and drug consumption, may also alter population projections. However, the single most important factor influencing the rate of population growth is the education of women.

Rapid growth in urban population has been evident in most countries for over 10 years. This has important implications for health and the environment. The concentration of people and economic production in urban areas brings many cost advantages in waste management. The per-capita cost of piped water, many kinds of sanitation, education, health care, and other services is likely to be less in some concentrated populations. Growing urban populations may also stimulate agricultural development and reduce the influx from rural populations. Urban growth, however, usually brings substantial health and environmental problems, especially for poorer groups. Without effective governmental policies, the potential advantages of urbanization may be outstripped by the many disadvantages.

The size, rate of growth, and age distribution of a population is only part of the demographic problem of a country or region. Movement of populations across borders also constitutes a major component of a demographic pattern. Migrants are usually driven by economic need toward countries where there is a greater potential for employment or the possibility of opening up new land. Increasingly, political refugees have contributed to migratory movements. Ecological change, such as drought, has also forced migration. While the total number of migrants represents a small fraction of the world's population, these people can have a major influence on the resources and structure of the host population, especially when unanticipated environmental or political events cause a large number of people to move to a neighboring country. These migrants are often confronted with severe health and environmental problems and seldom have access to basic health services and health insurance coverage. Their living conditions are usually inferior to those of the host population, resulting in a negative effect on their health.

Poverty

Poverty has been defined by the World Bank as the inability of an individual or household to attain a minimal standard of living. The level of prosperity in a country and the distribution of resources within it determine the level and nature of poverty. The association between poverty and health is strong and obvious. The poor usually have much lower life expectancy, higher infant mortality, and a higher incidence of disability. They suffer more from communicable diseases and a high proportion of their lives is spent in poor health.

The number of poor people in a given country is estimated from the number of people with incomes below a level defined as the poverty line. The World Bank estimates that in 1985 there were 1115 million people living below the poverty line, defined as $370 U.S. per person per year, or U.S. $1 per person per day. The extreme poverty line is set at $275 U.S. per person per year and there were 634 million people living at that level in the world in 1985 (see Table 1.9).

Defining poverty solely by level of personal income, however, cannot adequately represent all aspects of health. Also, setting a single international poverty line based on income per capita can be misleading since it cannot take sufficient account of differences between countries and the income needed to attain an adequate living standard. Furthermore, variations in living costs between areas

TABLE 1.9

WORLD BANK ESTIMATES OF THE SCALE OF POVERTY[A] IN DEVELOPING COUNTRIES, 1985

	Number of Poor (millions)	Head-count Index[b] (%)	Poverty Gap[c] (%)	Under-5 Mortality[d] (per thousand born)	Life Expectancy (years)	Net Primary School Enrollment Rate (%)
Sub-Saharan Africa	180	47	11	196	50	56
East Asia	280	20	1	96	67	96
China	210	20	3	58	69	93
South Asia	520	51	10	172	56	74
India	420	55	12	199	57	81
Eastern Europe	6	8	5	23	71	90
Eastern Mediterranean and North Africa	60	31	2	148	61	75
Latin America and the Caribbean	70	19	1	75	66	92
All developing countries	1116	33	3	121	62	83

[a]The poverty line in international dollars (using purchasing power parities) is $370 per capita a year for the poor.

[b]The headcount index is defined as the percentage of the population below the poverty line.

[c]The poverty gap is defined as the aggregate income shortfall of the poor as a percentage of aggregate consumption.

[d]Under −5 mortality rates are for 1980–85, except for China and South Asia, where the period is 1975–80.
Source: World Bank, 1990.

within countries are such that some people with income well above the poverty line may have inadequate living standards while someone living below the poverty line may have adequate standards.

A better way of calculating the number of people living in poverty is to evaluate the number that lack a minimum standard of living including adequate food, safe and sufficient supplies of water, secure shelter, access to education and health care, and, in high-density settlements, provision for the removal of domestic wastes. With these criteria it has been estimated that 2200 million people live in poverty in the developing world. According to the United Nations Development Program (UNDP) 1300 million live in absolute poverty, 840 million are undernourished (UNDP, 1997); 1400 million lack safe drinking water (UNICEF, 1997) and 900 million are illiterate (UNESCO, 1996), as discussed by the World Resources Institute (WRI, 2000).

In most cities in developing countries, between one-third and two-thirds of all inhabitants live in informal settlements with inadequate or no infrastructure or services. Even in the richest countries, a proportion of the population suffers the adverse health effects of physical deprivation and social exclusion. Particular cities or districts within cities that suffer most have not only high levels of unemployment, particularly among young people, but also high levels of poor-quality housing and social problems. They also tend to have significantly higher than average infant mortality rates and a lower life expectancy.

At the beginning of the chapter the overall increase in life expectancy was noted. But the gap in life expectancy between the least developed (43 years) and most developed (78 years) countries is widening; by the year 2000 the gap is projected to be 37 years. Also, even if improvements are made globally, changing conditions could result in dramatic setbacks in specific countries. The most striking example is the reduction in life expectancy in Russia following 1990 (WRI, 1996).

Consumption Patterns

One important obstacle to progress in resolving environmental health problems is the major difference in consumption patterns between different countries and between different groups within countries. The very high consumption of energy and natural resources by the richest countries and the richest groups within countries cannot be sustained. If the people of China achieved the same density of automobiles per capita as that in the United States, for example, the production of greenhouse gases, air pollution, and other traffic-related problems would create a major health crisis. Greenhouse gases also vastly increase the global problem of climate change (see Chapter 11, Climate Change and the Greenhouse Effect).

Rees and Wackernagel (1992) characterized the land area necessary to sustain current levels of resource consumption and waste discharge by a population as its *ecological footprint*. The ecological footprints of high income cities are hundreds of times larger than their politic or geographical area and are much larger than the ecological footprints of lower income communities.

Development is often seen as the poor reaching toward the lifestyle and economic level of the rich. Clearly, large gaps in health and well-being between population groups and countries are not equitable, but should the aim of development be for future generations to copy the rich? Or rather should it be to find a healthy and sustainable level of economic development? The challenge is for each society and the global community to establish limits of consumption that will make it possible to provide for the basic needs of all people, without sacrificing opportunities for personal improvements in lifestyle.

Technological innovations offer hope for expansion of "the good life" to everybody. Improvements in fuel efficiency of cars and the development of catalytic converters for pollution control are examples of such innovations. Electric cars may provide the next threshold of technological advance in relation to cars; however, the root problem lies in transport systems that encourage people to use cars instead of more cost-efficient and pollution-avoiding alternatives. Information technology may reduce the need for travel. Perhaps a whole new energy-efficient approach to living and working will develop.

Macroeconomic Policies

Macroeconomic policies have important direct and indirect effects on health and the environment. They influence the use and degradation of natural resources because they can affect consumer demand and the prices of natural resources. The effect of macroeconomic policies are felt most directly at the level of an individual's purchasing power. For example, they permit improvements in the quality and quantity of food and thus in nutritional status and susceptibility to disease. In an economic crisis, they may result in sharply diminished purchasing power and a lack of adequate nutrition.

Global economic changes, adverse changes in the terms of trade for some countries, and an increased debt burden driven by the rise of real interest rates have all contributed to periodic decline in the word economy. The International Monetary Fund (IMF) has required many countries to implement "structural adjustment programs" (usually cuts in public expenditures, including health and related services) before it provides loans to developing countries. Public works such as piped water supplies, sewers, and drains, which require a large capital investment, often receive the largest cuts. For example, in sub-Saharan Africa the social services budget fell by 26% between 1980 and 1985 and in Latin America by 18%. Health spending per person has declined in most countries since 1980. Most experts recognize that there may be adverse effects on nutrition and health. However, there is much uncertainty about the actual impact, and it is generally acknowledged that structural adjustment may adversely affect the environment and health.

Despite this pessimistic picture, there have been shorter periods of real growth, such as 1995–1998. The effect of macroeconomic policies cannot be considered in isolation. Trends in the global economy may also dictate personal income and what is possible for a country to attempt to do with macroeconomic policies. It should be kept in mind, however, that countries with better health status have more equitable social policies (Kawachi et al., 1999). It is not wealth *per se* but the distribution of prosperity in the society that seems to be the link between health and the social environment (Hertzman et al., 1994).

You Can Make A Difference

Confronted with all these problems and challenges, it is easy to despair over how little one professional can do to improve things. But there are good reasons for optimism. There are solutions to most, if not all, of these problems. This book can guide the reader toward such solutions. The role of environmental health professionals is to apply their knowledge and experience to help the community understand the environmental health hazards they face and to analyze the technical and social approaches to reducing or eliminating human exposure to environmental hazards and the resulting adverse health effects. On the basis of this analysis, other people in other jobs, some of them very far removed from environmental health, can take appropriate action to protect a community's health.

There are numerous examples of how one person, initially working alone or with a few colleagues, identified a problem, raised the alarm, and persisted in the necessary investigations and actions to get the problem solved. Joining forces at an early stage with people in all walks of life helps us to investigate and analyze the problem from all angles and to implement the solution as efficiently as possible.

This book will show the reader what to look out for and how to approach problem solving in environmental health. It cannot provide all the specific information required about each hazard, but it will indicate where to find the additional information. By observing, investigating, analyzing, and acting in partnership with other professionals and the community, every individual can make a difference.

The Multidisciplinary Team

Everyone should have some education in environmental health matters, as knowing about the environment is a part of living in the world. For any given aspect of environmental health, there are clearly different levels of expertise required, for junior assistants on up to the senior professional. All citizens need to know basic principles of environment and health protection. This knowledge is not just learned in school, but should be part of lifelong learning. Who should be trained at the professional level depends on the national needs in environmental health, present gaps in the workforce, and resources. Many of the following descriptions are adapted from *Guidelines on Planning Education and Training for the Control of Environmental Health Hazards: A Contribution to Capacity Building at National and Subnational Levels.* (Pisaniello et al., 1993).

Disciplines are intellectual tools that may be used to solve environmental health problems; *professions* are groups of workers, generally defined by discipline, that exist to advance the status of their discipline. In many developing countries, specialization may not be realistic, and one person may be responsible for tasks that call for skills from several disciplines. While the strength and character of the professions varies from one country to another, it may be helpful, whatever the setting, to appreciate the range of disciplines relevant to environmental health. Some examples are presented below, in alphabetical order, as no one discipline is more important than the other.

Although maintaining competence in one's own discipline is crucial, adopting a *transdisciplinary* perspective is also essential. Transdisciplinary thinking goes beyond the insights that come from different disciplines interacting, it allows new concepts to emerge that better solve real problems (Rapport, 1995b).

Environmental Health Officer Also termed *public health inspectors*, or *sanitarians*, environmental health officers are generally concerned with public health surveillance and the protection of the environment as it impacts health. Most environmental health officers are employed at the local government level and contribute to the control of infectious diseases, immunization, and enforcement of the law with regard to food establishments, food quality and safety, standards of habitation, and the safe disposal of domestic and industrial wastes. In times of crisis like floods or earthquakes, immediate action must be taken to prevent the outbreak of diseases that would inevitably follow the drinking of contaminated water or the disruption of waste disposal systems. The environmental health officer's multidisciplinary skills are invaluable in disaster management and prevention. Environmental health officers are in frequent contact with the public. Indeed, the basic training of these professionals usually involves a considerable period of salaried work experience, during which time they learn how to interface directly with, and respond to, public needs.

Environmental Health Technician These technicians have essentially the same tasks as the environmental health officer, but at a lower level of responsibility, and are supervised by a fully qualified environmental health officer. Specific titles may be given, e.g., food inspector, building inspector, pest control officer.

Environmental Inspector Environmental inspectors, who often have engineering or chemistry backgrounds, enforce environmental regulations and provide advice on following them. Such regulations usually cover atmospheric stack emissions, noise emissions, effluent discharge, wastewater disposal, waste treatment, and bulk chemical storage and transport.

Epidemiologist Environmental epidemiology can be conceived as the framework for approaching the task of protecting a population from environmental health hazards. At the national or provincial level, advanced expertise in environmental epidemiology is needed to plan and carry out major studies, give expert advice to government agencies and nongovernment organizations, and teach epidemiology in a variety of training schemes. At the local level, many public health officials need detailed knowledge about how to use epidemiology in their daily work. Environmental engineering staff, occupational hygiene and safety staff, primary health care staff, and other people with particular responsibilities (e.g., workers' health and safety representatives in industry) need at least a basic understanding of epidemiological principles. With regard to epidemiological research, it is important to stress that the collection of accurate, unbiased data is important, but not an end in itself. It is even more important to ask pertinent research questions and to put the findings into practice. An *epidemiologist* may be defined as a health worker who studies the occurrence of disease or other health-related conditions or events in defined populations. Epidemiologists need not be medically qualified, but they need to be able to creatively link their work with that of other disciplines, including medicine, biology, and the social sciences. Epidemiologists must be able to optimize the use of observational data and routinely collected information. In practice, the functions of the epidemiologist are broad and may include health and injury surveillance, collaborative research with clinical medical specialists and fieldwork, and the study of health-related behaviors in the home and at work.

Ergonomist Ergonomics integrates knowledge derived from the human sciences to match jobs, systems, products, and environments to the physical and mental abilities and limitations of people. Ergonomics emerged as a discipline during World War II when the human operator became increasingly the weakest link in modern sophisticated military systems. After the war, the discipline continued to grow to meet the challenge of civilian applications. Today, ergonomics encompasses a diversity of interests, including cognitive science, human reliability, occupational physiology, human–computer interaction, and organizational design and management. Because of the variety of these factors, people from many different backgrounds may be involved in ergonomic research and practice. These people, called ergonomists, can be physiologists, psychologists, engineers, physiotherapists, etc. Ergonomists usually work in multidisciplinary teams. For example, a physiotherapist and psychologist may work together with engineers to design a user-friendly instrument display and control panel for an aircraft or a large container ship.

Health Physicist Health physicists have detailed knowledge and experience in radiation safety matters. Usually these professionals have studied physics and have a background or training in the measurement of radiation. Those mainly concerned with environmental radiochemicals generally have a chemistry background, whereas nuclear safety engineers usually have a basic qualification in engineering. Technicians with no formal university qualification may operate in very narrow aspects of radiation protection in industry. In most countries, the radiation safety field is often heavily regulated. Consequently, a major function of these specialists is to oversee compliance with radiation regulations concerning personal and environmental radiation monitoring, inspection and record keeping, and instrument calibration. Health physicists cooperate with a number of other health professionals, e.g., physicians and hygienists, in the evaluation and control of ionizing and nonionizing radiation hazards.

Health Policy Analyst Often government agencies hire individuals specially trained to advise them about policies that need to be developed or adjusted to address current problems. These individuals may have backgrounds in economics, sociology, administration, law, or a variety of other disciplines relevant to policy making.

Laboratory Analytical Scientist Laboratory analytical scientists includes a broad group of professionals who deal with the analysis of environmental (food, water, soil, surface, air) and human tissue samples. This group may also include specialized technicians responsible for lung function testing and monitoring equipment maintenance and calibration. Scientists in the clinical chemistry laboratory measure chemical changes in the body to determine the diagnosis, therapy, and prognosis of disease. The main work of these technologists consists of the assay of various chemical constituents in blood, urine, and other fluids or tissues. In the environmental health context, this may mean conducting liver or renal function tests or enzyme alteration. Microbiology laboratories are chiefly concerned with issues such as food contamination with mycotoxins and bacteria and water contamination with protozoa. Analytical chemists are responsible for analysis of environmental samples, e.g., for asbestos, crystalline silica, and/or biological samples, e.g., for heavy metals and pesticides.

Occupational Hygienist Occupational hygiene (also called *industrial hygiene*), the discipline of anticipating, recognizing, evaluating, and controlling health hazards in the working environment is entrusted with the objectives of protecting workers' health and well-being and safeguarding the general community. In a number of countries, occupational hygienists deal increasingly with matters of environmental health outside the workplace. Although basically trained in engineering, physics, chemistry, or biology, the occupational hygienist has acquired, usually through postgraduate study and/or experience, a knowledge of the effects on health of various agents at various levels of exposure. The occupational hygienist is involved with the monitoring and analytical methods required to detect the extent of exposure and the engineering and methods used for hazard control. It has been estimated that there are at least 15,000 professional occupational hygienists worldwide, and although the law in many countries does not define the function of an occupational hygienist, regulations usually spell out the needed qualifications and roles of safety engineers, physicians, and nurses.

Occupational Health Nurse Traditionally, the role of the occupational health nurse has been one of primary care. Because of expanded training and an increase in the number of nurses, however their role has evolved and broadened considerably. Their various functions include rehabilitation of injured or ill workers, health education and counselling, treatment, environmental control and injury prevention, and health service administration. Of all the occupational and environmental health professionals, nurses make up the largest group. There are often various grades within the profession. Increasingly, greater emphasis is being placed on prevention of disease and injury through environmental control, although for most nurses, primary health care is still the most time-consuming activity.

Occupational and Environmental Health Physician Both occupational and environmental medicine are largely concerned with preventive medicine and health maintenance, and both have much in common. Indeed, in an increasing number of countries, the titles of relevant professional bodies have been changed to formally unite the two branches of medicine. Occupational physicians carry out health surveillance of workers and diagnosis, management, and investigation of occupational diseases (see Chapter 10). The work also involves health education of workers and management, the evaluation of occupational hazards, the recommendation of safety precautions, and statistical analysis of epidemiological data.

Occupational Health and Safety Inspector Traditionally, these inspectors were recruited from the ranks of tradespersons, e.g., boilermakers, electricians, etc., mainly for the purpose of enforcing safety regulations in the construction and manufacturing industries. While these functions are still carried out, there is a worldwide trend toward a more professional inspectorate—i.e., inspectors having tertiary educational qualifications, such as an engineering or science degree. In addition, inspectors in some countries may be expected to undertake personal exposure measurements or provide advice on exposure control.

Sanitary Engineer Sanitary engineering is a broad area of engineering that includes water supply, the collection, treatment, and disposal of wastes, air pollution control, and sanitary inspection of city planning. In a general sense, sanitary engineering is concerned with the adaptation of the environment by engineering means to the requirements of health. The sanitary engineer has a central role in the solution of environmental health problems related to water and sanitation.

Safety Professional Occupational safety is a multidisciplinary area. Safety professionals (also termed *safety engineers*) are drawn from a number of disciplines, e.g., engineering and psychology. They may serve as engineers, managers, or consultants, but they must have a thorough understanding of the causative factors contributing to accident occurrence and combine this with knowledge of motivation, behavior, and communication to devise methods and procedures to control hazards.

Statisticians Biostatisticians are concerned with applications of statistics (the science and art of collecting, summarizing, and analyzing data that are subject to random variation), to health issues. They collaborate with epidemiologists, registry personnel, and other environmental health professionals whose work involves the measurement, research, and analysis of data.

Toxicologist Toxicologists are biological scientists who study the adverse effects of chemical agents on living organisms. The specialist toxicologist acquires knowledge over many years and is often required to interpret animal experimental data and other laboratory-generated data for the purpose of predicting adverse human effects following exposure to toxin(s). Research toxicologists have skills in animal husbandry and handling, and in in vivo and in vitro testing and experimental design. Regulatory toxicologists advise government authorities on the regulation of public and occupational exposures. Often toxicologists are involved in risk assessment in field settings as well.

Study Questions

1. What proportion of people born in your country in the same year as you have already died, and what was the major cause of death?

2. Were any or many of these deaths related to the environment?

3. What will be the main health problems that you personally may encounter in the next 30 to 40 years, based on the typical situation for adults in your country?

4. Will any of these health problems be related to the environment?

5. How do human activities and human health relate to sustainable development?

6. What are the differences in health (and disease patterns) between developed and developing countries? What are the causes of these differences?

7. What differences are there between men and women in environmental risk? What is the role of women in sustainable development?

8. What are the environmental health issues of particular importance to aboriginal people in your country?

9. In your chosen professional role, which will be your most important environmental health concerns?

10. In the community where you live, which of the professions listed above are available as resource people for the community to consult? (make a list based on interviews, telephone directory, etc.)

2

NATURE OF ENVIRONMENTAL HEALTH HAZARDS

LEARNING OBJECTIVES

After studying this chapter you will be able to do the following:

- describe the difference between hazard and risk
- explain the logic of the various methods of classifying environmental hazards
- describe a scheme for identifying the level of hazard and toxicity
- explain why knowledge of the toxicology, microbiology, or physical properties of an environmental hazard is essential to determining the most appropriate approach to its risk assessment (i.e., using a different approach to carcinogens than to noncarcinogenic acute irritants)
- identify different experimental investigative methods
- explain the biological significance of biotransformation processes
- list the basic characteristics of chemical, physical, biological, mechanical, and psychosocial hazards

CHAPTER CONTENTS

HAZARDS AND RISKS

Defining Hazard and Risk

The assessment of health risks posed by specific environmental hazards is fundamental to protecting human health and the environment. A *hazard* is defined as "a factor or exposure that may adversely affect health" (Last, 1995); it is basically a source of danger. Hazard is a qualitative term expressing the potential of an environmental agent to harm the health of certain individuals if the exposure level is high enough and/or if other conditions apply. A *risk* is defined as "the probability that an event will occur, e.g., that an individual will become ill or die within a stated period of time or before a given age; the probability of a (generally) unfavourable outcome" (Last, 1995). It is the quantitative probability that a health effect will occur after an individual has been exposed to a specified amount of a hazard. A hazard results in a risk if there has been exposure— not if the hazard is contained or if there is no opportunity for exposure.

Types of Environmental Health Hazards

Environmental health hazards arise from both natural and anthropogenic (human-caused) sources. These include biological hazards (e.g., bacteria, viruses, parasites, and other pathogenic organisms), chemical hazards (such as toxic metals, air pollutants, solvents, and pesticides), and physical hazards (e.g., radiation, temperature, and noise). Health can also be profoundly affected by mechanical hazards (e.g., motor vehicle, sports, home, agriculture, and workplace injury hazards) and psychosocial hazards (e.g., stress, lifestyle disruption, workplace discrimination, effects of social change, marginalization, and unemployment).

On a global scale, environmental factors including overcrowding, migration, poor sanitation, and the broad use of pesticides intimately involved in the transmission of infectious agents have had a profound effect on the occurrence of disease. As discussed in Chapter 1, when infectious diseases are reduced, other environmental factors causing human diseases (e.g., chemicals, ionizing radiation, ultraviolet light) become increasingly important as determinants of ill health. Some traditional hazards, which are still predominant in less developed countries and rural areas, and modern hazards, which become more important with increasing urbanization and industrialization, are shown in Table 2.1.

TABLE 2.1

TRADITIONAL VERSUS MODERN HEALTH HAZARDS

Traditional Hazards	Modern Hazards
Disease vectors	Tobacco Smoking
Infectious agents	Transport hazards
Inadequate housing and shelter	Pollution from sewage and industry
Poor-quality drinking water and sanitation	Outdoor air pollution from industry and motorcars
Indoor air pollution from cooking	Overuse or misuse of chemicals
Dietary deficiencies	Industrial machinery
Hazards of child birth	Unbalanced diet
Wildlife and domestic animals	
Injury hazards in agriculture	

One can study environmental health hazards in various ways. Examining the *nature of the hazard*, which can be biological, chemical, physical, mechanical, or psychosocial, is one approach. Biological hazards can be divided into viruses, bacteria, parasites, etc. *Route of exposure* is also a useful organizing principle, e.g., via air, water, land. Each route can be further subdivided for purposes of separate discussion—e.g., indoor versus outdoor air, or groundwater versus surface water versus drinking water. Another approach is to focus on the *setting* where the hazard occurs, for example, home, work, school, hospitals, or by community. Table 2.2 provides one conceptual framework of biological, chemical, and physical hazards by routes of exposure and related factors.

Because environmental health is a huge field, it tends to be taught in fragments. (The nature-of-the-hazard approach is classic in academic settings. Microbiologists tend to teach the characteristics of biological hazards; toxicologists discuss the health effects of chemicals; health physicists teach the implications of radiation on human health; ergonomists discuss biomechanical hazards; and psychologists discuss psychosocial issues. It is, in fact, essential to have some understanding of the basic microbiological, toxicological, health physics, ergonomic, and psychosocial sciences in the practice of environmental health. To develop the public health perspective it may also be useful to focus on routes of exposure. Air pollution, for example, tends to be assessed and managed by a different group of public health professionals than water pollution or hazardous waste. This latter approach lends itself best to advocacy in the community at large. The middle chapters of this book present the hazards according to their routes of exposure (air, water, food).

The different hazards can also be described in the context of agriculture, settlements, and industry. This approach allows environmental issues to be dealt with as problems in community and economic development. The later chapters in the book analyze the health impacts and prevention methods of environmental issues in relation to settings and development issues (urbanization, energy use, industrialization, global concerns). This chapter introduces environmental health concerns according to the nature of the hazards, and outlines the basic issues in these areas. (The basic physiology needed to understand the effects of environmental hazards on human health can be found in standard physiology texts.)

TABLE 2.2
BIOLOGICAL, CHEMICAL, AND PHYSICAL HAZARDS BY ROUTES OF EXPOSURE

	Biological	Chemical	Physical
AIR			
Agent/source	Microorganisms	Fumes, dust, particles	Radiation, heat, noise
Vectorial factors	Coughing, exhalations	Contaminated air	Climate, unguarded exposures
Routes	Inhalation, contact	Inhalation, contact	Inhalation, direct penetration of the body
WATER			
Agent/source	Microorganisms, decayed organic material	Discharges, leaching, dumping	Radiation; heat in power station cooling water
Vectorial factors	Insects, rodents, snails; animals excreta; food chain	Contaminated food and water	Accidents; contaminated food and water
Routes	Bites, ingestion, contact	Ingestion, contact	Ingestion, contact
LAND			
Agent/source	Soil organisms	Solids, liquids	Radiation
Vectorial factors	Decaying organic matter, leading to vector breeding	Contaminated food and groundwater	Accidents; contaminated food and groundwater
Routes	Contact, bites	Ingestion, contact	Contact, ingestion

Adapted from Schaefer, 1991, with permission.

BIOLOGICAL HAZARDS

Types of Biological Hazards

Biological hazards include all of the forms of life (as well as the nonliving products they produce) that can cause adverse health effects. These hazards are plants, insects, rodents, and other animals, fungi, bacterial, viruses, and a wide variety of toxins and allergens. A recently discovered type of biological hazard has been called *prion* (disease-producing protein particle), which have been related to a number of diseases including Creutzfeldt-Jacob ("mad cow") disease (see Chapter 7.)

Environmental health is largely determined by the health effects of exposure to microorganisms and parasites, whose occurrence and spreading depend on environmental factors. The biological factors that play a role in the life cycle of the organisms are discussed below. Hazards associated with larger species will be treated as an issue of physical safety or as a hazard in transmitting infectious diseases.

Microorganisms of concern in environmental health include *bacteria, viruses*, and *protozoa*, such as amoebas. Most microorganisms and parasites that cause human illness need to grow inside the human body to cause it harm. Bacteria and protozoa may live and multiply outside other living cells, and they can survive and multiply for long periods in food items or water, as long as there are enough nutrients for them and the pH and temperature are within viability limits. Viruses, however, cannot multiply outside of other living cells, although some can survive for long periods and remain infective. To sustain their life cycle, viruses need to enter either human cells or the cells of an animal, insect, or plant. Many diseases caused by microorganisms are spread directly from one person to another. These diseases, considered person-to-person environmental health hazards, include tuberculosis (which is greatly increased by poor housing and crowded conditions) and many infectious childhood diseases. The five major infectious killers in the world are acute respiratory infections, diarrhea, tuberculosis, malaria, and measles (Table 2.3).

When a disease can spread from one person to another it is called an *infectious* or *communicable disease*. The spread can be *direct*, by contact between two

TABLE 2.3

ESTIMATED GLOBAL NUMBER OF DEATHS FROM INFECTIOUS AND PARASITIC DISEASES, 1993

Disease/Condition	Number of Deaths (thousands)
Acute lower respiratory infections under age 5 years	4110
Diarrhea under age 5, including dysentery	3010
Tuberculosis	2709
Malaria	2000
Measles	1160
Hepatitis B	933
AIDS	700
Whooping cough	360
Bacterial meningitis	210
Schistosomiasis	200
Leishmaniasis	197
Congenital syphilis	190
Tetanus	149
Hookworm diseases	90
Amoebiasis	70
Ascariasis (roundworm)	60
African trypanosomiasis (sleeping sickness)	55
American trypanosomiasis (Chagas' disease)	45
Onchocerciasis (river blindness)	35
Meningitis	35
Rabies	35
Yellow fever	30
Dengue/dengue hemorrhagic fever	23
Japanese encephalitis	11
Foodborne trematodes	10
Cholera	6.8
Poliomyelitis	5.5
Diphtheria	3.9
Leprosy	2.4
Plague	0.5
TOTAL	16,445

Source: WHO, 1995a.

persons, as happens with sexually transmitted diseases, or it can be *transmitted by air*, as with the common cold or tuberculosis. One infected person exhales the microorganism that causes the disease and another person inhales the contaminated air. The spread can also take place through *vehicles* other than air, in materials that have been contaminated by an infected person, e.g., food contaminated with worms (helminths) from another person. Finally, *vectors* (animals or insects that carry the microorganism or parasite and infect a person via a bite, e.g., malaria via mosquitoes) can spread disease as well.

Certain bacteria and parasites produce toxins that can cause disease through the poisonous action of the toxin, rather than an infection. Much food poisoning is this type of bacteria-produced toxic reaction. The difference between infection and a toxic reaction is important. Diseases that are caused by the toxins that bacteria produce are not contagious. That is, they do not spread from person to person, but are limited to the people who consume the contaminated food. Thus there is no subsequent risk to other people when the toxin causes the disease. Nonetheless, the precautionary measures taken to prevent both bacterial infection and bacterial toxins are similar (clean food preparation and adequate cooking).

Spread of Biological Hazards

Water polluted by human excreta is the main pathway for the spread of cholera, typhoid fever, dysentery, other diarrheal diseases, hepatitis, and schistosomiasis. Inadequate sanitation, the dumping of untreated sewage into surface water, and poor hygienic practices remain important targets for preventive actions in all countries. In developed countries with more or less complete sewage and water treatment, waterborne diarrheal diseases are efficiently prevented, but the cost of prevention is billions of dollars every year. Overcrowding and poorly ventilated housing contribute to the airborne transmission of tuberculosis, measles, influenza, pneumonia, pertussis, and cerebrospinal meningitis. Unhygienic animal husbandry helps to transmit *zoonoses* (animal diseases that can also afflict humans), e.g., plague and hydatids disease. Contamination of soil and water contributes to the spread of diseases borne by insect and rodent vectors, such as malaria, trachoma, schistosomiasis, filariasis, yellow fever, plague, typhus, and trypanosomiasis, while stagnant waters, unsanitary housing, and refuse dumps are sites that encourage insect reproduction and directly support disease vectors. This combination enables the spread of the most deadly vector-borne disease, malaria (Table 2.3).

Many parasites cause *tropical diseases*, which occur almost exclusively in tropical areas. For most of these diseases, the reason for their geographic confinement is that the disease spread is dependent on an insect vector, which can only survive in certain climates. Among the more important tropical parasite diseases are malaria, schistosomiasis, filariasis, and dracunculiasis (Guinea worm disease). However, many diseases such as tuberculosis are not considered tropical diseases, even though they are common in the tropics and contribute to the burden of disease in developing countries.

Environmental changes and disturbances to the balance of natural habitats may have profound effects on the spread of infectious diseases. New outbreaks such as the one reported in Congo in 1995 caused by the *Ebola* virus, have emerged lately when people encountered them by entering an unfamiliar or remote habitat. Others, such as hantavirus, Rift Valley fever, and cholera, have reemerged in association with environmental changes (see WRI, 1996 and Chapter 11 for further discussion).

Routes of Exposure

The main environmental exposure routes for biological hazards are air, water, and food. Some parasites enter the body by penetrating the skin (e.g., hookworm, schistosomiasis) and others enter a human body by insect bites (e.g., malaria). Bacteria and parasites may also spread from contaminated soil to the skin or via dust to the air, and eventually infect a person. Person-to-person contact is an important route for the spreading of biological hazards, but this route is not defined as environmental for purposes of this text.

The spread of microorganisms via air occurs mainly with respiratory diseases, and is often due to small droplets created while coughing or sneezing. A well-known example is the common cold. Although not always considered an environmental health concern, it could be put in that category, because environmental conditions such as crowding or lack of ventilation in confined spaces contribute to the spread of the virus via air. Other examples of microorganisms that spread via air exposure are tuberculosis bacteria and the Legionnaire's disease bacterium. The latter can grow in poorly maintained air conditioning systems (in the cooling water) and can spread to a whole building.

The single largest biological environmental health problem is the spread of fecal bacteria from an infected person to others via water. When the drinking-water supply for a community is contaminated with feces from one sick person, a large number of people drinking the water can fall ill and in turn spread the disease via their feces. *Cholera* is an example of a serious disease of this type. Very severe, watery diarrhea is a cardinal symptom of cholera; the person rapidly becomes dehydrated and may even die, unless treatment is given to replace the body liquid lost. A number of other bacteria and viruses in drinking water can also cause diarrheal diseases and are responsible for the high child mortality rates in developing countries. The potential for this environmental health hazard to cause serious disease also exists in developed countries, but the efficient filtration and disinfecting (chlorination) of drinking water protects these populations. To sustain protection, it is necessary to maintain systems for water supply and water purification at a considerable ongoing cost.

In cases of breakdown of water supplies due to natural disasters (such as the major earthquake in Kobe, Japan in 1995) or wars (such as the disruption of the water supply to Sarajevo, Bosnia-Herzegovina, in 1992 and 1995), the major concern is the risk of an outbreak of waterborne disease.

Another exposure route is ingestion of food, which, as mentioned earlier, is an important medium for growth of bacteria. Low noninfectious levels of bacteria in water can grow into higher infectious levels in food. The number of bacteria (or viruses, parasites) required to cause a specific disease in an individual is called the *minimal infectious dose*; exposures below this dose will not result in an infection. The growth of bacteria in the food is dependent on three factors: the type of foodstuff, the ability of the bacteria to grow in this foodstuff, and, most importantly, the temperature. Storing many foods at room temperature can lead to a dangerous buildup of bacteria. At temperatures below 4°C (40°F) or above 60°C (140°F), the growth is usually very slow. (Ideally, a refrigerator should keep the temperature below 4°C at all times.)

The main problem with biological hazards in or on soil is the problem of *helminths* (worms) from an infected person that defecates on soil. Intestinal worm infections are extremely common in poor areas of developing countries, particularly among children, who play on the soil and are not likely to take precautions. In poor communities where sanitary facilities are inadequate, it may be necessary (or more acceptable) to defecate outdoors on the ground, and the cycle of worm infection is maintained. Worm infections in pets or other animals can also be the source of this type of exposure. In addition, the reuse of sewage water for irrigation can cause infection problems among farmers tilling the irrigated land, unless special precautions are taken.

Distribution, Growth, and Defense Mechanisms

Many viruses, bacteria, and parasites also cause infections at the place of first contact with the body—e.g., the common cold virus is inhaled and causes upper respiratory tract infections, the staphylococcus bacteria may cause boils on the skin, and intestinal helminths cause worm disease in the intestines after being swallowed into the gastrointestinal tract. Others infect the body and cause disease at distant sites. Once a person has been exposed to a biological agent, or pathogen, this agent will be distributed via blood, lymph, or other body fluids to the parts of the body most favorable for it to grow. Certain bacteria are very specific in the sites where they can grow and cause damage—e.g., polio virus can grow in the intestines and cause diarrhea (this is the way the virus spreads), but it can also grow specifically in certain nerve cells in the spinal cord and cause paralysis.

Fortunately, the human body has a powerful defense mechanism against biological agents, the immune system. This system includes a number of specialized cells that identify the infectious agents as intruders that may cause harm and then engulf them or attack them with antibodies. Thus, any recognized infection is slowed or stopped by these mechanisms. In many cases the patient recovers spontaneously or doesn't develop symptoms at all because the immune system starts attacking the biological agent as soon as it has entered the body. A small number of viruses or bacteria would therefore be stopped in their tracks before infection and disease occur. Thus, until the minimal infectious dose is exceeded, the disease is not likely to occur. Dangerous diseases that spread rapidly, such as cholera and measles, often have a very small infective dose. The level of the minimal infective dose can vary substantially between individuals and is determined by physical condition and nutritional status, among other factors (also see Chapter 7).

Bacteria and parasites can be slowed down or killed by specific drugs, called *antibiotics*. When drugs are not available, the patient may still recover by means of the immune defenses, but for many diseases, the availability of effective drugs have made cures much more likely and much faster, e.g., for tuberculosis, streptococcus tonsillitis, and intestinal helminths. For some diseases, such as meningitis, the use of antibiotics is essential to saving the lives of patients.

An important aspect of the growth of bacteria is that some produce powerful toxins (chemical substances that cause health damage) when they grow. For instance, the most dangerous aspect of cholera is the very severe damage to the lining of the large intestines caused by toxins produced by the cholera bacteria. This damage produces a large loss of liquid from the body (watery diarrhea), which threatens the person's life unless intravenous replacement liquid is given. Similarly, when bacteria grow in food, toxins may be formed that are so powerful that the poisoning is a greater health risk than infection after the contaminated food has been eaten. For example, staphylococcus bacteria produce a toxin that causes diarrhea and vomiting. The most dangerous toxin formed in this way is that causing the deadly disease, botulism.

Health Effects

When a biological organism establishes itself in the body of a host, such as a person, and causes disease, it is called an *infection*. Infections may occur in any part of the body, but many organisms tend to cause infection only in certain organs and therefore cause distinctive diseases. Each year diarrheal diseases are responsible for a very high fatality rate among infants and children in developing countries. This is the result of the abundance of exposures to hazards enabling disease spread, the lack of knowledge at a family level about how to deal with a sick baby, and the lack of basic health services. In this age-group, a number of diarrhea-causing organisms can be involved and even common viruses that have little effects on adults can be fatal. For adults, cholera is the most dangerous disease, followed by typhoid, paratyphoid, salmonella, and shigella.

Respiratory infections are also very common diseases. Again, babies are particularly vulnerable. Many adults (particularly elderly people and people with suppressed immune systems, such as patients with HIV/AIDS) are at risk for tuberculosis and pneumonia. The common cold and a variety of influenza-like viruses have a great impact on our daily lives (e.g., days off work), but generally patients recover in a few days.

Sexually transmitted diseases have taken on a whole new importance because of the spread of HIV/AIDS. Although AIDS itself is not considered an environmental disease, it may well influence the occurrence of other environment-related infections. Because of the damage AIDS does to the immune system and the body's defense against other infections, AIDS has lead to a major resurgence of tuberculosis. Resistance to antibiotics has developed among many bacteria and parasites. Infections caused by the resistant organisms may be difficult to treat and may spread to others who would not be exposed if treatment were successful. Some cases of tuberculosis, for example, have been caused by inefficient treatment of patients with antibiotic-resistant tubercle bacilli who then infect others.

Investigation Methods

Microbiologists have developed laboratory methods to identify and quantify the occurrence of most viruses, bacteria, and parasites in any medium. These tools are constantly being refined on the basis of new knowledge about the microstructure of biological agents, particularly the structure of their DNA. In this way, samples of feces from a person with diarrhea can be tested to identify the specific agent responsible for the disease. If it is likely that the agent also occurs in blood, further analysis of blood can be carried out. Parasites can also be identified in blood. Some of them, like the malaria plasmodium, are easily detected using a microscope. The existence of antibodies against specific microbes can also show whether the person has had an infection in the past. To quantify the concentration of viruses in a material, samples are taken and inserted into living cells where the viruses grow and are eventually quantified. For bacteria, the growth before quantification can be generated in special growth media, such as *agar plates*. For larger parasites, direct counting of organisms under a microscope may suffice.

Normally the clinical health staff carry out these investigations on materials from patients. In environmental health investigations measurements of microorganisms are often taken from environmental materials, such as drinking water, foods, or soil. The same type of tools used for identifying and quantifying the occurrence of biological agents are used on these materials. One important difference in approach is the use of surrogate indicators of the biological agents of concern. For instance, for routine monitoring of drinking water, measurements of the *Escherichia coli* coliform organism's bacteria are taken to assess whether the water has acceptable quality or not. These bacteria do not normally cause disease, as they are the most common bacteria in the normal intestinal bacterial flora. The reason they are used as indicators of water quality is that they show whether the water has been contaminated by feces, which is the most important source of disease-causing bacteria in drinking water.

CHEMICAL HAZARDS

Hazard, Risk, and Toxicity

Approximately 10 million chemical compounds have been synthesized in laboratories since the beginning of the present century. About 1% of these chemicals are produced commercially and used directly (e.g., as pesticides and fertilizers); most chemicals are intermediates in the manufacture of end products for human use. There is virtually no sector of human activity that does not use chemical products, and these products have indeed created many benefits for society, such as the treatment of disease with pharmaceutical products and the use of fertilizers to increase food production.

All chemicals are toxic to some degree, with health risk being primarily a function of the severity of the toxicity and the extent of exposure. However, most chemicals have not been adequately tested to determine their toxicity.

Some international efforts have been made to rectify this situation. Specifically, in 1976 the United Nations Environment Program (UNEP) established the *International Registry of Potentially Toxic Chemicals* (IRPTC) (see website: irptc.unep.ch/irptc/databank.html), which now has a computerized central data file containing data profiles for hundreds of chemicals. Special files are available on waste management and disposal, chemicals currently being tested for toxic effects, and national regulations covering thousands of substances. In 1980, the WHO, UNEP, and International Labor Organization (ILO) set up the *International Program on Chemical Safety* (IPCS) to assess the risks that specific chemicals pose to human health and the environment. The IPCS publishes its evaluations in five forms: the detailed *Environmental Health Criteria*, which are intended for scientific experts; a short, nontechnical *Health and Safety Guide* for administrators, managers, and decision makers; the *International Chemical Safety Cards*, which are for ready reference in the workplace; the *Poisons Information Monographs* for medical use; and the *Concise International Chemical Assessment Documents*. (see www.who.int/pcs; for the Environmental Health Criteria, you may go directly to www.who.int/pcs/pubs/pub_list.htm)

It is important to distinguish hazard and risk from the term toxicity. The *toxicity* of a substance is defined as its inherent capacity to cause injury to a living organism (i.e., a person, animal, or plant). A highly toxic substance will damage an organism even if only very small amounts are present in the body. A substance of low toxicity will not produce an effect unless the concentration in the target tissue is sufficiently high. For the chemical to pose a risk there must be a real or potential exposure to it. A toxic chemical that is used in a totally enclosed process may in itself possess the capacity to induce adverse health effects, but may not pose a real health risk, since there is virtually no possibility of exposure. Factors that might be considered when assessing the risk posed by a toxic substance include the quantity of the substance actually absorbed (i.e., the dose), how the body metabolizes the substance, and the nature and extent of the induced health effect at a given level of exposure (dose–response or dose–effect relationship; see Chapter 3). The dose, in turn, depends on the route of exposure and the length, duration, and frequency of exposure. One must also consider individuals in the population who might be more sensitive to the toxin and whether the injury is permanent or reversible. Thus to identify and categorize chemical hazards, knowledge is needed of the following: (*1*) their physical and chemical properties; (*2*) their routes of entry; (*3*) their distribution and metabolism; and (*4*) the effects they have on body systems. Finally, it is necessary to know (*5*) how to identify chemical hazards in real settings (see Chapter 3).

Chemical Classification

There are numerous chemical classification systems available. For those without a basic chemistry background it is useful to be aware of the classification of chemicals into two major classes: (*1*) *inorganic chemicals* (which contain none or very few carbon atoms), and (*2*) *organic chemicals* (which have a structure based on carbon atoms). (The reader interested in the specific chemical structure of different compounds is referred to standard handbooks in chemistry or the IPCS *Environmental Health Criteria*).

Inorganic Substances *Halogens* are elements that form a salt by direct union with a metal. They include fluorine, chlorine, bromine, and iodine. At standard temperature and pressure, fluorine and chlorine are gases, bromine is a liquid, and iodine is a solid. When placed in water, reactions occur, yielding acids that irritate tissues. As individual elements and compounds, the halogens have their own inherent toxicity. The primary symptom of the inhalation of halogens (excluding organohalogens) is respiratory tract irritation, with the severity depending on concentration. Chlorinated and fluorinated hydrocarbons, which are formed during the reaction of halogens with organic compounds, will be further discussed in Chapter 11, where the impact of halogenated hydrocarbons on the depletion of the ozone layer and the implications for the global environment are addressed.

Corrosive materials include alkaline compounds such as ammonia, calcium hydroxide, calcium oxide, potassium hydroxide, sodium carbonate, and sodium hydroxide, among others. These cause corrosive local irritation of tissues such as the skin, eyes, and respiratory tract. These effects can also be caused by acids. Sulfuric acid and chromic acid are common industrial chemicals. Other compounds with corrosive or irritation effects include the common air pollutants ozone and nitrogen oxides. Ozone (O_3) is very irritating to all mucous membranes (e.g., eyes, nose, and mouth) whereas nitrogen dioxide is a moderate irritant. Both can trigger asthma attacks.

Metals such as cadmium, chromium, copper, lead, manganese, mercury, nickel, and arsenic are toxic and environmentally persistent. Of these, chromium, copper, and manganese are *essential metals* in that they are required by living organisms. Both the environmental fate and the level of toxicity of metals depend strongly on their physical and chemical form. Living organisms are capable of changing the chemical form and thereby altering health risks related to exposure to these chemicals. For example, bacteria can convert mercury ions to methyl mercury, which is fat soluble and may therefore accumulate in fish and enter the human food chain. Similarly, some forms of organic lead (methyl and ethyl derivatives such as tetraethyl lead) are soluble in organic solvents and are used as anti-knock agents in gasoline. Because lead compounds are neurotoxic, their use is being phased out in many countries. For most of these chemicals, IPCS Environmental Health Criteria have been developed.

Organic Compounds *Hydrocarbons* are basically a string of carbon molecules with hydrogen attached to the carbon molecules. *Aliphatic hydrocarbons*, either short-chain or paraffin (long-chain), come almost exclusively from petroleum and can be *saturated*, implying that no further atoms (especially hydrogen atoms) can be added to the molecule. These hydrocarbons include (from the smallest to the largest molecules) methane, ethane, propane, butane, pentane, hexane, heptane, and octane, among others. Methane and ethane are gases and are relatively inert biologically, while hydrocarbons bigger than ethane (i.e., propane, butane etc.) are central nervous system depressants asphyxiants and flammable. Mucous membrane irritation increases from pentane to octane. *Olefins*, or saturated aliphatic hydrocarbons, are molecules having one or more double bonds between molecules that potentially could be broken so that hydrogen atoms could be added to the molecule. They are thus not saturated with hydrogen atoms. These hydrocarbons are also formed as by-products of petroleum breakdown. Specific unsaturated aliphatic hydrocarbons include ethylene, propylene, 1,3 butadiene, and isoprene.

Saturated and unsaturated hydrocarbons may also exist in an *alicyclic* (i.e., circular) form, e.g., cyclohexane, methylcyclohexane, and turpentine. Here, the hy-

BOX 2.1

Xenoestrogens

Estrogens form a class of steroid hormones synthesized both in males and females. These hormones play an important role in human reproduction, including sexual differentiation, development of female secondary sex characteristics, and development and functioning of the testes. Hormones exert their action by binding to a specific receptor. When a hormone binds to a cellular receptor to form a hormone–receptor complex, a number of reactions take place that eventually result in a physiological effect. To develop and function normally, hormonal blood levels have to be regulated very accurately. This regulation of hormone levels is determined by the rate of synthesis and elimination by metabolism. This mechanism of regulation can be disturbed, however, when humans or other organisms are exposed to environmental chemicals that are also capable of binding to the estrogen receptor. In principle, there are two possible reactions. (*1*) The binding of the environmental compound to the estrogen receptor results in the same cellular response; this is called an *estrogen-mimicking effect.* (*2*) Binding to the receptor does not result in the normal response. This may indicate that the xenoestrogen, not normally present in the body, has (permanently) blocked the receptor, making it unable to interact with endogenous estrogens.

Humans may be exposed to xenoestrogens in many different ways. The human diet may contain large amounts of phytoestrogens such as lignans and isoflavones. Estrogen-blocking effects have been demonstrated in women who ate a isoflavones-enriched diet. However, most phytoestrogens are metabolized and excreted in urine in the same way as endogenous estrogens and therefore do not accumulate in the body. The opposite holds true, however, for some other xenoestrogens, including polychlorinated biphenyl (PCBs), dioxins, and furans. Exposure to some PCB congeners has been correlated with reduced sperm motility and density. Furthermore, after in utero exposure, increased fetal loss, reduced birth weight, and behavioral and developmental effects were reported after severe poisoning accidents in Japan and Taiwan. Occupational exposures to estrogenic compounds (like Kepone) have also resulted in decreased sperm count and motility, and abnormal sperm morphology.

Other xenoestrogens to which humans can be exposed are alkylphenols, phthalate esters, and bisphenol-A. Considerable concern about these compounds has

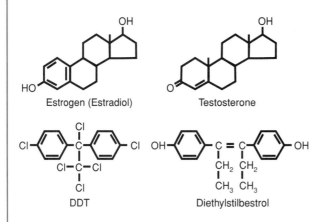

Figure 2.1 Chemical structure of estradiol, testosterone, diethylstilbestrol, and DDT. From Colburn et al., 1996, with permission. *(continued)*

(continued)

been raised because they are so pervasive in the environment. In particular, intake of phthalates, which may amount to several hundreds of μg/kg/day, mainly by consumption of food, may result in estrogenic effects. The most obvious exposure to xenoestrogens is, of course, the direct administration of synthetic hormones, such as diethylstilbestrol (DES), the effects of which are well documented in the offspring of women who took it. In some countries, the same hormones may be present in meat and dairy products. The similarities in chemical structure between endogenous estradiol and the xenoestrogens DES and dichlorodiphenyl-trichloroethane (DDT), are shown in Figure 2.1

Whether xenoestrogens in the environment are having an effect on people in general is unknown and certainly unproven. The data on falling sperm counts among men are not consistent from one place to the next and there is little evidence of a rise in breast cancer rates among women when age and birth history is taken into account. The risks associated with environmental xenoestrogens are better documented for animals than for people. For example, it is not clear that exposure to xenoestrogens, which tend to be weakly estrogenic in environmental exposure, can match the direct exposure to estrogen that women have today from living longer and healthier.

---

drocarbon chain bends around so that the last carbon molecule is attached to the first to form a circle. In general, the longer the carbon chain (whether saturated, unsaturated, or cyclic), the more lipid (fat) soluble. Unsaturated hydrocarbons are more reactive and usually more toxic than saturated ones. The *aromatic hydrocarbons* are also circular molecules containing one or more benzene rings. A *benzene ring* is a circular six-carbon hydrocarbon with alternating single and double bonds.

For various reasons, a benzene ring is a very stable structure (i.e., a lot of energy is needed to break a benzene ring). This category of chemicals is further classified depending on the number of benzene rings and the type of linkage between them in the molecule. These groups are (*1*) *benzene* and its aliphatic and alicyclic derivatives; (*2*) *polyphenyls*, i.e., two or more noncondensed rings; and (*3*) *polycyclic rings*, or two or more condensed rings. Examples of aromatic compounds include benzene, toluene, styrene, and naphthalene. Aromatic hydrocarbons act as primary irritants to the mucous membranes and cause central nervous system depression. In addition, some have particularly toxic and carcinogenic properties. For example, benzene has long been known for its toxicity to the hematopoietic (i.e., blood) system and its ability to cause leukemia. In general, the more benzene rings in the molecule, the less soluble and more persistent it is in the environment (i.e., it doesn't break down easily). Because of these last two features, these chemicals are more likely to be carcinogenic or ecotoxic, although other characteristics of the molecule (such as its three-dimensional shape) may also contribute to its toxicity.

Certain types of organic compounds have *estrogen-like activity* (see Box 2.1). Such action by exogenous chemicals is believed to occur because of the spatial (geometric) resemblance between the toxicant and the natural (endogenous) estrogen hormone. Links to breast cancer and male infertility have been hypothesized for these estrogen-like substances (Davies et al., 1995; Sharpe and Skakkeback, 1993). Similar concerns about specific disease causation have been raised for chemicals that disrupt the endocrine system (*endocrine disruptors*), thought by some to be the heralding of a new wave of environmental concern (Colborn et al., 1996).

Halogenated hydrocarbons (i.e., hydrocarbons with at least one atom from the halogen group of atoms [fluorine, chlorine, bromine or iodine] attached) are among the most commonly encountered industrial chemicals. Examples include chloromethane, dichloromethane, chloroform, and carbon tetrachloride. Chemicals in this group are extensively used for dry cleaning or as industrial solvents (e.g., trichloroethylene) and in the production of plastics (e.g., polyvinyl chloride [PVC]). In general, the larger and more chlorinated the compounds are, the more the compounds cannot be broken down, and therefore they remain in the environment. Chlorinated cyclic hydrocarbons are environmentally damaging because they persist for long periods and are consumed and accumulated by wildlife. Besides being persistent in the environment, the bioaccumulation of these compounds and their excretion in human and animal milk pose high risk to infants. (Bioaccumulation will be discussed in Chapter 7. Persistent organic pollutants are discussed further in Box 2.2.) Toxic signs of human exposures are central nervous system alterations, developmental delay in children, immune system suppression, and a persistent skin rash called *chloracne*. Some environmental polychlorinated hydrocarbons such as dioxins originating from waste incinerators are frequently discussed in relation to their carcinogenic potential. A model compound, 2,3,7,8-tetrachlorodibenzo-para-dioxin, is known to be carcinogenic to humans (IARC classification group 1). However, other polychlorinated dibenzo-para-dioxins are not classifiable as carcinogenic to humans (group 3).

Alcohols are hydrocarbons in which at least one or more hydrogen atoms are substituted by a hydroxyl (molecule composed of an oxygen and a hydrogen atom) group. Specific alcohols include methanol, ethanol, and propanol, which are toxic to several organs, most notably to the central nervous system. For example, fetal alcohol syndrome is a recognized disorder in which ethanol ingestion by the mother damages the child before birth. The chronic effects of methanol ingestion include blurred vision and ultimately blindness; this situation is most common when alcohol is drunk from illegal and contaminated liquor distillation. Higher-molecular-mass (i.e., bigger) alcohols can produce a dermatitis (i.e., a skin rash).

Glycols and derivatives, such as ethylene glycol, have two hydrogen atoms substituted by hydroxyl groups. They are used as anti-freezing agents and in humans to produce anesthetic and dermal effects. Other types include ethers, which contain carbon-oxygen-carbon linkages; epoxy compounds, which are cyclic ethers; ketones, aldehydes, and organic acids; anhydrides, esters, and organic phosphates; cyanides and nitrites; nitrogen compounds; and miscellaneous organic nitrogen compounds. Toxicological information is available about all these classifications of chemicals through the IPCS Environmental Health Criteria. (see www.who.int/pcs/pubs/pub_list.htm)

Organic solvents are widely used in industry and pose a potential risk of high exposure to workers. Many of these chemicals are toxic, persist in the environment, and are known or suspected to be carcinogenic (e.g., benzene, trichloroeth-

BOX 2.2

Persistent Organic Pollutants

Persistent organic pollutants (POPS) constitute an important group of chemicals of environmental concern. They are branched-chain or ringed organic compounds, are often highly chlorinated, and are resistant to biological, chemical, and photolytic breakdown. Consequently, POPs remain in the environment for many years. They are fat (lipid) soluble, accumulate along food chains, and are often toxic to living organisms. Health effects may involve disturbances of the nervous or immune system, or increases in the risk of certain cancers. The POPs include the first generation of organochlorine pesticides (e.g., chlordane, DDT, heptachlor, minex, and toxaphene); polycyclic aromatic hydrocarbons such as pyrenes and anthracenes, which are generated in the combustion of coal or other (fossil) fuels; dioxins and furans, which are by-products of certain chemical processes (e.g., in the pulp and paper industry) or waste incineration; and PCBs, which were produced on a large scale for use as dielectric and hydraulic fluids, among other applications. Some of the POPs mentioned constitute large chemical families of related compounds called *congeners;* for example, there are 209 PCBs and 670 or more toxaphenes (see Chapter 11).

Contributed by Evert Nieboer, McMaster University, Canada.

ylene). Some of these compounds, such as benzene and toluene, are also present in combustion products of organic material, such as when tires are burned. Paints used to include organic or inorganic hydrobarbon solvents, but increasingly, water is being used as a solvent, which has significantly reduced the health risks of painters.

Routes of Exposure

Chemicals can be released into the environment in many different ways. These include the naturally occurring chemicals released during natural geological processes and from mining and dredging, as well as wastes from many industrial, agricultural, commercial, domestic, and manufacturing sources. Chemical pollution may also occur by the unintentional release of chemicals during production, storage, and transportation of products such as household products. Air, soil, fresh waters, and oceans are all subject to chemical pollution. Contamination of food involves absorption of chemical residues in the food chain as well as the use of chemicals in food processing. Natural toxins (aflatoxins, ochratoxins, pyrrolizidne alkaloids) also cause a variety of illnesses.

Exposure to chemical hazards may occur via all types of exposure: inhalation, oral ingestion, absorption through the skin, absorption through the eyes, placental transfer from a pregnant woman to the fetus, inoculation and direct penetration to target organs, and from mother to child through breastfeeding. In the nonoccupational environment, ingestion of substances containing chemicals is the most common route of exposure. In the workplace, because of the nature of exposure, duration of the workday, and character of the compounds, inhalation is the most significant route of entry, followed by skin absorption and ingestion.

Distribution, Metabolism, and Elimination

Once a chemical has entered the body, it may be metabolized, excreted, or accumulated. Figure 2.2 shows the routes of absorption, distribution, and excretion of potentially toxic substances. Usually, absorption is most rapid from the lungs, less rapid from the gastrointestinal tract, and least rapid through the skin. Different chemicals follow different pathways. In the case of metal exposures, all pathways may be of relevance. The materials potentially useful for biological monitoring are marked in Figure 2.2 with dotted lines.

After inhalation of particulate matter, the size of particles determines where in the respiratory tract they are deposited and therefore also where they exert their toxic effect. Gases have effects in the respiratory tract depending on their solubility in water. Gases that do not dissolve easily in water can reach the alveoli relatively easily, and may therefore cause health effects throughout the respiratory system. Exposure to particulate matter is common in industrial settings, resulting in well-defined diseases, for example, silicosis (lung restriction and obstruction) due to inhalation of crystalline silica; asbestosis (lung inflammation/

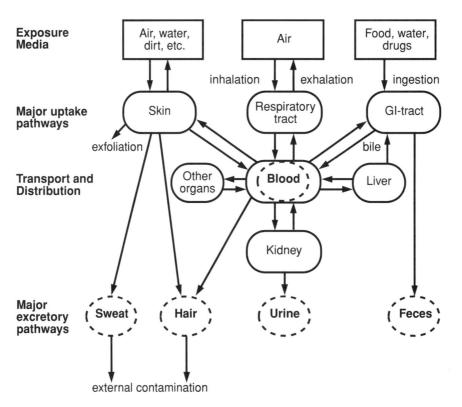

Figure 2.2 Routes of absorption, distribution, and excretion of potentially toxic substances. Dotted lines indicate materials potentially useful for biological monitoring. Modified from Clarkson et al., 1988, with permission.

fibrosis) as a consequence of the inhalation of asbestos fibers; and lung cancer due to exposure to asbestos, nickel oxides, and sulfides, chromium compounds (chromates), and arsenic trioxide. For the development of these chronic diseases, high levels of exposure of long duration are usually required (typically 10–20 years). Furthermore, particulate air pollution of diameters less than or equal to 2.5 μm (the $PM_{2.5}$ fraction) appears to be linked to increased mortality from lung cancer, cardiopulmonary disease, and other respiratory causes. These effects have been quite strongly correlated with suspended sulfates and contributions from metals are also suspected (see Chapter 5).

Once chemicals are absorbed from the lungs, the skin, or the rectum (suppositories), they may enter the general blood circulation directly and be rapidly spread through the body in an unmodified form. Chemicals absorbed from the stomach and intestines (the gastrointestinal [GI] tract) enter the blood and are transported by the hepatic portal system to the liver where they may be modified by a series of reactions. This modification process in the liver and, to a lesser extent, in other organs is referred to as *biotransformation*. These reactions have also been referred to as *detoxification*, when the transformation causes reduced toxicity, or *bioactivation*, when it causes increased toxicity.

Biotransformation can be divided into two distinct phases: phase I and phase II. In general, the biotransformation process converts hydrophobic (water-hating) or lipophilic (fat-loving) compounds into more hydrophilic (water-loving and therefore water-soluble) ones. During phase I, the molecule is altered by the introduction of electrostatically charged (polar) groups (e.g., −OH, −COOH, and −NH2) (Fig. 2.3). The phase I reactions may also lead to the unmasking of such groups in the original compound. These changes may take place as a result of oxidation, reduction, or hydrolysis. In phase II, substances are combined with hydrophilic endogenous compounds. The result is a substance with a sufficiently hydrophilic character to allow rapid excretion. These so-called conjugation reactions can occur with a variety of substances—usually intermediates in metabolism, such as glucuronic acid, sulfate, glycine, and glutathione. Sometimes the process of biotransformation, especially phase I, results in a more active chemical compound that may react with DNA or other important structures in the cell. Some very important carcinogenic chemicals, such as benzene, require phase I transformation to become reactive. Because some of these exist for only a very short time, just long enough to induce damage, they are usually difficult to detect or measure (Box 2.3).

Chemicals that undergo phase I and phase II reactions are normally those that are fat-soluble (lipophilic) and tend to accumulate in body fat and milk if not converted to an excretable form (Fig. 2.4). If this fat is mobilized under stress conditions, the substances may return to the blood and cause acute intoxication. Some of these substances may be broken down to components by bacteria in the gut, from where they are then reabsorbed to undergo phase II reactions. Water-soluble substances (and dissociated polar, electrostatically charged, substances) go directly to the blood circulation, from which they may be lost in expired air from the lungs (if they vaporize readily), to the kidneys and urine (following ultrafiltration), and/or be actively secreted in other secreted fluids such as tears, saliva, milk, or sweat.

Bioactivation of Benzene

Many carcinogenic chemicals require bioactivation for their action. For instance, during metabolism of aflatoxins, vinyl chloride, benzo[a]pyrene, and benzene, highly reactive intermediates, *epoxides,* are formed. These epoxides exist for only a very short period of time because of their high instability and reactivity. Since the epoxides are electrophilic, they react with nucleophilic groups, including those in biomacromolecules like proteins and DNA. As a result of this reaction, cellular processes can be disturbed and the genetic code may be modified. As will be discussed later, changes in the genetic code may eventually result in tumor formation and cancer. The chemical formation of the epoxide from benzene is illustrated, in Figure 2.3. After the formation of phenol, this end product of the phase I reaction is conjugated (coupled) with glucuronic acid, an endogenous compound, to form phenylglucuronide during phase II. To show the structural resemblance between different types of chemicals that are converted to reactive epoxide intermediates during phase I reactions, the structures of vinyl chloride as well as its epoxide are also shown in Figure 2.3.

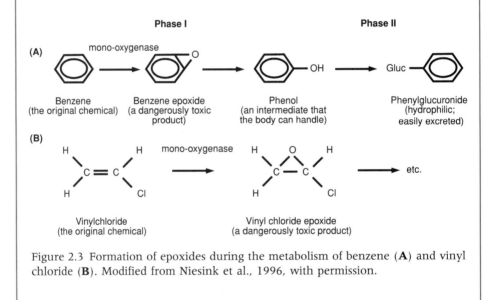

Figure 2.3 Formation of epoxides during the metabolism of benzene (**A**) and vinyl chloride (**B**). Modified from Niesink et al., 1996, with permission.

Systemic and Organ-Specific Toxicity

Toxicity was defined previously as any harmful effect of a chemical or a drug on a target organ. *Systemic toxicity* can be expressed as an effect on the body system after a chemical has been absorbed and spread by the blood throughout the body, as opposed to simply a *local reaction*, which affects only the organ where the chemical first made contact with the body. Some toxicants exert their effects on specific organs, such as the liver, kidney, or nervous system (see Box 2.4). They

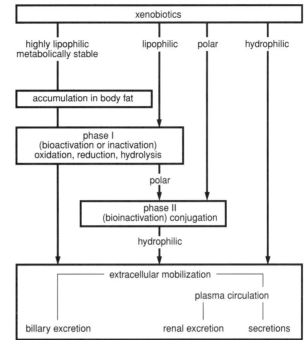

Figure 2.4 Metabolism and excretion of potentially toxic substances. Adapted from Niesink et al., 1996, with permission.

may also create allergic diseases through altering the immunologic system, or they may alter the DNA to cause cancer or birth defects. Whether the toxic effects are systemic or local, they can be acute or chronic, and temporary or permanent.

Reproductive and Developmental Toxicity

Various toxic chemicals have effects on both male and female reproductive systems. Exposures of concern may occur before or after conception. They may affect fertility, sexual function, and libido, but of particular concern are the potential effects on the fetus, which may include genetic abnormalities, interference with normal development, and poisoning of the fetus before birth. The results of those processes may include congenital defects, failure to thrive and develop normally, low birth weight, and miscarriages (spontaneous abortions). The nature of the outcome depends on the type and extent of exposure as well as the timing of exposure with respect to fetal development. Figure 2.5 shows the critical periods of fetal development by organ system. It is important to realize that birth defects and all the other negative outcomes may happen even without exposure to toxic chemicals; often the only clue to the presence of a reproductive risk is that the frequency of such adverse birth outcomes is increased. The extent to which toxic chemicals contribute to our present level of reproduction-related health problems is completely unknown, but the frequency of birth defects overall does not seem to be rising.

Genotoxicity and Carcinogenicity of Chemicals

Chemical, physical, and biological agents can interact with DNA, resulting in structural and/or functional changes that might lead to the alteration of genetic

Major Patterns of Health Effects that May Be Caused by Toxic Substances

1. *Systemic toxicity*. Toxic effects that result from absorption of a chemical and its spread to different body systems. Examples of common systemic toxicity include the serious, sometimes fatal, poisoning that may occur from contact with certain organophosphate pesticides (parathion) and inhalation of organic solvents.
2. *Organ-specific toxicity*. Certain chemicals have a target organ specificity (i.e., they harm a certain organ rather than others) often because of biotransformation or bioconcentration. The route of exposure might also be responsible for specific organ injury.
3. *Liver toxicity*. Most chemicals are metabolized in the liver. Therefore, the liver becomes the target organ for many chemicals. Organic solvents ($CC1_4$, chloroform, ethanol) and certain trace metals (copper, cadmium) may cause extensive liver damage, characterized by fatty changes, necrosis, fibrosis, and alteration of the structure.
4. *Kidney toxicity*. Many xenobiotics are removed by glomerular filtration and tubular excretion, while essential elements are reabsorbed in the tubuli. Chemicals with kidney toxicity include metals (e.g., mercury, cadmium, lead).
5. *Skin toxicity*. Skin rashes are a common reaction to chemicals. Allergic reactions can occur in sensitive individuals whereas skin irritation can occur in anyone exposed to a wide variety of irritating chemicals. Certain chemicals produce a characteristic type of skin reaction, which provides a clue as to the exposure the person may have experienced. Most, however, do not.
6. *Neurotoxicity*. Most toxic substances act on the central or peripheral nervous system. Functional or organic alterations of neurotransmitters can cause excitative symptoms or paralysis (through exposure to organophosphates, chlorinated organic compounds, metals).
7. *Immunotoxicity*. The function of the immune system ensures (*1*) nonspecific defense mechanisms against agents for which no previous sensitization has occurred, and (*2*) specific, adaptive mechanisms directed against specific agents to which the organism has previously been sensitized or with which it has been infected. The body has very complicated mechanisms to defend itself against attack by viruses and bacteria and these can be impaired by exposure to certain chemicals. One result of such exposure may be a subtle increase in the frequency of viral illnesses, such as influenza or colds. Impaired immunological reactions can lead to allergy. Molecules can react with other body components, altering their properties and hence their biological functions. This may result in the immune system treating these components as foreign. Antibodies may be produced that bind to abnormally altered body components and trigger inflammation, tissue breakdown, and other harmful effects.

codes and information. This complex process involves gene mutation, chromosomal alteration (structural and numerical), and/or gene rearrangements, all of which are described briefly in Box 2.5.

Cancer arises as a consequence of multiple genetic and nongenetic events that

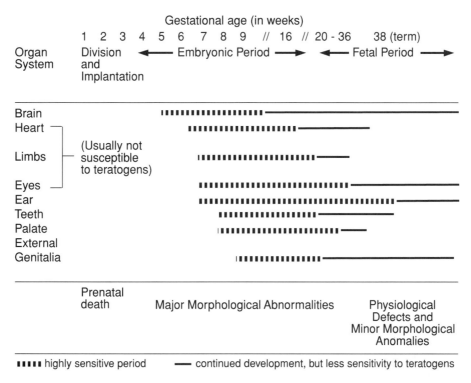

Figure 2.5 Critical periods of fetal development by organ system. From Jedrychowski and Krzyzanowski, 1995, with permission.

might lead to uncontrolled proliferation of cells. Although the individual steps are difficult to distinguish, there are two major classes of carcinogenic agents: agents primarily reacting with the DNA, and agents that have primarily nongenetic reactivity, acting through nongenetic mechanisms. In reality, carcinogenesis is a complex process, involving several stages in which genotoxic and nongenotoxic mechanisms take place. The multistage process of carcinogenesis can be characterized by three major steps: (1) initiation, which leads to (2) promotion, which develops into (3) progression.

Initiation Mutagenic chemicals, ionizing radiation, and viruses may cause changes in the DNA, creating an initiated cell. The initiated genotype is regarded as a potentially malignant state, which may be converted to a cell with the capacity for unrestricted proliferation. Initiation is thought to be *dose related*, which means that an increasing dose leads to greater numbers of initiated cells or cells with multiple crucial mutations. It occurs only in a small proportion of the target cell population and with greater frequency if the cells in the tissue are rapidly dividing. This can be explained by the fact that the DNA in the dividing cell is less protected and therefore more susceptible to chemical alterations. Furthermore, rapidly dividing cells have less time to repair initial damage, e.g., enzymatic removal of DNA base adducts, before they become irreversible mutations as a result of DNA replication. This process is called *mutation fixation*. Initiated cells show no recognizable biochemical or behavioral changes from their normal state, as the damage is not expressed as a new phenotype. However, the damage will be converted to a permanent change unless the DNA is rapidly repaired.

Promotion A *promoter* is a substance that does not cause tumor development itself but which, by its action, transforms the initiated cell into an abnormal, activated cell that may be the first cell of a tumor. This transformation results in local cell proliferation leading to usually benign tumor formation. As with everything in toxicology, dose and duration of exposure are key factors, so under certain circumstances, a promoter can also be tumorigenic in and of itself. At this stage, the tumor is not yet malignant. Some tumors may be benign, but others take the next stage of progression and become malignancies.

Progression In this stage, the tumor cells become malignant and the unrestricted proliferation results in invasion of adjacent tissues and metastases. *Metastases* occur when cells from the tumor break off and are transported elsewhere in the body to give rise to new tumor masses. These may grow even more rapidly than the original tumor, which is called the *primary tumor*.

The carcinogenic potential of a given agent is assessed primarily by human epidemiology and experimental animal studies. Genotoxicological short-term tests can also render data that might be helpful in assessing carcinogenicity. In 1974, the International Agency for Research on Cancer (IARC) started to systematically assess the carcinogenic risk of substances and exposures to humans. To date more than 500 evaluations have been carried out. The IARC's categorization, based on the accepted evidence for carcinogenicity, is probably the most widely recognized and widely used one by regulatory agencies. These categories are listed in Table 2.4.

Examples of different groups of carcinogens are shown in Box 2.6. Most chemicals that cause cancer are organic, such as polycyclic aromatic hydrocarbons (B naphthylamine, benzidine) benzene, bis-chloromethyl ether, and nitrosamines. Most chemical carcinogens tested appear to act as electrophiles (electron-deficient), which react covalently with nucleophiles (electron-rich) within the target cell. Apart from alkylating agents such as sulfur mustard, *N*-methyl *N*-nitrosourea, ethyl methane sulfate, and nitrosamides, chemicals often require enzymatic conversion to electrophiles. Even nitrosamides need hydrolyzing to active alkylating agents. The conversion by enzymes provides one explanation for the often tissue-specific nature of carcinogens, i.e., the necessary enzymes may have low activity or be nonexistent in the unaffected tissues.

The variations in how individuals metabolize carcinogens may explain differences in susceptibility to cancer. One theory is that individuals can differ in their rate of absorption from entry site and/or in the mechanisms they have to repair DNA, and that this could be responsible for the differences in risk experienced by different individuals, families, or other groups.

Toxicity Testing in Experimental Animals

A large number of different tests are available to determine the toxicological profile of a chemical. These tests may either assess acute, subchronic, and long-term toxicity or focus on specific areas of toxicity, covering a range of end points (see Table 2.5). The construction of the toxicological profile and the dose–response relationship are the first stages in risk assessment, as will be discussed in Chapter 3. When animal testing is used, the ethical issues associated with it must be considered.

Acute Toxicity Studies Acute animal studies are most commonly used to predict human effects of short-term, high-level exposures, such as may occur following an

TABLE 2.4
CARCINOGENIC CATEGORIZATION BY THE INTERNATIONAL AGENCY FOR RESEARCH ON CANCER

Accepted Categories

1. There is sufficient evidence for carcinogenicity in humans
2a. An agent is probably carcinogenic to humans
2b. An agent is possibly carcinogenic to humans
3. There is inadequate evidence for carcinogenicity to humans
4. Not carcinogenic

accident, and these studies can provide a measure of the toxic potential of different compounds. Metabolic and pharmacokinetic studies are used to determine the absorption, distribution, and elimination of the test compound, its biotransformation, and the rates in which these processes occur.

When toxicity is described in quantitative terms, the concepts lethal dose at 50% (LD_{50}) and effective dose at 50% (ED_{50}) are often used. The ED_{50} is the dose that would cause the effect in 50% of the test population; the LD_{50} is the dose that would kill 50%. The LD_{50} or ED_{50} is determined according to the dose–response relationship. Lethal doses by inhalation of chemicals in the form of a gas or vapor can also be tested. In this case, the concentration of gas or vapor that kills half the animals is known as the lethal concentration for 50% (LC_{50}). Although the LD_{50} and the LC_{50} only give information about the death of animals, they are very widely used as an index of toxicity. The criteria in Table 2.6 are often used for purposes of classification of acute toxic effects in animals.

The LD_{50} and LC_{50} are relatively reliable and in most cases correlate with levels of human toxicity. However, they are not sufficient to fully characterize the toxicity of chemicals, and it is impossible to assess health risks on the basis of

TABLE 2.5

RANGE OF TOXICITY STUDIES AVAILABLE FOR CONSTRUCTION
OF A TOXICOLOGICAL PROFILE

Study	Comments
Acute toxicity	Emphasis on acute effects and clinical signs, including lethality (LD_{50})
Subchronic toxicity	Often used to determine a dose without effect, generally of 28 or 90 days duration; also referred to as subacute studies
Chronic toxicity	Generally of approximately 2 years duration when rodents are used. May be designed as carcinogenicity studies, chronic toxicity studies, or both types combined.
SPECIALIZED STUDIES	
Reproduction studies	*Multigenerational studies* are used to investigate effects on reproductive performance, effects on fertility, fecundity, prenatal and perinatal toxicity, lactation, weaning, and postnatal development and growth. *Teratology studies* are used to investigate the ability to induce defects during pregnancy and fetal/embryo toxicity.
Genotoxicity studies	Investigation of the ability to induce mutations, chromosomal aberrations, and other end points indicative of heritable genetic damage having predictive relevance for carcinogenicity or the induction of inheritable defects
Skin and eye irritation tests	To determine the effects of skin and eye contamination, e.g., in occupational exposure
Skin sensitization	To investigate the potential to produce allergic sensitization
Immunotoxicity	To investigate the specific effects on the immune system, e.g., on the thymus, lymph nodes, bone marrow, and corresponding cellular and humoral (antibody-producing) effects
Neurotoxicity	To investigate the specific effects on the peripheral and central nervous systems, e.g., with compounds known to be neurotoxic, such as organophosphorous compounds. Also, behavioral toxicity tests may be required to investigate neurotoxicity.
Inhalation	To investigate the specific effects on the lung and upper respiratory tract or toxicity that occurs when the agent enters the body through the lungs or pathogens of exposure that result from inhalation or any combination of these. Inhalation studies are particularly challenging to standardize and interpret

Adapted from Niesink et al., 1996, with permission.

LD_{50} or LC_{50} alone, especially for carcinogens. (For instance, we are not particularly interested in the dose that will kill 50% of the human population.) Moreover, the LD_{50} and LC_{50} give no information about the mechanism or type of toxicity of the chemical or its possible chronic effects. Thus the LD_{50} and LC_{50}

TABLE 2.6

CLASSIFICATION SYSTEM FOR ACUTE TOXIC EFFECTS IN ANIMALS

	Oral LD_{50} Rat (mg/kg)	Dermal LD_{50} Rat or Rabbit (mg/kg)	Inhalation LD_{50} Rat (mg/m^3 hr)
Very toxic	<25	<50	<500
Toxic	25–200	50–400	500–2000
Harmful	200–2000	400–2000	21,000–20,000

are very crude indices of toxicity. Other more specific tests give more specific information. One example of a specific short-term test is the short-term irritancy test known as the *Draize Test*. The chemical being tested is applied to the animal's skin, and the area is examined over the next few days for signs of a rash or flared response. This test can also be carried out on the animal's eyes. (As noted below, animal testing is now discouraged when other possibilities exist.)

Subchronic Tests In subchronic toxicity tests, animals are usually exposed repeatedly to a given chemical over a relatively long period (28 days or longer), normally 10% of the lifetime of the selected animal. This means that inhalation or ingestion studies last about 90 days for rats and approximately 1 year for a dog. Crude studies simply call for examination of the general condition of the animals based on weight, food intake, activity and behavior, as well as examination of the organs for gross abnormalities to the naked eye. More sophisticated studies include functional tests such as kidney and liver function, histopathological examination of organs and other tissues, and chemical analysis of blood or urine samples.

Chronic Toxicity Testing The purpose of lifetime or chronic bioassays is to determine whether chemicals have any health effects that may take a long time to develop. Cancer is often the long-term health effect of greatest concern, but other effects on organs such as the kidney are also often studied. These studies are performed by exposing animals, by ingestion or inhalation, to the chemical being tested for the whole of the animal's lifetime. In rats, this may be 2 years; in mice, a little less than 2 years. In a typical test, 50 mice or rats will be exposed to a high but nonlethal dose of a chemical under study. The test animals are compared throughout their lifetime with a similar number of control animals. A good study will expose different groups of animals of both genders to different doses of the chemical. These studies may include very large numbers of animals and are then referred to as *megamouse studies*.

Reproductive Studies Studies in animals to check for adverse effects of a chemical on any aspects of reproduction involve exposing one or both parents to the chemical being tested, prior to mating, then observing the effects on any offspring. Sometimes just the pregnant female animal is exposed. Reproductive effects are classified according to whether the offspring are fewer in number, lower in birth weight, or deformed or damaged in some way. Sometimes multigenerational studies may be necessary to determine effects that may be passed on to future generations.

Other Types of Toxicity Testing

Each type of toxicity testing has its own challenges and scientific problems. For example, inhalation studies are among the most difficult studies to perform in toxicology. It can be very challenging to control the exposure of animals and the effects are often subtle or confined to certain tissues. Interactions are common and extrapolation to human disease may be uncertain. As a result, large-scale inhalation studies on animals are usually conducted in a small number of laboratories with proper equipment and experienced personnel.

Genotoxic Short-Term Tests Genotoxic activity of a given agent can be assessed by short-term tests for gene mutation and chromosome alterations both in vitro and in vivo. Over 50 tests have been developed over the last 20 years, of which some 6–10 tests have been validated satisfactorily for the prediction of germinal mutational effect and carcinogenic activity. The introduction of in vitro metabolic activation systems, enabling the conversion of chemicals to nucleophilic reactives, has made the approach suitable to test a wide variety of chemicals. The most commonly used and best-validated tests are the *Salmonella* revertent test (AMES)/mammalian microsome test, the chromosome aberration *in vitro* test, and the bone marrow cell test (chromosome aberration or micronucleus) *in vivo*.

Human Studies Information on toxic effects in humans can be obtained from either clinical studies or epidemological studies that investigate health effects after exposure in occupational settings or other environments. *Clinical studies* usually focus on the detailed study of individual cases of disease, whereas *experimental studies* are carefully controlled experiments in healthy humans, using low doses otherwise considered to be safe. In view of the ethical aspects, only relatively minor and reversible health effects, such as subtle changes in reaction time, behavioral functions, and sensory responses, can be studied in experiments. Epidemiological research methods and the use in the health risk assessment process will be discussed in Chapter 3.

Structure–Activity Relationships For many years it has been hoped that by applying knowledge of the physical structure and chemical characteristics of a substance one could predict its biological activity. Much information has been collected for various classes of compounds on the correlation between chemical structure, in terms of functional groups and special orientation, and parameters of toxicity. Short-term tests for assessing toxicity and maximum permissible concentrations for occupational and ambient air pollutants have been developed on the basis of such studies. However, the toxicological mechanism of all chemical structures is not understood and there are many compounds that do not react as expected, based on the structure–activity relationship. At the current level of knowledge, structure–activity relationships are useful indicators of potential toxicity and may help to priorize toxicological research, but they require corroborating evidence and should not be relied on solely in the decision-making process.

Information on Toxicity

Product identity is, of course, crucial in hazard identification. A product may have a common trade name that is used for advertising and marketing purposes. The *Chemical Abstracts Service* (CAS), a section of the American Chemical Society, assigns a CAS registry number to every chemical. Most product information sheets contain CAS numbers, which are useful in researching the toxicity of the chemical in question. The *Registry of Toxic Effects of Chemical Substances* (RTEC) number is also important, as it is linked to a list of scientific articles on the health effects of chemicals. This registry is operated by the National Institute for Occupational Safety and Health (NIOSH) in the United States.

TABLE 2.7

TWO CLASSIFICATION SYSTEMS FOR HAZARDOUS CHEMICALS

Canadian Categories of Controlled Substances		Categories of Dangerous Substances as Defined by the Council Directive of European Communities
Class	Definition	
A	A compressed gas	Explosive
B	Flammable and combustible material	Very toxic/toxic
C	Oxidizing material	Oxidizing
D	Poisonous and infectious material	Extremely flammable/highly
D1	Immediate and serious	Flammable/flammable
D2	Other toxic effects	Harmful
D3	Biohazardous	Corrosive
E	Corrosive material	Irritant
F	Dangerously reactive material	Sensitizing
		Carcinogenic/mutagenic
		Toxic for reproduction
		Dangerous for the environment

Right-to-know legislation in many jurisdictions has helped considerably in the identification and control of hazards. In Canada, for example, the *Workplace Hazardous Materials Information System* (WHMIS) requires provision of Material Safety Data Sheets (MSDS) on every substance, the labeling of controlled products according to categories as listed in Table 2.7, and the training of workers in the understanding of the MSDS and appropriate use of the substances. Similar legislation exists in many other countries, but certainly not all jurisdictions. In the countries of the European Community, several signs and sentences indicating the potential risk (R sentences) and safety precautions (S sentences) are used and it can be expected that these will be used increasingly in other European countries as well. Combinations of different R and S sentences provide adequate safety precautions for handling hazardous substances and preparations.

All the above information is usually supplied as a precondition for marketing in most countries. An example of an International Chemical Safety Card is shown in Figure 2.6. These cards are published by the IPCS and are available in many languages for more than 1000 chemicals.

PHYSICAL HAZARDS

Types of Physical Hazards

Physical hazards are forms of potentially harmful energy in the environment that can result in either immediate or gradually acquired damage when transferred in sufficient quantities to exposed individuals. Physical hazards may arise from forms of energy that occur naturally or are anthropogenic. A variety of different energy types can pose physical hazards, for example, sound waves, radiation, light energy, thermal energy, and electrical energy. Mechanical (kinetic) energy, which results in injury when a sufficient amount is transferred to an individual, will be discussed separately in Mechanical Hazards, below. The release of phys-

NITROGEN DIOXIDE			ICSC: 0930

NITROGEN DIOXIDE

CAS#   10102-44-0   Nitrogen peroxide
RTECS# QW9800000   (cylinder)
ICSC#   0930 NO_2
UN#   1067 (liquefied) Molecular mass: 46.0
EC#   007-002-00-0

ICSC: 0930
HAZARD SYMBOLS
Consult national legislation

TYPES OF HAZARD / EXPOSURE	ACUTE HAZARDS / SYMPTOMS	PREVENTION	FIRST AID / FIRE FIGHTING
FIRE	Not combustible but enhances combustion of other substances. Supports combustion of carbon, phosphorus and sulfur.	NO contact with all combustible materials including clothing.	Shut off supply; if not possible and no risk to surroundings, let the fire burn itself out; in other cases extinguish with powder, dry chemical.
EXPLOSION	Elevated temperature may cause cylinders to explode.		In case of fire: keep cylinder cool by spraying with water. Combat fire out of sheltered position.
EXPOSURE			IN ALL CASES CONSULT A DOCTOR!
• Inhalation	Cough, headache, nausea; symptoms may be delayed; see Notes	Ventilation, local exhaust, or breathing protection.	Fresh air, rest, half-upright position, and refer for medical attention.
• Skin	Redness	Protective gloves, protective clothing when liquefied gas.	Remove contaminated clothes, rinse and then wash skin with water and soap, and refer for medical attention.
• Eyes	Redness, pain.	Safety goggles, or, when liquefied gas, face shield, or eye protection in combination with breathing protection	First rinse with plenty of water for several minutes (remove contact lenses if easily possible), then take to a doctor.
• Ingestion		Do not eat, drink, or smoke during work.	

SPILLAGE DISPOSAL	STORAGE	PACKAGING AND LABELLING
Evacuate danger area, consult an expert, ventilation use water spray to knock down vapour, neutralize running water with chalk or soda, do NOT absorb in saw-dust or other combustible absorbents (extra personal protection: complete protective clothing including self-contained breathing apparatus).	Separate from combustible, organic oxidizable substances; ventilation along the floor.	UN haz class: 2.3 UN subsidiary risks: 5.1 FURTHER INFORMATION ON LABELLING: Consult national legislation

IMPORTANT DATA	PHYSICAL STATE: APPEARANCE REDDISH BROWN COMPRESSED LIQUEFIED GAS OR YELLOW FUMING LIQUID, WITH PUNGENT ODOUR. PHYSICAL DANGERS: The gas is heavier than air. CHEMICAL DANGERS: The substance decomposes on heating above 160° producing nitric oxide and oxygen which increases fire hazard. The substance is a strong oxidant and reacts violently with combustible and reducing materials. Reacts violently with anhydrous ammonia, chlorinated hydrocarbons, petroleum, ordinary fuel and rocket fuel. Reacts with water forming nitric acid and nitric oxide. Reacts with alkalie to form nitrates and nitrites. Attacks many metals in the presence of moisture. OCCUPATIONAL EXPOSURE LIMITS (OELs): TLV: 3 ppm: 5.6 mg/m^3 (ACGIH 1990 - 1991) PDK: 2 mg/m^3 (USSR 1984)	ROUTES OF EXPOSURE: The substance can be absorbed in the body by inhalation. INHALATION RISK: A harmful concentration of this gas in the air will be reached very quickly on loss of contaminent. EFFECTS OF SHORT-TERM EXPOSURE: The substance irritates the eyes, the skin and the respiratory tract. Inhalation of this gas may cause lung oedema, (see Notes). The substance may cause delayed effects on lungs. EFFECTS OF LONG-TERM OR REPEATED EXPOSURE The substance may have effects on the lungs. Accelerating capacity was seen in a group of lung-tumor susceptible mice.
PHYSICAL PROPERTIES	Boiling point: 21°C Melting point: -9.3°C Relative density (water = 1): 1:45 (liquid) Solubility in water reaction Vapour pressure, kPa at 20°C: 96 Relative vapour density (air = 1): 1.58	
ENVIRONMENTAL DATA		

NOTES	
The commercial brown liquid under pressure is called nitrogen tetroxide. Actually this is an equilibrium mixture of NO_2 and the colourless N_2O_4. Nonirritant concentration may cause lung oedema. The symptoms of lung oedema sometimes do not become manifest until 24 - 36 hours have passed and they are aggravated by physical effort. Rest and medical observation are therefore essential. Turn leaking cylinder with the leak up to prevent escape of gas in liquid state. Corrosive to steel when wet, but may be stored in steel cylinders when moisture content is 0.1% or less	Transport Emergency Card: TEC (R)-109 NFPA Code: H 3; F O; R O; oxy

Figure 2.6 International chemical safety card. Source: International Program on Chemical Safety, WHO, Geneva.

ical energy may be sudden and uncontrolled, as in an explosive loud noise, or sustained and more or less under control, as in working conditions with long-term exposure to lower levels of constant noise.

Noise, radiation (including light), and temperature factors are the most common examples of physical hazards. They can cause health effects in natural exposure situations, such as when ultraviolet (UV) radiation from the sun causes eye cataracts or when heat waves kill the frail, the young, and the elderly. For environmental health management, human-made exposure situations are of the greatest importance, such as the loud noise that millions of people are exposed to in their workplaces. Other examples include the ionizing radiation isotopes spread from the accident at the Chernobyl nuclear power plant, which exposed 5 million people to excessive doses and made large land areas uninhabitable for many years.

Noise and Vibration

Noise is defined as an unwanted sound. Sound travels as waves in air (or pressure changes) that make the eardrum vibrate. The eardrum passes these vibrations on to three bones in the middle ear, which in turn pass the vibrations to the fluid contained in the cochlea (in the inner ear). Within the cochlea are tiny nerve endings commonly known as hair cells. They respond to the fluid vibrations by sending neural impulses to the brain, which then interprets the impulses as sound or noise. Intense sound produces higher-amplitude waves than less intense sound. The intensity of a sound is determined by the height (or amplitude) of a sound wave. Higher waves carry more energy and produce greater vibrations. These higher waves produce greater vibrations within the ear, which can damage the hair cells. Sometimes the damage is temporary and is naturally repaired after a few minutes or days. The ringing in the ear that one experiences after attending a loud music concert is a common symptom of this temporary damage. At high noise intensity, however, the damage is permanent because hair cells, like all nerve cells, cannot be replaced and have very limited capacity to repair themselves. Each year, millions of industrial workers lose significant proportions of their hearing capacity because of high noise exposures in their workplaces. High noise levels may also occur in the general environment, but mainly in conjunction with traffic and transport systems. The noise level on a sidewalk of a busy street or in a speeding subway train with open windows can reach levels that may damage hearing.

At lower intensity levels, noise can cause disturbed sleep, stress, and reduced well-being. The problem of community noise and its disturbance effects is increasing, as more and more people live in cities where noise from traffic, neighbors, and industry is seldom brought under any control—at least not at the first stages of urbanization. Increasingly, as a result of community protests against the noise, sound protective barriers are being erected along motorways and railways.

Sound intensity is measured in *decibels* (dB). The sound intensity is determined by the changes in the pressure of the sound wave. The intensity of a sound observed by the human ear also depends on the frequency or tone of a sound. The frequency is determined by the number of sound waves per second and is expressed in Hertz (1 Hz equals 1 sound wave per minute). Therefore, sound levels are commonly adjusted to the observation of the human ear, i.e., using the

TABLE 2.8
SOUND LEVELS OF SOME FAMILIAR SOUNDS

Sources	Aural Effect	Sound Level dB(A)
Shotgun blast Jet plane (at take-off) Firecrackers, exploding	Human ear pain threshold	140
Rock music, amplified Hockey game crowd Thunder, severe Pneumatic jackhammer	Uncomfortably loud	120
Powered lawn mower Tractor, farm type Subway train, interior Motorcycle, snowmobile	Extremely loud	100
Window mounted air conditioner Crowded restaurant Diesel powered truck/tractor	Moderately loud	80
Singing birds Normal conversation	Quiet	60
Rustle of leaves Faucet dripping Light rainfall	Very quiet	20
Whisper	Just audible	10

"A" scale: dB(A). Sound intensity is measured by an instrument called a *sound level meter*. Table 2.8 outlines some familiar sounds and their dB(A).

Increasing sound intensity increases the risk of hearing loss. Risk of incurring hearing loss begins with prolonged exposure to sound of approximately 75 dB(A) (WHO, 1980a). Many countries use 85 dB as the noise safety limit in workplaces. As a rule of thumb, if a loud voice is not understandable at a distance of 1 meter because of excessive background noise, the background noise level is above 85 dB and likely to be dangerous. Even if the sound level is not noticeably uncomfortable, hair cells in the inner ear can be damaged. As intensity increases, the length of exposure time that causes hearing loss decreases. For example, approximately 15% of individuals exposed to 90 dB(A) for 8 hr per day during a whole working life (40 years) will experience significant hearing loss. At 85 dB(A) the risk is 10%.

Noise-induced hearing loss can be prevented by a program of both noise control and monitoring of workers for early detection of hearing loss by looking for the temporary threshold shift and implementing changes before hearing loss becomes permanent. Noise control is a highly technical specialization that may involve acoustical engineering, plant design, engineering controls, and containment or isolation of noise sources. However, most problems involving excessive noise can be handled effectively and inexpensively using basic principles.

Hearing conservation programs should include regular monitoring of the workplace, baseline and annual audiograms for all exposed workers, in-service

BOX 2.7

The Basics of Radiation

The *atom* is the simplest unit into which matter can be broken down yet still retain its identity as a distinct element, including all of its chemical characteristics. Each atom consists of two components: a *nucleus* (containing protons and neutrons) and orbiting *electrons*. The number of *protons* in the nucleus of the atom, also indicated as the atomic number, determines the identity of element. There is an equivalent number of electrons in the atom unless it is ionized or incorporated into a molecular bond. The atomic number determines the chemical characteristics of the element—how many electrons, how they are arranged, and how atoms of the element bond to one another and other elements.

Unstable atoms, which possess too many or too few neutrons, try to become more stable by emitting particulate and/or electromagnetic radiation (energy). The type of radiation emitted (alpha, beta, or gamma radiation) depends on the type of instability. When alpha or beta particles are emitted, the atoms of one element actually convert to atoms of another element. The emission of radiation from an unstable atom is called *decay* or *disintegration*. Each type of unstable atom has a known half-life, which represents the length of time required for half the atoms to decay, to emit radiation. Examples of half-lives are as follows:

uranium-238	4.5 billion years
plutonium-239	24,390 years
cesium-137	30 years
strontium-90	29 years
tritium	12.5 years
iodine-131	8.5 days
radon	3.8 days

A unit of radioactivity is called a *becquerel* (Bq). It is equivalent to one atom decaying per second. The amount of damage caused by this radioactivity depends on a number of factors, especially the radiation type and the actual dose, measured as Gray (Gy) or Sievert (Sv). The types of radiation can be broken down as follows:

1. *Alpha radiation.* An alpha particle is a heavy particle (actually a helium nucleus) with a charge of +2, which gives up energy in short distance, mostly through ionization. It is not very penetrating and is easily shielded against when the source is external to the body. For instance, alpha radiation cannot penetrate the skin surface. However, when particles emitting alpha radiation are inhaled or ingested, they can ionize atoms in living cells, leading to significant damage.
2. *Beta radiation.* This radiation is the result of the emission of electrons from the nucleus. Electrons are smaller and lighter than alpha particles and also pose a hazard if the source is inhaled or ingested. Compared to alpha radiation, it has a higher penetration (depending on energy and density of the material) but has a lower rate of ionization than alpha radiation. Usually beta radiation is shielded against by using plastic or light metals because it can produce gamma radiation when passing through lead, which is often used for shielding against radiation.
3. *Gamma radiation.* This radiation is a form of electromagnetic energy emitted from the nucleus, often together with emission of beta particles. This electromagnetic radiation with high energy and frequency can penetrate relatively easy but has a lower rate of ionization. Both internal and external sources can pose a hazard.

(continued)

(continued)

For example, X-rays are machine-made gamma rays, whereas cosmic rays are gamma rays from space.

4. *Neutron radiation.* Free neutrons can be a form of radiation when they are released from the atomic nucleus. They can induce significant cell damage by ionization because the heavy particle carries a high amount of energy. Material through which they pass may become radioactive, absorbed by nuclei of atoms in the material, which then become unstable and decay themselves; this is called *neutron activation.*

and preservice worker education regarding hearing conservation, systematic record keeping, worker notification when problems are detected, and the provision of hearing protection to all exposed workers. Many programs in industry include referral of affected employees to specialists, administrative controls to limit the duration of assignments in noisy areas, and noise control measures. (As an example of a risk management strategy, a workplace-based hearing conservation program will be described in Chapter 4.)

In addition to noise, which can be regarded as a vibration transmitted by air to the ear, vibration energy can also be transmitted directly to other parts of the human body. The use of many tools or hand equipment can result in adverse health effects as a result of arm and hand vibration. The most characteristic effect of prolonged exposure to vibration of the hand is *vibration vasculitis*, or *white finger disease*, a form of spontaneous or cold-induced blood vessel constriction that results in reduced sensation to fine touch, vibration, or temperature, and causes marked pain. It is named for the white appearance of the fingers when the blood vessel constriction occurs. Vibrations can also be transmitted to the entire body when driving vehicles like bulldozers, excavators, trucks, and cars on rough lands or bumpy roads. These vibrations may damage the musculoskeletal system.

Ionizing Radiation

Radiation hazards can be divided into those from ionizing and nonionizing radiation. (Nonionizing radiation and light as one specific form of nonionizing radiation are discussed in Noniodizing Radiation, and Light and Lasers, below.) The basic principles and the different types of radiation are described in Box 2.7. *Ionizing radiation* emerges when an electron is removed from a neutral atom and a pair of ions are produced—a negatively charged electron and a positively charged atom. It is the ionization of atoms in the human body that causes harmful biological effect. The ions are highly reactive and damage critical cell structures, including proteins and DNA. Ionizing radiation is, in fact, defined as electromagnetic radiation (see next section for definition) with sufficient energy to displace an electron from an atom.

Knowledge about the nature and probability of adverse health effects of ionizing radiation is based on animal experiments and observations of the effects of human exposures at high doses, such as the studies of survivors of the atomic bombings of Japan and of people exposed in radiation accidents. Studies of patients exposed to radiation for medical treatment as well as occupational health studies have also demonstrated important effects (e.g., miners exposed to radon have been found to have a higher incidence of lung cancer). The effects of ionizing radiation are divided into two basic types; *threshold effects* (also known as *nonstochastic*, or *deterministic*) and *nonthreshold effects* (*stochastic*). The nonstochastic effects follow a dose–effect relationship in a single individual, as in the ingestion of a toxic substance (see Chapter 3, Relationship Between Dose and Health Outcome). Stochastic effects occur as an all-or-none outcome with a certain probability following exposure. For example, following exposure to high levels of radiation, a person may have a high risk of developing cancer but any one person will not get more of a cancer with higher exposure.

Exposure to radiation from natural sources, such as cosmic radiation, and indoor exposure, including radiation from building materials and radon exposure, account for more than half of the annual dose people usually receive. The total dose depends on the geographical area where people live. In addition to the natural background radiation, people can be directly exposed to ionizing radiation during medical treatments, for instance, radiation therapy for cancers and X-rays for imaging of internal organs. Strict precautions have to be taken to protect both patients and hospital staff. The health risk as a result of medical application of ionizing radiation can be kept at a minimal and acceptable level. Some consumer articles also contain minute amounts of radioactive materials, such as smoke detectors, light switches, or illuminating watches and clocks. The contribution of these sources to the total background exposure is very low (<0.5%). Other sources of ionizing radiation are nuclear accidents (Chernobyl), nuclear testing, and nuclear power plants. There are many nuclear power stations in different countries around the world, and in some countries they produce the bulk of electricity used in the country (e.g., France). Again, strict precautions need to be taken to prevent accidents, but when an accident happens, as in Chernobyl, the health effects can be very serious. The causes and consequences of the accident in Chernobyl will be discussed in Chapter 9.

When people incur exposure to high doses of radiation that exceed a certain threshold, the deterministic health effects include skin burns, damage to the bone marrow, sterility, acute radiation sickness, and death. These effects have been observed in atomic bomb survivors, patients treated by radiation, and in workers accidentally overexposed, as in the case of workers at the Chernobyl power station at the time of the accident. The effects occur at doses of a few tenths of *Sieverts* (Sv), the common measure that takes into account the absorbed dose and the type of radiation. (It replaces the old unit called a *rem*; 1 rem = 0.01 Sv). The deterministic effects occur at doses much higher than those that would occur to workers in normal operations or to the public from normal environmental discharges from nuclear power production, in which case, doses may be in the order of millionths of a Sievert (i.e., microsieverts). The stochastic or nonthreshold-related effects, including cancer and genetic effects, are believed to occur as the result of low as well as high doses.

The basic question in assessing this risk for workers and members of the public concerns the nature of the dose–response relationship at low doses and dose rates. According to the International Commission on Radiological Protection (ICRP), it is prudent to regard the dose–response relationship for cancer risk from radiation as linear down to zero dose. The probability of the occurrence of fatal cancers over a lifetime in a population exposed to radiation at low doses has been estimated by the ICRP to be about 5/100 per person-Sieverts; or if 100,000 people were exposed to a dose of 1 mSv each, then 5 would die of cancer. The cancers of greatest concern with respect to radiation are lung cancer, leukemia, and cancers of the skin, breast, and thyroid. Generally, there is a long latency: approximately 5 years for thyroid, 10 years for leukemia, and 20–30 years for the other cancers. The human embryo and the fetus are particularly sensitive to radiation, and the risk of cancer induction is likely to be higher for fetuses than in the general population, while the risk of genetic damage is probably at least as high. As a result of the observation of malformations in animal studies, it is recommended that occupational exposure of pregnant women be controlled such that the dose to the fetus does not exceed 1 mSv during the course of the pregnancy.

Radon is a gas present in rock, groundwater, and soil in some geographic areas. It is a product of the natural decay of radium, a solid material found in the earth's crust in many locations. It has been linked to increased lung cancer in miners (particularly uranium miners). It can seep into basements of houses and expose the inhabitants. There is increasing concern that residential radon may also be contributing to an increased risk of lung cancer in some countries (see Chapter 4).

Nonionizing Radiation

All forms of nonionizing radiation are part of the electromagnetic spectrum. *Electromagnetic radiation* is a form of energy that consists of an electric and a magnetic component. The energy is transported by the propagation of disturbances in electric and magnetic fields that are always at right angles to each other. The two fields vary in phase with one another in the form of a wave motion.

The waves travel at the speed of light, which is in vacuum approximately 3×10^8 m/sec. Figure 2.7 shows the complete electromagnetic spectrum, which spans from wavelengths shorter than 10^{-10} (gamma rays) meter to longer than 1 meter (up to 100 km) for radiowaves. Electromagnetic radiation with a wavelength above 10^{-10} meter does not have enough energy to cause ionizations. Therefore, this part of the spectrum is referred to as *nonionizing radiation*.

As indicated in Figure 2.7, nonionizing radiation includes UV radiation from the sun, which can cause eye cataracts that in turn can lead to blindness, as well as skin cancer and immune system damage. In recent years, there has been considerable concern about this hazard, because the depletion of stratospheric ozone layer has led to an increase in UV radiation exposures (see Chapter 11 and WHO, 1994a). Another type of nonionizing radiation to which millions of people are exposed is *electromagnetic fields* (EMF). These develop around electric power lines, electric machinery, electric installations in home radio transmitters, and portable telephones. In most situations the doses are too low to cause any adverse health effects. However, a number of suspected adverse health impacts, including cancer, have been reported, but research data have not given a clear picture yet. Light is in itself a type of radiation that can cause blindness if the eye is directly exposed to very high–intensity light, such as when a person looks straight at the sun for too long (see Light and Lasers, below).

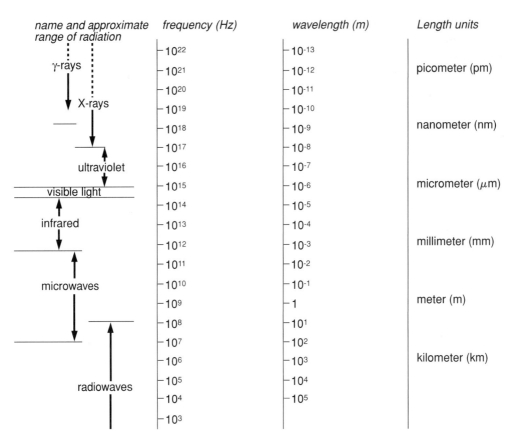

name and approximate range of radiation	frequency (Hz)	wavelength (m)	Length units
γ-rays	10^{22}	10^{-13}	
	10^{21}	10^{-12}	picometer (pm)
X-rays	10^{20}	10^{-11}	
	10^{19}	10^{-10}	
	10^{18}	10^{-9}	nanometer (nm)
ultraviolet	10^{17}	10^{-8}	
	10^{16}	10^{-7}	
visible light	10^{15}	10^{-6}	micrometer (μm)
	10^{14}	10^{-5}	
infrared	10^{13}	10^{-4}	
	10^{12}	10^{-3}	millimeter (mm)
	10^{11}	10^{-2}	
microwaves	10^{10}	10^{-1}	
	10^{9}	1	meter (m)
	10^{8}	10^{1}	
	10^{7}	10^{2}	
	10^{6}	10^{3}	kilometer (km)
radiowaves	10^{5}	10^{4}	
	10^{4}	10^{5}	
	10^{3}		

Figure 2.7 Range of the electromagnetic spectrum.

Exposure to UV radiation occurs mainly from sunlight, but it can also occur from electric welding arcs and from UV lights used in laboratories. Sunlight contains UV-A, UV-B, and UV-C, but normally only UV-A reaches the earth's surface in significant amounts. UV-B and UV-C are more damaging to health but they are normally reflected away from the earth by the stratospheric ozone layer. In case of damage to the ozone layer, which has now been shown to occur because of contamination of the atmosphere with chlorofluorocarbon (CFC) chemicals, people may be exposed to an increasing intensity of UV-B. UV-C does not reach the earth's surface.

The most well-documented health effect of UV radiation exposure is skin cancer. People with light skin are at greater risk, particularly if they work outside in occupations that do not provide much protection from the sun. An example is the very high risk of skin cancer among outdoor workers (including farmers) in Australia and New Zealand. Excessive sun-bathing is another exposure that adds to the risk of skin cancer. Skin cancer is now becoming increasingly common in countries with light-skinned people, such as the United Kingdom and Scandinavia.

Another important health effect of UV radiation is cataract (lens opacity) of the eye. Cataracts may lead to blindness and are increasingly common at older ages. This effect is caused by direct exposure of the lens to UV radiation. In India, for example, many farmers work in the fields in the blazing sun all day long without wearing any protection of the eyes. In this country alone, 2 million people develop blindness each year; half of these cases are caused by cataracts. Ultraviolet ray–related cataracts are not dependent on skin color, so this health effect may be even more critical in tropical countries than in Europe. The intensity of UV radiation at ground level in tropical areas, on average throughout the year, is many times greater than that in temperate areas (e.g., Europe).

A third potential health effect of UV radiation is changes in the immune system, but so far this has only been demonstrated in animals. If high UV exposure reduces the function of the immune system in people, it could increase the occurrence of infectious diseases in exposed people, and it could decrease the effectiveness of immunizations against communicable diseases, such as measles and hepatitis, in children. Currently, we do not know if this is a real problem.

Concern about exposure to EMF has been raised by studies that suggest a small increased risk of cancer with prolonged exposure. As mentioned earlier, exposures occur close to high-voltage power lines, particularly near the above-ground power lines with super-high voltages, which have become increasingly common in recent decades along with the use of electrical appliances in the home and the increasing presence of electricity in urban life. Exposure can also occur in homes with electric wiring systems of a particular type and in workplaces where electric machinery is placed in close proximity to workers. There is not sufficient scientific evidence to support a definitive statement about whether EMF is an important health concern. Nevertheless, in many countries, limit values have been set for exposure to extremely low frequency fields.

Light and Lasers

Visible light is one type of nonionizing radiation. It is not as powerful as UV radiation and mainly causes damage to the eye after overexposure. *Laser* (which stands for light amplification by stimulated emission of radiation) is light that has been synchronized such that the radiation is of one specific frequency and the light waves are all traveling in phase in pulses. This delivers much larger energy directly to the eye than normal light. Laser light of high energy can therefore be extremely damaging to the eye and can even burn the skin or other materials. Although laser light is an occasional hazard in occupational settings, the lack of sufficient lighting, particularly in the work environment, is a much more general problem. Poor lighting increases the risk of injuries in factories as well as on roads, and increases eye strain in people who have to read or perform precision tasks in their work. Eye strain can led to headaches and various psychosomatic symptoms. The lighting needed for fine tasks increases significantly with age, because of the natural deterioration of eyesight with age. A 40-year-old person needs twice as much light as a 20-year-old person to see an object with the same clarity. However, because lighting consumes energy and this increases costs, many factories and homes are poorly lit, especially in poor countries.

Pressure

Barometric pressures above or below one atmosphere (the normal pressure at sea level) are part of the conditions of work in special environments, such as under water or at high altitude. The absolute pressure is usually less critical than the changes experienced by the worker. The direct adverse effects of these pressure changes are called *barotrauma* and are of particular interest in aerospace and undersea medicine. There are also a number of problems that result from the dissolving of gases into body fluids or, conversely, the release of gases out of body fluids.

Health problems associated with compression generally occur only when there is no way to equilibrate pressures in an enclosed space. Decompression effects are more common and can be severe as a person emerges from a pressurized environment. They occur when a diver returns to surface too quickly or when workers who are in compressed chambers, such as caissons, have been depressurized too abruptly. All commercial and amateur divers are instructed in the use of diving tables, a set of graphs and tables that provide guidelines for ascent after diving to a given depth and remaining there for a given period of time. Failure to adhere closely to these tables, through inattention or during an emergency, may result in potentially serious effects, including decompression sickness, air emboli, and aseptic necrosis (death of small areas) of bone.

Effects associated with ascent to high altitude and reduced barometric pressure are dealt with in the literature of aerospace medicine and are too highly specialized and uncommon to describe here in detail. However, it should be remembered that already at 2000 meters altitude the reduction of oxygen pressure by inhaled air can cause shortages of breath in people not accustomed to this altitude, and above 4000 meters nausea and unconsciousness may occur unless precautions are taken.

Extremes of Temperature

Hazards associated with extremes of temperature can be divided into exposure to heat and exposure to cold. In most countries, the climate changes from cold to warm once a year, or a change in seasons brings torrential rainfall or hurricanes. Heat and cold affect the well-being and health of millions of people each year. Adaptation to the climate, and type of housing, clothing, and other precautions will determine the impact on health.

Internal temperature regulation in the presence of temperature variation in the environment is necessary for human life. Problems arise when one of three conditions occurs: (*1*) temperature variations are so extreme that they exceed the considerable ability of the body to adapt; (*2*) mechanisms of adaptation, such as vasodilatation or sweating, are impaired; or (*3*) exposure to extremes of temperature is concentrated on a particular body part, as in frostbite or thermal burns. The human body regulates temperature through the central nervous system from a control center in the hypothalamus, a small structure in the center of the brain. This center receives neural impulses from thermal receptors on the skin and receptors sensing the temperature of blood in deep body structures. It responds by activating mechanisms controlled by the autonomic nervous system that dissipate heat (vasodilatation and sweating) or that increase the internal generation of heat (shivering) and conserve heat (vaso). It also sends signals to the cortex of the brain that make one aware of being hot or cold, initiating behavioral changes, such as changes in dress, seeking shelter, or modifying activity. This center can become disoriented from factors including infection, vasodilation associated with alcohol and autonomic dysfunction, or potentially lethal extremes in bodily temperature, and as a result, it prompts inappropriate responses.

The body regulates average temperature in the deep body within a narrow range centered on about 37°C. Although core temperature is maintained approximately constant, there is continuous variation in the heat flux needed to maintain this constancy in the body. Heat is generated by metabolic processes and by work performed by the muscles. Heat is also taken into the body from the environment if the external temperature is warmer than the body core. Heat is lost to the environment by four means: radiation from the surface of skin (as infrared radiation), evaporation in the form of sweating, conduction by contact with a cooler surface, and convection by air movement carrying heated air away from the surface of the skin or expired air from the lungs. Expired air from the lungs is saturated with water vapor and is therefore able to carry much more heat than dry air, so it is another mechanism of heat loss through evaporation and convection. Heat cannot be lost as efficiently from the body when there is interference with these mechanisms. Radiation and conduction may be reduced by insulation, as with padded clothing, which reduces evaporation and convection, thus restricting air circulation close to the skin. Evaporation is also reduced when humidity of the air is elevated. In contrast to homeostatic temperature regulation, perception of heat and cold is highly subjective and a matter of individual preference. Current norms and standards for heat and humidity are based on comfort for the largest proportion of workers but may be perceived as uncomfortable for some.

Cold is particularly dangerous because it may also reduce awareness of an injury. Temperature and air movement, called *windchill,* can severely affect and even kill a person who is not properly protected. Both severe heat and severe cold are particular hazards for the very young and very old. Local cold damage results in frostbite while cold affecting the whole body results in hypothermia. *Frostbite* is the local freezing of tissue that may result in irreversible damage. Extremities such as fingers, toes, and the tips of ears and noses are particularly vulnerable. Amputation of the affected area may be required in severe cases. *Hypothermia* is the condition of low body temperature. It is usually fatal if not recognized and treated by warming the patient.

Extremes of heat can also have local or systemic effects. Local heat can result in burns. Less extreme but prolonged heat results in systemic effects such as *heat stress*, a problem that is not limited to tropical climates or jobs involving proximity to a heat source. It can also occur as the result of excessive heat retention due to the combination of heavy clothing and strenuous exercise or in combinations of heat and humidity that interfere with evaporative cooling. Evaporation or artificial cooling must balance the heat gained from convection and radiation when the surroundings are hotter than the person. If heat loss does not equal heat gain and heat generation, then heat accumulates and the core temperature rises.

There are several medical conditions that can develop as a result of heat stress. Of these, *heat stroke* is the most serious. This potentially fatal condition occurs when a person can no longer adapt to the heat and collapses with failure of the circulation. It may occur in the workplace in jobs where exposure to intense heat is uncontrolled. Heat stroke is more common among people who are not used to heat and is most likely to occur during occasional heat waves, especially in cities. As a consequence of increasing urbanization, more and more people are living in urban agglomerations where heat can accumulate during sunny, hot periods. Cities are usually warmer than the surrounding countryside and are often more humid. In unprotected populations, heat stroke may occur during heat waves, especially when it is very humid. The resulting fatalities occur most often among the elderly, the chronically ill, and people who are not eating well or drinking enough fluid. Compounding this is the fact that peaks of air pollution from car exhaust and ozone production at ground level often coincide with heat waves because they often occur during the summer months. The combination of air pollution and extreme temperatures can be serious. Heat in the workplace and general environment also has an effect on work capacity. Traditional methods of house construction in hot countries are largely effective in protecting against the hazards of extreme heat, but modern house building methods may require air conditioning or artificial cooling systems, and when these systems break down or cannot be afforded, people are at increased risk.

Localized extreme heat resulting in *burns* can occur in variety of ways. Direct exposure to fire results in many serious burns, but contact with hot substances is also very common. Hot substances include liquids (common during cooking), hot solid objects such as stovetops or machinery, or hot gases. More house fire deaths occur due to suffocation from smoke inhalation than from burn injury. Nevertheless, burn injuries both at work and in the community are important causes of morbidity and mortality. Burns that occur at home will be discussed in Home and Recreational Injuries, below. Burns can also be the result of exposure to electrical hazards, which occur both in the workplace and in the community. Most deaths from electrocution occur immediately at the scene as a result of cardiac arrest. Victims who survive are at risk of significant disability, as loss of limb frequently results, especially following high-voltage contact. Injuries that do not seem very serious initially can worsen progressively over 2–4 days, manifesting damage to deeper tissues.

MECHANICAL HAZARDS

Understanding Mechanical Hazards

Mechanical hazards are those posed by the transfer of mechanical or *kinetic energy* (the energy of motion). The transfer of mechanical energy can result in immediate or gradually acquired injury in exposed individuals. The terms *injury* and *trauma* are often used interchangeably to refer to the harm that may result from mechanical hazards. The events and circumstances that result in injury have commonly been referred to as *accidents*. This term is no longer used by those working in injury control. In many languages it implies that injuries are random, unpredictable, chance types of events. Environmental health specialists believe that most injuries are predictable and preventable, and can be studied using epidemiological methods, just like any illness or health effect.

Cultural attitudes toward injury are important. Where injury deaths are culturally viewed as determined by fate, there will not be a receptive response to an injury control initiative. Many cultures glorify risk-taking behavior involving dangerous acts of physical ability. Risky behavior is often considered brave or adventuresome in contrast to cautious behavior which may be seen as cowardly or dull. These have positive and negative connotations. Children raised with access to television are exposed to these cultural values from a very young age by characters who engage in exciting, risk-taking behaviors without any connection to real consequences.

Socioeconomic factors are also important to consider when addressing the problem of mechanical hazards. Injury rates are linked with poverty within both developed and developing nations. Much of the world's population lacks the resources to provide optimal safety in their immediate environment. The necessity of obtaining food for the family by riding a broken-down bicycle through crowded, poorly maintained streets without a helmet is an example of this. Governments and industry are tempted to compromise safety for economic reasons, leading to tragedies such as the collapse of a public building. Many transportation accidents involving trains, ferries, and buses are the result of inadequate resources provided for the safe upkeep and regulation of roads, rails, and vehicles.

Mechanical hazards cannot be considered in isolation from other hazards and realities of day-to-day life. Perceived injury risks are mentally weighed against other environmental hazards, necessities of survival, and perceived benefits of accepting a risk. Consider the risk of sleeping in a poorly constructed shack that would collapse in an earthquake versus the risk of having no shelter at all; the risk of traveling through an unsecured zone of conflict to obtain food versus the risk of starving; and the risk of driving on a crowded freeway to work rather than taking safer public transit for the benefit of saving time and preserving independence. In approaching any injury control issue, the cultural and socioeconomic context must be appreciated.

Impact of Injury on the Individual and Society

Injury is a major cause of mortality throughout the world and has been described as the most underrecognized major public health problem. For example, injury is the single greatest killer of North Americans between the ages of 1 and 44; in Canada, injuries are responsible for 63% of all deaths between the ages of 1 and 24 (Shah, 1994). A similar pattern exists in most developed countries. The importance of injury is becoming increasingly recognized in developing countries, as injury mortality is high in developing countries and generally decreases with development. The only exception is traffic accident deaths, which increase in line with the growth of motor vehicle use in a country. While traditional health problems of infectious diseases and malnutrition remain important causes of mortality in developing nations, increased urbanization and the influx of automobiles (often on roads not designed for them) has led to increased mortality from injury.

Surveillance systems for nonfatal injuries are relatively new and are subject to underreporting. Thus accurate morbidity incidence data are difficult to obtain. However, many local and national reporting systems are able to capture injuries for which hospital care was required. Some surveys and cohort studies have been done to obtain community estimates. It is estimated, for instance, that each year, one out of three adults and children experience a nonfatal injury such that they seek medical care or are unable to carry out their usual activities (NCIPC, 1989). For every death of a child caused by injury it is estimated that 45 injuries require admission to hospital, 1270 are treated in an emergency room and are released, and likely twice that many do not require hospital care (Guyer and Gallagher, 1985). Beyond the acute event, injuries contribute greatly to the morbidity of long-term disability and chronic disease. Trauma is estimated to be responsible for 78 million disabled individuals worldwide, which is 15% of the world's disabled population (WHO, 1982). In the United States, one-quarter of permanent disability results from trauma, and highway trauma alone is considered responsible for 20,000 new cases of epilepsy annually (Waller, 1986).

One way to describe the prematurity of death is the calculation of *potential years of life lost* (PYLL). The age at which a death occurs is subtracted from a standard age (usually 65) and the difference is the number of premature or productive years of life that were lost because of the young death. For example, a traffic fatality at age 20 results in 45 years of PYLL, whereas a similar death at age 60 only results in 5 PYLL. While this approach is not intended to judge the value of a lost human life, this measure is used to describe the loss to the individual and to society of the potential contributions an individual may have made. Injuries account for an enormous amount of PYLL even in comparison to other leading causes of death (cardiovascular disease and cancer) that tend to occur in older age-groups. In the United States, the PYLL due to injury in 1985 was more than cancer and cardiovascular diseases combined (NCIPC, 1989).

When calculating the cost of injury, one must take into consideration initial rescue and transportation costs, medical care costs, rehabilitation costs, and the cost of long-term support and lost productivity for those disabled. These costs are far-reaching in addition to the cost of human suffering. The direct cost of all injuries occurring in the United States in 1985 was estimated at $45,000,000,000. Lifetime cost per death for injuries was significantly greater than cancer and cardiovascular lifetime costs combined in the United States (Kraus and Robertson, 1992). This largely reflects the early age of injury and long period of treatment, support, and rehabilitation. Even minor injuries are costly, as injuries are the leading cause of physician contact in some countries (Waller, 1986). The impact of injuries clearly reaches beyond injured individuals to families, employers, health care systems, and communities.

Vulnerable Groups

Children, the elderly, and disadvantaged groups have higher rates of injury than the overall population. Peak ages for fatal injuries are ages 1–4, 15–25, and over 70. Deaths in the 15–25 year range are mostly motor vehicle related. At all ages, males have higher injury death rates than females.

The rates of child injury mortality have been falling in many countries over the last few decades; since 1960 injury mortality in boys aged 5–14 years has fallen 60% in Australia, 53% in Canada, and 33% in the United States (Pless, 1994). However, these figures have not decreased at the same rate as deaths from other causes. In 1930, deaths from diseases were eight times as common as deaths from injuries in Canadian children aged 1–4 years. Disease and injury death rates reached equivalence by 1980, as disease death rates had shown dramatic reductions while injury death rates had decreased by only half (Baker et al., 1984). Currently, injury takes more lives of Canadian children than the next nine leading causes combined, including cancer, circulatory diseases, infectious diseases, congenital anomalies, and diseases of the nervous and respiratory systems (Guyer and Gallagher, 1985).

Elderly people are particularly vulnerable to injuries from falls. Elderly women who fall are particularly subject to fractures due to *osteoporosis* (thinning bones). Hip fractures cause more deaths and disability and are more costly than all other fractures due to osteoporosis. Hip fractures result in death in 10%–20% of victims, often not because of the intrinsic nature of the injury, but because of the resulting sequelae. Falls are the leading cause of injury mortality in the elderly, whereas falls are the leading cause of morbidity but not mortality at other ages. Most falls occur among the elderly. Additionally, suicide rates are highest among the elderly. Suicide will be discussed in Intentional Injury, below.

Disadvantaged groups have also been noted to have higher rates of injury, as noted in Chapter 1. Minority groups are noted to have higher injury mortality rates, which is thought to be related to income and living conditions. Poverty has also been associated with increased rates of injury. This may be due to greater exposure to environmental hazards, as poor, untrained, and undereducated people may perform the most dangerous jobs and live in poorly maintained housing in urban areas with high rates of violence (Kraus and Robertson, 1992). Alcohol use is also associated with increased injury rates, and alcohol use is also more prevalent in low-income populations.

Injury Settings

Historically, injuries that occur at work and injuries that occur in other settings have been considered separately, more for practical reasons than for conceptual reasons. Work environments often present a high level of exposure to mechanical hazards both in terms of the magnitude of risk (working with dangerous machinery) and the length of exposure (40 hr a week for 30 years). Legislation has been passed in many jurisdictions to control and regulate the workplace for the protection of workers, as discussed further in Chapter 10. In some jurisdictions, compensation systems exist to cover the financial burden of injury on the worker through payment generally charged back, at least partially, to the employer where the injury occurred. The cost of workers' compensation to employers has added further incentive to explore preventive options. The emphasis on injury prevention has also contributed to the training of physicians, nurses, ergonomists, and other professionals with expertise in the prevention and treatment of work-related injuries. The work and research of these professionals have greatly advanced the understanding of injuries in the workplace.

In contrast, injuries that occur elsewhere, such as in the home, on the road, and in various places of recreation, have not received an equal amount of attention. The situations in which injuries occur are diverse, and no one health professional or body has been charged with the overall responsibility of community injury prevention. Additionally, safety regulation of the general community, such as seat belt legislation, sometimes runs into opposition on the grounds of civil liberty infringement. As a result, community injury prevention is a relatively new field that began in the 1960s and has made rapid advances since the 1980s. Currently, there is a network of communities around the world, sponsored by the WHO, that is devoted to reducing trauma from all causes. The participating communities in this Safe Community Network have developed strategies for making activities of daily life safer in road traffic, at work, recreation, and school yard play, and in sports, travel, and household activities.

Conceptually, there is a great deal of overlap between workplace injuries and other injuries. Someone using a power tool at work or a power tool at home is exposed to the same biomechanical hazard. Even more striking is the family farm where the workplace and home are one and the same. Since this traditional distinction still exists, further discussion of specific types of injury will be organized around the setting in which injuries occur. The one departure from this is intentional injury, which can occur in any setting. Intentional injury includes assault and suicide (violence), as opposed to most other injuries, which are nonintentional. Some countermeasures have been effective in reducing both intentional and nonintentional injuries. For example, high fences on the roofs of tall buildings prevent nonintentional falls, suicides, and homicides.

Occupational Injuries and Ergonomics

Occupational injuries represent a serious cost to industry and to society, and they tend to affect people during their most productive years, when they have families to support. Injury at the workplace results in significant working time loss, disability, and fatalities. As mentioned earlier, the mechanism of injury does not differ from that of injuries sustained elsewhere, but the exposure may be great in some worksites. Forestry, construction, mining, and fishing are occupations with high rates of work-related trauma. Agricultural injuries are often very severe, occur in rural locations where medical care may not be easily accessible, and may affect family members, including children, who are working and living on the farm. Ironically, healthcare is another sector in which injury rates are high. Back injuries are the most common type of work-related injury. Musculoskeletal injuries account for the vast majority of time loss claims for workers' compensation. Injuries that result from *cumulative trauma*, known also as *repetitive strain injuries*, are particularly costly (Yassi, 1997; Yassi, 2000).

As industrialization develops in a country, new and serious work-related mechanical hazards emerge. The tragic experience of many injured workers has caused the most enlightened industries to develop and apply effective safety measures to protect workers against injury from moving parts of machinery, heavy falling objects, and slippery or uneven floors (including obstructions on the floor) (see NIOSH, 1995 and ILO, 1998). Nonetheless, millions of workers will lose their limbs and lives in future years because of lack of awareness of and interest in their safety at many worksites and because industrial/factory safety norms are not in place.

The elements of a work-related incident can be viewed using the *host–agent–environment triangle*, which includes the *person* susceptible to injury (the host), the *hazard* that is capable of inducing the injury (the agent), and an *environment* where both coincide in the workplace. Together these elements create a situation that is the context for the incident. A person may decide whether to take a risk on the spur of the moment and may not perceive the hazard, giving it faulty appraisal. This person may be distracted, not trained to recognize the hazard, or make a decision that in retrospect was not reasonable. There is a very critical period just before the incident when these factors come together into a particular incident-predisposing situation. Most of these situations will develop into a near-miss—an injury that could have happened but does not occur. But there is a certain probability that these elements will come together and the injury will occur.

In theory, at least, there are factors common to each type of injury that can be modified. Proper equipment must be purchased, with care given to the physical layout of the worksite to ensure appropriateness. Workers must be trained to recognize the hazard and to use safety equipment properly. Policies and procedures must be developed to empower workers to use proper techniques, with the consequences of not doing so also specified. The workplace culture must foster senior management commitment and full worker participation to ensure that the policies and procedures are feasible and will be enforced. *Ergonomics* is most commonly discussed within the context of the workplace environment, although it can be applied to the wider environment. The prevention of injuries is one major objective of the practice of ergonomics, as are good workplace design and increased efficiency. Ergonomics is devoted to designing a workplace that can be modified and adapted to the needs of individual workers. Whenever possible, it is preferable to change the environment rather than to find a worker with specific characteristics to do the job. Tasks requiring upper body strength to pull levers may be redesigned for women by using foot pedals, for example. Changes in the workplace environment will be more reliable, protect a greater number of workers, and be more conducive to a healthy and productive work environment than measures which rely on changing the behavior of workers or selecting certain workers for distinct tasks.

Information processing is made much easier and more accurate when presented to the senses in a way that facilitates rapid perception and cognitive interpretation. Instruments can be clustered and designed such that deviations from the expected are immediately obvious. The selection of type fonts, colors, coding schemes, visual cues, and labels is an inexpensive but highly effective way to increase efficiency and reduce errors in performing complex tasks. Likewise, readouts can be designed so that unusual or urgent information is easily and rapidly visible by color-coding or by visual displays, rather than being presented on a meter. Additionally, the application of ergonomic principles makes it possible, usually at low cost, to accommodate the needs of disabled or recuperating workers and to ensure their continued employability.

Traffic-Related Injuries

Motor vehicle–related crashes are by far the leading cause of serious injuries in most countries. Unfortunately, high rates of injuries are usually tolerated by society and accepted as an unavoidable cost of transportation. This is quite unnecessary as injuries can be prevented by improved design of roads, improved design and regular maintenance of cars and trucks, education of drivers, and enforcement of traffic rules.

The annual number of traffic deaths globally is estimated to be 500,000 and is increasing. Of these, 350,000 occur in developing countries (WHO, 1992a). While these developing countries have lower rates of vehicles per population, this is offset by a higher rate of fatality per vehicle and a high proportion of motorcycles, which are particularly hazardous compared to cars. The anticipated growth of motorcars in developing countries and newly independent states in the coming decades creates a real challenge for public health. If effective preventive measures against crashes and injuries are not taken, traffic injuries could become one of the most severe epidemics. As discussed previously, the cost of traffic injuries is staggering. In developing countries motor vehicle crashes are estimated to cost between 1% and 2% of gross national product (GNP) (WHO, 1992a).

The highest rates of traffic fatalities occur among young adults, and among males more than females. Traffic injury is also a leading cause of hospitalization in people under 45. It is estimated that globally 30 million people are disabled as a result of traffic injuries. This accounts for 5.8% of all disability and 38% of all disability from trauma (WHO, 1982). Alcohol use is involved in a high proportion of fatal crashes. Heavy drinkers are 4.4 to 5 times more likely to have a motor vehicle crash than the general population.

Traffic mortality and injury rates have declined in developed nations. This trend has paralleled safety initiatives such as improved roads, driver education, seat belt legislation, infant car restraints, and improved vehicle design. There is much work yet to be done to fully apply known technologies (e.g., optimum vehicle design, including airbags, and crash-friendly roadways) and to develop further technologies and strategies to combat this important public health problem.

Bicycle injuries are also very common worldwide. Although bicycle helmets are thought to prevent 85% of head injuries and 88% of brain injuries, the use of helmets is still low. Some Canadian provinces and other countries (e.g., Germany, Sweden, and New Zealand) have passed mandatory helmet laws, either for the whole population or for children.

Home- and Recreation-Related Injuries

Home- and recreation-related injuries cover a broad range of settings and types of injury. Home-related injuries affect primarily children and the elderly and can be very serious. Other than work, the home is the most common place for fatal injuries. Recreation- and sports-related injuries tend to affect primarily young people. Although these injuries tend to be less serious in general, they are often troublesome, costly to treat, and may occasionally be fatal. They are also a common cause of lost time from work.

Drownings, burns, poisoning, and falls are critical causes of pediatric morbidity and mortality. Young children can drown in only a few centimeters of water in a matter of seconds and should never be left unattended near water or in the bath. Backyard pools and natural open water are hazards for young children who may wander unattended into the water. Pools should have adequate fencing and locks to protect against this hazard. Young children may be the victims of fire as often they are not able to remove themselves from a burning building. Properly functioning smoke detectors are effective in alerting a family in time to remove children from a burning home. Innovative programs supplying smoke detectors to families of newborns at hospital discharge have been implemented in an attempt to make this countermeasure more widely adopted. Smoking is related to many deaths—either parents' cigarettes cause the fire or matches and lighters are within children's reach. Lighters are now required to be child resistant in some countries. Regulations prohibiting flammable sleepwear have also been adopted by some countries, thus decreasing burn injuries. Hot water scalding is a major cause of home burn injuries in young children and the elderly, who have more vulnerable skin and are often not able to remove themselves quickly enough from a situation of inadvertent exposure. Hot water tanks are often set at levels at which scalding can readily occur. It is thus recommended that hot water tanks be preset to prevent scalding, and families with young children be warned to be particularly vigilant in this regard. The practice of cooking over an open fire, common in many areas of developing nations but also a practice in many poorer communities of the developed world, can result in serious burns in young children.

Inadvertent poisoning is a major cause of childhood morbidity and mortality. Families with young children are advised to store medications and household chemicals out of children's reach and lock cupboards as needed (an active strategy). More effective measures have been passive ones, such as child-resistant pill bottles and limits on the dispensing of children's analgesics to nonlethal amounts.

Choking, suffocation, and strangulation can be lethal in the home or recreational environment. Foods associated with high risks of choking are peanuts, unsliced sausages or wieners, hard candy, and hard, crunchy food such as carrots. Toys with small parts and plastic bags have caused inadvertent suffocation. Waterbeds are also known to pose a suffocation hazard for young babies. Strangulation deaths have resulted when loose clothing, necklaces, drawstrings, or skipping ropes become entangled during play. Cribs are now regulated to avoid spaces between slats or the frame and the mattress that can permit strangulation.

Falls are a critical cause of pediatric injury. Serious and lethal falls from high-rise windows have prompted some communities in the United States to apply window locks to all excessively high apartment dwellings, with good results. Baby walkers were associated with particularly severe injuries when the walker inadvertently fell down the stairs. Such walkers have been removed from many markets.

Many countries provide playgrounds for children in school and community parks, and it has become increasingly recognized that the playground equipment provided can be associated with a significant injury burden—mostly upper arm fractures and head injuries. Many countries, including England, New Zealand, Australia, Canada, and the United States, have developed guidelines over the past decade to influence the safer design of playground equipment. Most injuries occur when children fall from excessive heights to hard ground. The combination of decreasing the height and providing impact-absorbing material beneath the equipment is an example of a passive environmental approach to an identified hazard.

Another area of concern involves the use of off-road vehicles, which are used mainly for recreation but also in farming. All-terrain vehicles (ATVs) are known to be particularly hazardous; injuries also occur with the use of dirt bikes, snowmobiles, dune buggies, and go-carts. Although these injuries mostly involve men in their mid-20s, children and teenagers are also injured. The design of ATVs renders them unstable and results in many rollover injuries.

Intentional Injury

Intentional injury is a particularly difficult problem. War, civil unrest, homicide, suicide, and assault all reflect deeply rooted social problems. Although they are usually beyond the scope of the environmental health professional's duties, the control of intentional violence is a fundamental problem combining human rights, social development, international cooperation, peacekeeping, and law enforcement.

Intentional injury can be directed toward oneself (suicide) or toward others (murder, assault and child abuse). Suicide represents a significant proportion of PYLL. Even though most suicides occur among people below the age of 40, the highest rates of suicide in individual demographic groups occur in the elderly, and particularly among elderly men. Suicide rates have remained stable for most age-groups but are rising among teenagers and young adults. Disadvantaged minorities also experience higher rates of suicide. In general, although females make more suicide attempts, males are more successful in their attempts and so have a higher suicide mortality rate. Firearms, hangings, and poisonings by gas (e.g., carbon monoxide) or medication overdose are the most common means used to accomplish suicide in most developed countries.

Assault is particularly prevalent in crowded urban areas where criminal activity is widespread. Youth gang violence in association with illicit drug activity is increasing in many countries and many young lives have been tragically lost. The availability of guns in a society is predictive of the lethality of crimes and of domestic violence. Unintentional shooting injuries also increase with the availability of firearms, and the victims are often children.

Child abuse is a particularly tragic form of violence. Often the social disruptions of unemployment, alcohol or drug abuse, or mental illness are taken out on the most vulnerable. Scalding, cigarette and other burns, drownings, blows, tight grips, and violent shaking are typical intentional injuries. Sexual abuse of children is becoming increasingly recognized and is known to be underreported. Often disclosure occurs much later in adult life once tremendous damage and suffering have occurred.

In some areas of the world experiencing war and conflict, violence is an all too familiar part of life. Recent tragedies in Rwanda, Bosnia, Sierra Leone, Liberia and Kosovo painfully illustrate the toll of conflict. Land mines continue to maim countless innocent people. Massive loss of life and injuries from terrorist attacks represent another much-feared aspect of political violence. Environmental health professionals need to appreciate the necessity of peace as a prerequisite to health (see Chapter 11, Health Consequences of War).

Concepts in Injury Prevention

To approach any of the injury problems mentioned above, it is necessary to understand a few key concepts in injury prevention. One such concept is the distinction between active and passive approaches to injury control. The distinction lies in the level of effort or action required on the part of individuals for the strategy to be effective. *Active strategies* are those requiring initiative (such as seat belt

TABLE 2.9
THE HADDON MATRIX APPLIED TO MOTOR VEHICLE–RELATED INJURIES

| Phases | Factors | | |
	Human	Vehicle	Environment
Preinjury	Prevent drunk driving	Ensure braking capacity	Ensure visibility of hazards
Injury	Use seat belt	Avoid sharp or pointed surfaces	Provide barriers that prevent head-on crashes
Postinjury	Prevent hemorrhage	Maximize rapidity of energy reduction	Facilitate emergency medical response

Source: Haddon, 1980.

use) whereas *passive strategies* lie at the opposite end of the continuum—little or no action is required (such as automobile airbags). The consensus within the injury prevention field is that passive strategies should be employed wherever available, and when active strategies are necessary, they are most effective when mandated. The need for a flexible combination of strategies has been recognized.

Another key tool in injury prevention is the *Haddon matrix*, which is based on the concept that injury events can be broken down into preinjury, injury, and postinjury phases. This phase concept is combined with the traditional causation concepts of host, agent, and environment, resulting in a way of breaking down an injury situation and thinking about possible points of intervention. This matrix approach has been embraced by injury prevention researchers and applied in various forms to numerous injury prevention situations. An example of how this can be used is shown in Table 2.9, where Haddon's matrix is applied to analysis of motor vehicle injuries. It is generally accepted that control programs that modify the vehicles, vectors, or environment are more effective than those that modify the host.

A further contribution to injury prevention analysis is Haddon's ten countermeasure strategies for reducing injuries. These are generic measures that can be applied to any type of injury prevention initiative, including the physical hazards discussed previously. These are listed in Table 2.10 in abbreviated form.

Safety measures should be integrated into a comprehensive package so that they are mutually reinforcing, backed by public policy, specific to local hazards,

TABLE 2.10
HADDON'S TEN COUNTERMEASURE STRATEGIES FOR REDUCING INJURIES

Injury Reduction Strategy

1. Prevent the creation of the hazard in the first place.
2. Reduce the amount of hazard brought into being.
3. Prevent the release of an existing hazard.
4. Modify the rate or spatial distribution of release of the hazard from its source.
5. Separate, in time or in space, the hazard and that which is to be protected.
6. Separate the hazard and that which is to be protected by interposition of a material barrier.
7. Modify the basic qualities of the hazard.
8. Make that which is to be protected more resistant to damage from the hazard.
9. Counter damage already done by the environmental hazard.
10. Stabilize, repair, and provide rehabilitative and cosmetic surgery.

Source: Haddon, 1980.

clear and explicit, and aimed toward realistic, obtainable objectives that everyone understands. Project coordinators should be able to evaluate progress.

PSYCHOSOCIAL HAZARDS

Psychosocial Hazards and Stressors

Uncertainty, anxiety, and a lack of a feeling of control over one's own life situation or environment lead to what is popularly called *stress*. The word stress is sometimes used to describe a stimulus: a specific event or situation that causes a mental or physiological reaction. To keep the terminology straight, it is best to speak of *stressors* rather than stress in this meaning. *Stress* can thus be defined as a human response to stressors. This definition of stress indicates the state of pressure that a person experiences. Another definition emphasizes the fact that stress is a process, resulting from the interaction between humans and the environment. The stress process consists of two stages: the first involves deciding whether an event (stressor) indeed poses a hazard; the second involves appraising the possibilities of dealing with the situation. As long as an individual can cope with the stressors, there is no problem. However, when coping strategies are no longer adequate, adverse stress reactions will occur.

For many people in both developed and developing countries, stress is a part of daily life, and it may lead to a variety of serious health effects, including depression, suicide, substance abuse, violence against others, psychosomatic diseases, and general malaise. Psychosocial hazards are those that create a social environment of uncertainty, anxiety, and lack of control. This may include the anxiety about mere survival from violence, as in the case of war-torn countries, or the uncertainty about future health effects of radiation exposure, for example, after the Chernobyl accident.

The occupational environment is another setting in which health can be damaged by a high mental burden. The well-known *Karasek model* is used to document how jobs with a low degree of decision-making authority (low control) and a high degree of physical or mental demands are particularly stressful. The increasing demands on workers and office staff as companies go through restructuring for increased efficiency (meaning fewer employees having to produce more) are a major psychosocial hazard. Women are generally exposed to additional stressors as they often must try to strike a balance between their roles as employee and homemaker. Five categories of potential sources of work-related psychosocial stress can be distinguished: factors intrinsic to the job, the role of the worker in the organization, career development, interpersonal relationships at work, and organizational structure and climate (Kalimo et al., 1987; Chapter 10 will also address this further). The major determinants of health at work are indeed those workplace organizational factors that determine psychosocial well-being of workers (Polanyi et al., 2000; Sullivan et al., 2000). In the private social environment, the death of a close friend or family member, divorce, or other family-related events can also be seen as psychosocial hazards.

The urban environment has its own characteristic psychosocial hazards. Poor or nonexistant urban planning, overcrowded residential areas, lack of sufficient recreational areas, disrupted social structures, and social isolation are some of the major examples (Chapter 7 will address these further). The exact impact of each individual hazard is difficult to establish, however, since a mixture of urban stressors and socioeconomic factors is usually involved. Finally, potential environmental health hazards of any kind (waste incinerators, emissions from chemical industry, or natural disasters) may induce psychological stress responses.

Health Effects of Stress

The modern perception of stress is that it is a negative or adverse reaction. The evolutionary perspective is different, in that stress is considered to be an important mechanism to prepare the human organism for urgent action, both physically and mentally. The physiological characteristics of the stress reaction include increases in heart rate, blood pressure, respiration, and blood transport to skeletal muscles and a simultaneous decrease in digestive activity. Increased production of stress hormones, such as epinephrine and cortisol, also play an important role in this reaction. All of these reactions prepare the individual for defensive actions—attack or flight. They thus improve the individual's chance of survival and can influence the success of a given species.

If an individual is continuously exposed to environmental stressors and has no adequate coping strategies, adverse health effects are a likely outcome. Cardiovascular diseases such as arterial hypertension and ischemic heart disease may be associated with stress. Other medical conditions such as peptic ulcer disease, bronchial asthma, and rheumatoid arthritis are influenced by psychological factors, although the prevalence of these diseases is less than that of cardiovascular diseases.

Since cardiovascular and other stress-related diseases take many years to become clinically significant, there is an opportunity to prevent these diseases at an early stage. This requires methodologies to quantify environmental or occupational stress. Since psychological factors are more difficult to measure than physical factors and may vary substantially among individuals, attempts have been made to identify physiological stress indicators. Useful screening measurements may include the ratio of epinephrine to norepinephrine in urine or blood, the ratio of potassium to sodium in urine, or levels of lipoproteins (cholesterol and triglyceride) in blood. As an example, it has been demonstrated that individuals living near the nuclear power station at Three Mile Island, where an accident was narrowly averted in 1979, had higher urinary levels of epinephrine and norepinephrine 1 year after the event than controls living further away. It should be realized, however, that all individuals may react differently to environmental stressors and that many other variables of personality, experience, and mood may influence the measured stress indicators. Results of these studies should therefore be interpreted with caution.

Study Questions

Give examples of reproductive effects caused by each of the following: a chemical, a physical agent, a biological agent, a mechanical hazard, and a psychosocial hazard. What type of evidence led you to the conclusion that each of the hazards you cited causes the effect in question.

3

RISK ASSESSMENT

LEARNING OBJECTIVES

After studying this chapter, you will be able to do the following:

- define the elements of risk assessment
- describe the types of information needed for each element of risk assessment
- describe how hazards can be identified in the field
- describe extrapolation methods used for the assessment of human dose–response relationships
- explain the difference between threshold and non-threshold effects, and to indicate the importance of this difference in risk assessment
- discriminate between different types of markers of exposure and provide several examples of useful markers of exposure
- describe how estimates of the magnitude of the potential risk are made, including the assessment of exposure
- describe the application of toxicology to the assessment of human health risks
- illustrate the difference between direct and indirect approaches of exposure assessment
- describe potential errors in environmental sampling

THE HEALTH RISK ASSESSMENT AND RISK MANAGEMENT FRAMEWORK

The ultimate goal of studying the relationship between environmental hazards and health is to take some action to reduce or eliminate those hazards or to reduce the harm that may result from their effects. This is called *risk management*. But before anything can be done, the risks themselves must be identified and thoroughly characterized. This process of analysing the possible effects on people of exposure to substances and other potential hazards, such as radiation, is known as a form of *risk assessment*. The steps typically taken in this process are shown in Figure 3.1. Because of different laws and approaches to regulation in different countries and different institutions, the terminology used in various reports on risk assessment varies, even in the same countries. The one used here is commonly found in WHO, ILO, and UNEP documents.

The first step in risk assessment is to identify hazards based on results from the relevant toxicological and epidemiological studies. This hazard identification step may also involve describing how a substance behaves in the body, including its interactions at the organ, cellular, and molecular levels. Such studies may also identify toxic effects that are likely to occur under experimental conditions. *Hazard identification* may be considered a qualitative description of potential health effects. Some of the research methods used to identify environmental hazards (e.g., toxicological tests) were introduced in Chapter 2. In the section Epidemiological Methods we will deal with epidemiological methods to identify hazards, and in the section Hazard Identification in the Field will discuss how hazards are identified in field studies.

In the next step of risk assessment, research data have to be used to describe and quantify the relationship between exposure or absorbed dose and its related health risk. This second step is known as a *dose–response assessment*. It is vital that the methods used to extrapolate data (e.g., from high to low exposure levels, from animal studies to humans, or from short-term to chronic exposure) are appropriate. The dose–response assessment should describe and justify the methods of extrapolation used. It should also describe the statistical and biological uncertainties of these methods. The dose-response relationship will be discussed further in the section Relationship Between Dose and Health Outcome.

The third step, called *exposure assessment*, is to measure the exposure itself, identifying the sources of exposure, estimating intake into the body by the various routes, and obtaining demographic information to define the exposed population. Field measurement data provided by monitoring and surveillance sys-

Research	Risk Assessment	
Laboratory and field observations (including epidemiological studies) of adverse health effects from exposure to particular agents. ⇨	**1. Hazard Identification** (Which are the health effects that this agent can cause?)	
Quantitative dose-response studies and extrapolation from high to low dose and from animals to humans. ⇨	**2. Dose-Response Assessment** (What is the relationship between dose and occurrence of health effects in humans?)	**4. Risk Characterization** (What is estimated occurrence of the adverse effect in a given population?)
Field measurements estimating exposures in defined populations. ⇨	**3. Exposure Assessment** (What exposures are currently experienced or anticipated under different conditions?)	**5. Risk Management** (Development, evaluation and implementation of regulatory options, aimed at risk reduction and control)

Figure 3.1 Steps in risk assessment.

tems are obtained, when possible, to assess the environmental quality. If no measurement data are available, emissions may be calculated or estimated at the source and exposure levels may be estimated on the basis of mathematical models showing how these emissions are carried by air, water, or in the ground. Integration of these data provides an estimation of the most likely exposure levels for individuals who may come into contact with the contaminants. This part of the risk assessment process is addressed in greater detail in the section Human Exposure Assessment.

Risk characterization is the integration of the first three steps in the risk assessment process. Ideally, it should produce a quantitative estimate of the risk in the exposed population, or estimates of the potential risk under different plausible exposure scenarios. Typically, a range of estimates is developed, using different assumptions and statistical methods that determine how sensitive the estimates are to basic assumptions in the model. If different health effects are likely to occur, the risk of each should be characterized. Other exposures or factors contributing to the health effects should also be characterized. This process will be described in the section Health Risk Characterization.

The literature on environmental health risk assessment can be confusing, as the same terms are used to refer to both generic risk assessments (often regulatory agency–based) and specific field risk assessments. Generic risk assessments characterize a hazard in general scientific terms on the basis of anticipated exposures and hypothetical population characteristics. However, when there is suspicion of a risk in a specific situation, it must be ascertained if people really are sufficiently exposed for health effects to occur.

Risk assessment has its limitations. In practice, crucial data are frequently lacking, and reasonable assumptions are made to arrive at a quantitative risk estimation. Most risk assessments contain one or more of the many sources of uncertainties that may accompany a risk assessment, listed in Table 3.1, and it is essential to evaluate their impact on the assessment. This process, usually referred to as *sensitivity analysis*, may be quite complex.

In many situations, only a qualitative risk assessment may be appropriate. In this approach, reasoned judgment is used, taking into account what information

TABLE 3.1

SOURCES OF UNCERTAINTY IN A RISK ASSESSMENT

Use of an experimental study involving an inappropriate route of exposure

Differences in biokinetics and/or mechanism of toxicity between species

Poor specification of exposure in experimental study, i.e., concentration, duration, route, chemical species

Extrapolation of high-dose to low-dose situations

Difference in age at first exposure or lifestyle factors between experimental data and a risk group

Exposure to multiple hazards in epidemiology studies

Potential confounding factors

Misclassification of the health outcome of concern

Adapted from Hallenbeck, 1993, with permission.

is known. When there is little likelihood that an exposure could be harmful, a qualitative risk assessment may be all that is necessary. If it is possible that a serious adverse effect may occur and that people may be affected, a quantitative risk assessment is usually preferred.

When the health risk of a specific environmental hazard or situation has been characterized, decisions must be made regarding which of the various control actions should be taken. Regulatory agencies may develop regulatory options, evaluate the (public health, economic, social, and political) consequences of the proposed options, and/or they may implement agency decisions. These actions and decisions form the core of the *risk management* process, discussed in Chapter 4.

EPIDEMIOLOGICAL METHODS

Data from epidemiological studies may be used directly to identify hazards and dose–response relationships. The types of studies used in epidemiology each have their own benefits and limitations.

Steps in Epidemiological Field Investigations

A framework of epidemiological concepts and techniques through which environmental health investigations may be carried out is presented in Figure 3.2. A methodical program of research to control a particular disease or health problem might follow the sequence described in Figure 3.2. Efforts to reduce mortality and ultimately prevent diarrhea in children have followed this framework. In the beginning, it is essential to define a case, identify the population at risk, and obtain a measure of the excess risk. The first phase involves *descriptive studies*, which are conducted to describe the current problem, e.g., how many children have diarrhea and to what extent it affects their health. These are followed by *analytical studies* to gain further information on possible causal factors, intervention studies (to evaluate possible treatments or prevention approaches), and development of surveillance. The aim of analytical studies is to determine if any environmental factors (or other risk factors) are indeed associated with the problem (or outcome of interest). Alternatively, enough data may exist to warrant implementing controls. The follow-up then would be to determine if control of the suspected environmental hazard would reduce morbidity or mortality. An ongoing sur-

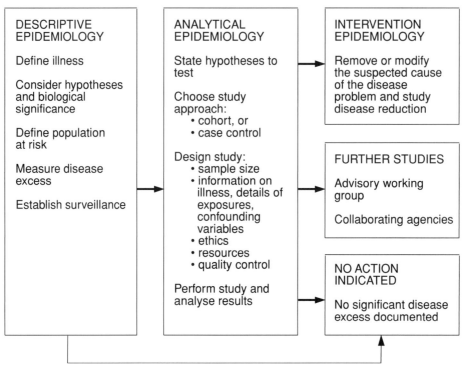

DESCRIPTIVE EPIDEMIOLOGY	ANALYTICAL EPIDEMIOLOGY	INTERVENTION EPIDEMIOLOGY
Define illness	State hypotheses to test	Remove or modify the suspected cause of the disease problem and study disease reduction
Consider hypotheses and biological significance	Choose study approach: • cohort, or • case control	
Define population at risk	Design study: • sample size • information on illness, details of exposures, confounding variables • ethics • resources • quality control	FURTHER STUDIES Advisory working group Collaborating agencies
Measure disease excess		
Establish surveillance	Perform study and analyse results	NO ACTION INDICATED No significant disease excess documented

Figure 3.2 Logical development of epidemiological field investigations. From WHO, 1991a, with permission.

veillance program may be required to monitor progress and identify changes in the pattern of the disease outcomes or causes.

Study Methods

Epidemiological study types differ considerably in their strengths and weaknesses. Table 3.2 summarizes the main features of the traditional types of epidemiological studies. Note that in each of these types of studies, the individual person is the unit of analysis. Ecological studies, in which the community or region is the unit of analysis, will be discussed later.

Descriptive studies may be longitudinal (often) or cross-sectional. Historical studies provide trends over time in an exposure or in the health effects of interest. Cross-sectional descriptive studies provide a snapshot of the exposure or the effects at a given time, or both. Researchers conducting descriptive studies do not try to draw associations between an environmental exposure and a health problem; instead, they simply try to describe the ways things have been or currently are. However, both historical and cross-sectional studies can compare an exposure or an environmental exposure prevalence to a health problem's prevalence in a study group and a control group, to establish whether a link may exist between a risk factor and an outcome. The study designs used most often in analytical epidemiology are cohort studies and case–control studies. These two study designs differ fundamentally from each other because they approach the questions of causation (or more precisely, association) from opposite ends of the cause-

TABLE 3.2

STUDY DESIGNS IN ENVIRONMENTAL EPIDEMIOLOGY THAT USE THE INDIVIDUAL AS THE UNIT OF ANALYSIS

Study Design	Population	Exposure	Health Effect	Confounders	Problems	Advantages
Descriptive study	Community or various subpopulations	Records of past measurements	Mortality and morbidity statistics; case registries; other reports	Difficult to sort out	Difficult to establish exposure–effect relationships	Cheap, useful to formulate hypotheses
Cross-sectional study	Communities or special groups; exposed vs. nonexposed	Current	Current	Usually easy to measure	Current exposure may be irrelevant to current disease	Can be done quickly; can use large populations; can estimate prevalence
Prospective cohort study	Community or special groups; exposed vs. nonexposed	Defined at outset of study (can change during study)	To be determined during study	Usually easy to measure	Expensive, time consuming; exposure categories can change; high dropout rate possible	Can estimate incidence and relative risk; can study many diseases in one study; can describe associations that suggest cause–effect relationships
Historical cohort study	Special groups, e.g., workers, patients, insured persons	Records of past measurement	Records of past or current diagnosis	Often difficult to measure because of retrospective; nature; depends on quality of previously obtained data	Need to rely on records that may not be accurate	Less expensive and quicker than prospective study; can be used to study exposures that no longer exist
Case–control study	Usually small groups; diseases (cases) vs. non-diseases (controls)	Occurred in past, determined by records or interview	Known at start of study	Possible to eliminate by matching for them	Difficult to generalize due to small study groups; some incorporate biases	Relatively cheap and quick; useful for studying rare diseases
Experimental (intervention study)	Community or special groups	Controlled/known already	To be measured during study	Can be controlled by randomization of subjects	Expensive; ethical considerations; study subjects' compliance required	Well-accepted results; strong evidence for causality or efficacy of intervention

Source: WHO, 1991a.

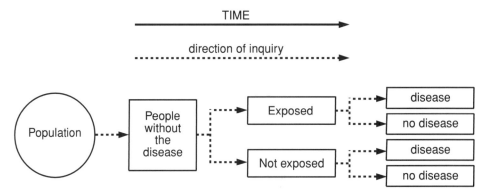

Figure 3.3 Design of a cohort study. From Beaglehole et al., 1993, with permission.

and-effect spectrum. *Cohort studies* start with a population that has been exposed to the risk factor, then the frequencies of disease in the exposed and unexposed populations are compared as they occur over time (see Fig. 3.3). *Case–control studies* start with people who have the disease, then frequencies of exposure that occurred in the past in the population with the disease and the population without the disease are compared (see Fig. 3.4). Researchers using analytical epidemiology must look out for bias in the information, or *confounders*, factors that are not causal but may be associated with the exposure and the disease for other reasons.

Case–control studies can provide powerful and accurate estimates of risk ratios and are usually economical in terms of both cost and study duration. An example of the use of a case–control study in testing the association between an acute epidemic disease and a particular exposure is the toxic food oil syndrome investigation that took place in Spain (see Box 3.1). Case–control studies can also be used in examining chronic, long-latency, hyperendemic problems and are especially useful in studying rare diseases, as noted in Table 3.2.

Cohort studies have the advantage of being able to directly measure the risk of a disease and calculate the actual population illness rate, the occurrence of ill-

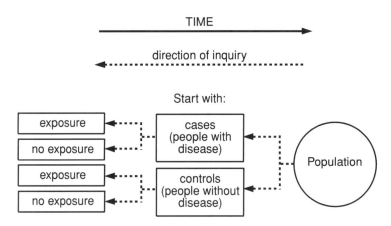

Figure 3.4 Design of a case–control study. From Beaglehole et al., 1993, with permission.

BOX 3.1

Toxic Oil Syndrome in Spain

In May 1981, a previously unknown disease appeared in Madrid, Spain. It subsequently spread rapidly to the provinces northwest of the city. Symptoms of the disease included respiratory distress, fever, rashes, nausea, and vomiting. Over 20,000 people were affected, and over 340 deaths occurred.

Many potential causes of the syndrome were investigated. Initial descriptive studies implicated a black market cooking oil as a possible cause for the syndrome. In a subsequent case–control study, food ingestion histories of 124 people with the syndrome (the cases) were compared with 124 people without the syndrome (the controls). Both groups were from similar socioeconomic backgrounds. One hundred percent of people with the syndrome had reported consumption of the illegally marketed cooking oil, but only 6.4% of the control group (those who were not sick) had consumed the clandestine oil (as it was called in Spain).

Cases (with syndrome)	$\longrightarrow$	100% had consumed the oil
	$\longrightarrow$	0% had not consumed the oil
Controls (without syndrome)	$\longrightarrow$	6.4% had consumed the oil
	$\longrightarrow$	93.6% had not consumed the oil

In a similar fashion, within case families, the estimated amount of oil consumed per person correlated with the severity of the symptoms of the disease. The syndrome became known as *toxic oil syndrome* (TOS) and was probably caused by imidazoline-thiol components, derivatives of isothiocyanate.

This is an example of a case–control study, as investigators started with individuals with and without the disease, and looked for an association to exposure before the symptoms started, in this case, ingestion of the cooking oil. Case–control studies can be used in this manner to investigate the cause of an unknown disease epidemic. If there is a statistically higher level of exposure in the cases than in the controls, then the exposure *may be* the causative agent. (In this situation, with 100% of cases having consumed the oil, and 0% of cases not having consumed it, the odds ratio, as discussed in the section Quantifying Risks, would be infinity.)

Within 2 months of the date when the initial case was recorded, the number of persons contracting the syndrome had reached its peak and the incidence declined. This decline corresponded with public education about the oil and the replacement of the oil with uncontaminated cooking oil.

Source: WHO, 1990c.

ness in a defined population over a period of time is measured. However, cohort studies can be costly, especially if the disease under study is rare. Large population groups may be needed to achieve statistically meaningful results. Cohort studies allow for the assessment of many competing risk factors, thereby providing a distinct advantage over case–control studies. Cohort studies are often used to study occupational diseases, an example of which is provided in Box 3.2.

A *prospective cohort study* is one that starts with a group currently exposed to a potential hazard or risk factor and an unexposed group. The groups are then

BOX 3.2

Vinyl Chloride and Cancer: An Example of the Historical Cohort Study

The vinyl chloride monomer (VCM) is a gas produced largely through chlorination of ethylene, a product of the petroleum industry. When polymerized, it forms polyvinyl chloride (PVC), one of the major polymer plastics widely used today. It has been produced commercially since the 1930s and its production has steadily increased. It is widely used in floor tiles, seat covers, toys, water pipes, and other common products. Once considered a relatively inert gas, VCM was widely used for a time as a propellant in spray cans.

In 1967, the U.S. National Institute for Occupational Safety and Health (NIOSH) was notified that 4 cases of a rare liver cancer, angiosarcoma of the liver (ASL), had occurred in a workforce of only 500 workers. Shortly thereafter, further observations were reported, including an Italian study on rats, that supported the association between VCM and the development of ASL. The NIOSH decided to conduct a historical cohort mortality study of workers at PVC polymerization plants to compare observed cause-specific mortality rates among these workers with that expected in the U.S. population. Four plants were selected for the study based on length of operation, accessibility of records, and probable ease of follow-up. The total person-years at risk for disease were calculated. Follow-up was virtually complete (1287 out of 1294 workers) with 10-year latency. Thirty-five cases of cancer had occurred. Expected numbers of deaths were calculated according to the ages of the people at risk. From the expected number of deaths in this workforce by age category and the standardized mortality ratio (SMR) (for the workers with 10-year latency), it can be seen that the cancer mortality is significantly increased. As the numbers are small, only the excess in liver tumors is statistically significant. Excess numbers for leukemia and lung and brain cancer should be noted as deserving further study.

Cause of death	Observed	Expected	SMR	95% confidence intervals
Cardiovascular	57	54.7	104	79–135
Cancer	35	23.5	149*	104–207
Pulmonary	12	7.7	156	80–272
Liver/biliary	7	0.6	1167**	467–2404
Leukemia/lymphoma	4	2.5	160	51–386
Brain	3	0.9	333	85–907
Other	9	11.8	76	35–145
Cirrhosis of liver	2	4.0	50	8–165
Pulmonary disease (excluding cancer)	6	3.4	176	64–384
Violent deaths	13	14.2	92	49–157
All other causes	22	26.5	85	52–126
Unknown cause	1			
TOTAL	136	126.3	108	90–127

*$p = 0.05$; **$p = 0.01$.
Source: Falk and Heath, 1986.

compared to see who gets the disease and who does not over time. A *historical cohort study* starts with information about who had been exposed to a potential hazard and then determines their disease rates since the time of that exposure. Both types of cohort studies start by defining an exposed population with the goal of determining disease rates that follow.

Variants of cohort studies and case–control studies are *proportional morbidity studies* and *nested case–control studies*. In the former, all deaths are classified according to cause. The proportion of the study group dying of the cause of interest (e.g., cancer) is compared to the proportion of an age-matched (standardized) general population dying of this cause. This approach works well for uncommon diseases but is subject to distortions then applied to common conditions such as heart diseases. A nested case–control is the second phase of a cohort study. Here, the causes of the disease in the exposed group are further investigated by comparison to controls.

Quantifying Risks

There are a few standard equations used in epidemiology to determine if the study population is at an increased risk or has an increased number of cases of the disease in question compared to a standard population. The rate of disease, the most fundamental measure (Fig. 3.5), can be measured in terms of incidence (new cases) or prevalence (existing cases). To determine if the observed rate is excessive, a risk ratio, or relative risk should be calculated. These are usually calculated from cohort studies.

A risk ratio of 1.0 means that the rate of the problem (or outcome of interest) in the group being studied is not different from the rate of the occurrence in the general population. A risk ratio of >2 or 3 is usually considered evidence of an important risk. For example, a risk ratio of 5 would mean that the population with the risk factor (e.g., those who are exposed to asbestos) are five times

RATE OF DISEASE: $\dfrac{\text{Number of cases of disease in population at risk}}{\text{Number of persons in population at risk}}$

Expressed as: $\dfrac{\text{Number of Cases}}{\text{100 or 1000, 100,000 (usually) etc. persons at risk}}$

Example: $\dfrac{\text{50 Cases}}{\text{2500 persons at risk}} = \dfrac{20}{1000}$

RISK RATIO: $\dfrac{\text{Rate of disease in population with the risk factor}}{\text{Rate of disease in population without the risk factor}}$
(comparison population)

Expressed as: A numerical ratio (1.5, 3.0 etc. indicating that risk of disease in the exposed (or at risk) population is 1.5, 3.0, etc. times greater than that in the unexposed (or not at risk) population

Example: $\dfrac{20 / 1000}{10 / 1000} = 2.0$

Figure 3.5 Definition and calculation of rates of disease and risk ratios.

more likely to have or get the disease (e.g., lung cancer) than the population without the risk factor (e.g., those who were not exposed to asbestos).

A *risk ratio*, the most widely used form of risk measure, is defined as "the ratio of the risk of disease or death among the exposed to the risk among the unexposed" (Last, 1995). Data from case–control studies approximate the relative risk by a calculation known as an *odds ratio*. Other measures of risk, which can be derived from epidemiological studies, are defined in Box 3.3. The *risk difference* is "the absolute difference between two risks" (Last, 1995). It demonstrates the excess risk of the health problem in the exposed population, by subtracting the risk of the unexposed population from the risk of the exposed population. This is also known as the *incremental risk*. The *attributable fraction (exposed)* describes the proportion of new cases of a disease in the exposed population that are due to the exposure—i.e., "the proportion by which the incidence rate of the outcome among the exposed would be reduced if the exposure were eliminated" (Last, 1995). The *attributable fraction (population)* describes the proportion of new cases of a disease in the whole population that are due to the exposure—i.e., "the proportion by which the incidence rate of the outcome among the entire population would be reduced if the exposure were eliminated" (Last, 1995).

A commonly used method of evaluating mortality in a group of people is to calculate the *standardized mortality ratio* (SMR) for the group, which is the ratio of the observed deaths in a group divided by the number of deaths that would normally be expected in a group with a similar age distribution. The SMR is expressed as follows:

$$SMR = \frac{\text{Observed number of deaths (or events) in the study population} \times 100\%}{\substack{\text{Expected number of deaths (or events) if the study population had the} \\ \text{same age and gender specific death rates as the comparison} \\ \text{(e.g., national) population}}}$$

The denominator of the SMR (e.g., the expected number of deaths) is computed as follows:

1. A calculation is made of the person-years at risk in the cohort for each age/gender group (the sum of the number of years that each individual in the cohort has been followed).
2. The figure obtained is multiplied by the expected age/gender specific mortality rate for the disease(s) being considered based on national health statistics.
3. The expected number of cases is the sum of cases in the age/gender groups.

An SMR of 130 for a particular cause of death indicates that there was a 30% greater mortality of that disease found than was actually expected.

Since these measurements of risk are statistical, we cannot be sure that the observations in a study did not occur by chance. The statistical variation of these measures is usually expressed as the *confidence interval*. The 95% confidence interval is the range within which the true value lies, with 95% probability. The

BOX 3.3

Common Measures of Risk Derivable from Epidemiological Studies

$$\text{Risk difference} = E - U$$

$$\text{Risk ratio} = \frac{E}{U}$$

$$\text{Attributable fraction (exposed)} = \frac{(E - U)}{E} = \text{(through mathematics)} \ \frac{(RR - 1)}{RR}$$

$$\text{Attributable fraction (population)} = \frac{I - U}{I} = \frac{[p \, (RR - 1)]}{[p \, (RR - 1) + 1]}$$

where U = incidence (or mortality) in the unexposed group; E = incidence (or mortality) in the exposed group; p = prevalence of exposure at a designated time prevalence in the total population; I = incidence in the total population; and RR = risk ratio.

When the size of the total population at risk is not known, e.g., in case–control studies, the RR can be estimated by calculating the odds ratio (OR). Consider the following notation for the distribution of a binary exposure and a disease in a population divided into four groups: individuals with disease and exposed (A), with disease and unexposed (C), without disease and exposed (B), and without disease and unexposed (D). The OR would be calculated as follows:

	Disease	
Exposed	Yes	No
Yes	A	B
No	C	D

Thus

$$OR = \frac{A/C}{B/C}$$

true effect is most likely to be the mean or central tendency of the confidence interval but it may be larger or smaller; 95% of the time, however, it will fall within the range calculated as the confidence interval. There is also a 5% chance that the true value lies outside the confidence interval; that is, it is higher or lower than either extreme value of the confidence interval. The width of the confidence interval depends on the number of cases observed, the size of the population in the study, and the variability of the comparison or expected rates. These issues are discussed at greater length in *Basic Epidemiology* (Beaglehole et al., 1993) and other standard epidemiology texts.

Study Difficulties and the Determinants of Causation

In determining the degree of weight that should be placed on the evidence obtained from an epidemiological study, it is necessary to distinguish between the concepts of *association* and *causation*. Association means that the risk factor occurs often (more than expected) where the disease appears. Causation means that the risk factor plays a role in the events leading to the disease. A causal relationship implies that the disease has been shown to be actually induced by the environmental agent. There are numerous reports in the scientific literature alleging links between environmental agents and disease outcome that have turned out to be spurious. Therefore, guidelines are needed to assess the likelihood that the association is a cause-and-effect relationship (The most widely accepted were originally conceived by British statistician Sir Austin Bradford Hill, and are shown in Table 3.3). These guidelines are not absolute but are useful in achieving consensus about whether a known risk factor is likely a true cause of the disease in question. It takes several studies to prove causal relationships. Because epidemiological studies cannot be controlled in the same way as laboratory experiments, they are always subject to greater uncertainty and require useful interpretation.

A major limitation of most studies is the statistical possibility that a real association will be detectable in the study. The study has to be large enough to allow for a sufficient statistical power. For example, to detect a twofold increase in major congenital malformations (with 95% certainty that an increase found was not a chance finding, i.e., $a = 0.05$, and with an 80% chance of finding a true increase if it is indeed present, i.e., $b = 0.20$), more than 300 live births would have to be studied, as shown in Table 3.4. Guidelines for the calculation of statistical power have been published by the WHO (Lemeshov et al., 1990).

Cluster Investigations and Ecological Studies

In their daily practice, health services staff are regularly confronted with clusters of disease that raise concerns about possible relationships to environmental factors. A *cluster* of disease is the occurrence of an unexpectedly high number of cases in a given geographical area, period of time, and/or population. An example of a geographic cluster is the relatively high occurrence of childhood leukemia in a

---

TABLE 3.3

TESTS OF CAUSATION

Temporal relation: Does the cause precede the effect? (essential)
Plausibility: Is the association consistent with other knowledge?
Mechanism of action: Is there evidence from experimental animals?
Consistency: Have similar results been shown in other studies?
Strength: What is the strength of the association between the cause and the effect? (relative risk)
Dose–response relationship: Is increased exposure to the possible cause associated with increased effect?
Reversibility: Does the removal of a possible cause lead to reduction of disease risk?
Study design: Is the evidence based on a strong study design?
Judging the evidence: How many lines of evidence lead to the conclusion?

Source: Beaglehole et al., 1993 (these are modified criteria of causation from those originally developed by Bradford Hill).

TABLE 3.4

SAMPLE SIZE REQUIRED TO DETECT A DOUBLING OF BACKGROUND
INCIDENCE IN REPRODUCTIVE OUTCOME

Reproductive Outcome	Size of Each Group Required[a]
Infertility	161 couples
Spontaneous abortion	161 pregnancies
Stillbirth	161 pregnancies
Low birth weight	293 live births
Major birth defects	316 live births
Infant deaths	928 live births
Severe mental retardation	4493 live births
Chromosome abnormalities	8951 live births

[a]With alpha = 0.05; beta = 0.20.
Source: NIOSH, 1988.

rural community using well water contaminated with pesticides. The increased occurrence of respiratory problems during a summer smog period can be seen as a cluster in time. An increased occurrence of lung disease in workers at a particular workshop is a cluster in the population.

Clusters thought to relate to environmental factors sometimes receive a lot of publicity. However, many clusters are actually not real, because the presumed diagnoses are incorrect or misunderstood. Others are just chance events. For other clusters, there may be explanations other than a common environmental exposure because the exposure cannot account for the cluster.

A basic approach has been developed to investigate reported clusters as efficiently as possible. The objective is to verify expediently (*1*) if a cluster truly exists or if it is a coincidence or merely false; (*2*) if human exposure to a possible environmental hazard actually exists; and (*3*) if the relationship between these two merits further investigation and/or action. Even if the answer to the first two questions is yes, it still remains to be determined whether there is a causal relationship between the increased number of diseased individuals and the relatively high exposure levels. Each question needs to be pursued independently, because each requires further action if positive, even if the other is negative.

An *ecological study* is one in which the unit of analysis is the population group or region, rather than the individual. Typically, regions involve persons living in a geographic area such as a census tract, country, or province. For each group or region the average exposure level to the agent in question and the rate of disease in question are determined independently. It is not known whether the individuals who have been exposed are the same individuals who developed the disease. Because the exposure levels of individuals are not linked to the disease occurrence in the same individuals, ecological designs are incomplete as evidence for causal association, although they may be very useful for generating new hypotheses or proposed associations that can be tested in other studies. Ecological studies are also an inexpensive option for linking available health data sets or record systems to environmental data. Other important variables are often available in these studies, such as sociodemographic and other census variables. Figure 3.6 illustrates the findings of an ecological study of the relationship between

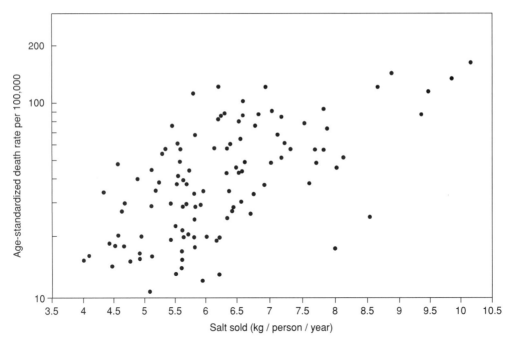

Figure 3.6 Study of the relationship between salt sold in Chinese counties and esophageal cancer mortality rates. From Beaglehole et al., 1993, with permission.

salt sold in a county (local government area) and esophageal cancer mortality rates. Ecological studies can be classified into five basic design types that differ according to the method of study selection and methods of analysis: exploratory studies, space–time cluster studies, multiple groups studies, time trend studies, and mixed studies.

HAZARD IDENTIFICATION IN THE FIELD

From toxicological and epidemiological data, potential health effects of hazardous substances can be estimated. Recognizing hazards in a specific industrial pollution situation, however, requires a different approach. This is commonly done by conducting *health hazard evaluations* and *hazard audits*, both of which involve walking through the plant (or community facility) and investigating all operations. The difference between the two is that in a health hazard evaluation the walk-through is intended to identify the cause of a particular problem but in a hazard audit all potential hazards are systematically examined.

Occupational Environment

In the workplace it can be relatively easy to make an inventory of all potential hazards. This is made easier by an accurate registration or tracking system of all chemicals that are frequently used or stored, which unfortunately is not always available. To make an inventory of chemical hazards, product identity is, of course, crucial. From knowledge of which product is used, one may then learn what is in it and what constituents are hazardous. Identifying the chemicals in a product may be difficult if the manufacturer is not required by law to list ingredients or if the material is not labeled properly (see Chapter 2, Information on Toxicity), or if the composition of the product is protected as a trade secret.

General Environment

When a point source of pollution is suspected, such as a specific industrial plant, the hazards may be established on the basis of the type of materials used and the industrial processes involved. The identity of chemical hazards is usually difficult to determine in uncontrolled environments, such as illegal dumping sites or abandoned industrial locations. For example, the chemical hazards at a suspected soil contamination may be from almost anything. One approach is to check whether there is information within the community regarding former industrial or other activities at the suspected location. Depending on the results of such an inquiry, further research can be streamlined in a specific direction. However, if no records exist or no industrial activities can be described by former workers, the situation becomes far more difficult. In such a situation, chemical analysis of samples will have to be conducted to determine the nature of the contamination. Since it is too costly to screen for all possible contaminants, chemical analysis has to be concentrated on specific marker components. For instance, analysis of benzopyrene may be used as a marker for contamination with polycyclic aromatic hydrocarbons, dieldrin for pesticides, and toluene for volatile organic compounds. All such screening methods have their limitations.

RELATIONSHIP BETWEEN DOSE AND HEALTH OUTCOME

Dose–Effect and Dose–Response Relationships

The terms dose-response and dose-effect are occasionally used interchangeably. Strictly speaking, however, a *dose–response* relationship is one between the dose and the proportion of individuals in an exposed group that demonstrate a defined effect (Fig. 3.7). A *dose–effect* relationship describes that between the dose and the severity of a health effect in an individual (or a typical person in the

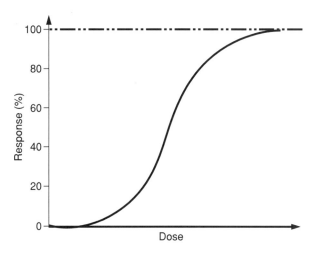

Figure 3.7 Dose–response relationship. From Beaglehole et al., 1993, with permission.

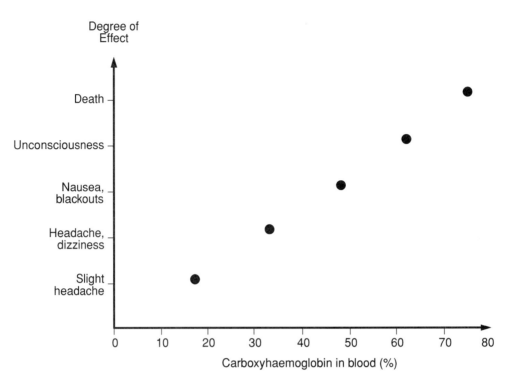

Figure 3.8 Dose–effect relationship. From Beaglehole et al., 1993, with permission.

population) (Fig. 3.8). A hierarchy of effects on health can be identified for most hazards, ranging from acute illness and death to chronic and lingering illnesses, from minor and temporary ailments to temporary behavioral or physiological changes, as shown in Table 3.5. Dose–response relationships are considerably different for non-carcinogens (thought to have a threshold) and carcinogens (thought to be non-threshold) as discussed further below.

Calculating Risks for Threshold Effects

Many environmental hazards have a specific effect on individuals only when the dose reaches a certain level, i.e., a *threshold* for that effect. Figure 3.9 illustrates the dose–response relationship for various health effects of lead concentrations in blood in children. Sometimes the number of years of exposure has to be used as an indicator of dose, when duration and levels of exposure are not known. When concentration and dose are known, a dose index can be calculated. This was done for workers in a Swedish battery factory (Kjellström, 1986b). Figure 3.10 illustrates how increased years of exposure to cadmium and average exposure level (mg/m^3) relate to high levels of β_2-microglobulin in the urine (>290 μg/liter), a measure of kidney dysfunction.

Dose–response relationships can also be obtained for physical hazards. Figure 3.11 illustrates the relationship between sound levels at work and the percentage of those with impaired hearing according to the age of the workforce. This figure shows that the dose–response relationship is different in the different age-groups.

TABLE 3.5

RANGE OF EFFECTS ON HUMAN HEALTH DUE TO ENVIRONMENTAL EXPOSURE

Premature death of many individuals
Premature death of any individual
Severe illness or major disability
Chronic debilitating disease
Minor disability
Temporary minor illness
Discomfort
Behavioral changes
Temporary emotional effects
Minor physiological changes

Dose–response relationships also apply to injuries. As shown in Figure 3.12, speed is used as an indicator of dose. With an increase in speed there is an increased risk of nonfatal injury in car drivers in a collision. This figure also shows that using seatbelts reduces the risk of injury by about 50%.

The concept of the dose–response relationship extends to psychological distress as well. As shown in Figure 3.13, the greater the noise level, the greater the percentage of people annoyed by it. At a given noise level, a higher level of annoyance was found in a U.S. Environmental Protection Agency (EPA) study, than that found by another investigator.

Thresholds and Other Important Benchmarks

A *no observed adverse effect level* (NOAEL) is the point on a dose–effect curve at which a threshold is reached. Before this level, there are either no symptoms or our technology is not sufficient to detect a problem (depending on the situation). These levels are often determined in animal studies. Similarly, a *lowest observed adverse effect level* (LOAEL), is the lowest level at which some symptoms are found

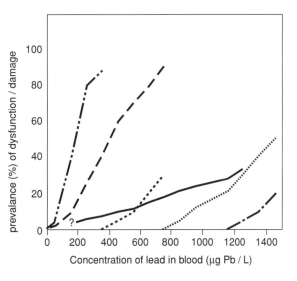

Figure 3.9 Dose–response curve for various health effects of lead in children. — - - decreased α-ALA D activity; – – increased ZPP; ······ anemia; ——— effect on the CNS; - - - - - decreased nerve conduction velocity; — - — palsy, colic pain, encephalopathy. From Elinder et al., 1994, with permission.

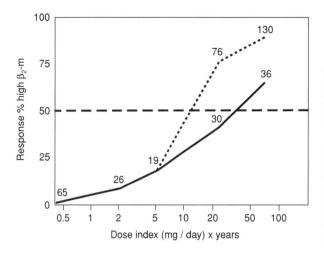

Figure 3.10 Dose–response relationship for cadmium exposure and prevalence of high urinary levels of β_2-microglobulin (β_2-m >290 μg/liter) The dotted line indicates a maximum possible response if all retired and deceased workers with dose index above 12.5 had a high β_2-microglobulin. From Kjellström, 1986b, with permission.

(see Fig. 3.14). A *no observed effect level* (NOEL) is the level at which no effect, either good or bad, is detected.

Because all individuals are constantly exposed to certain levels of environmental chemicals, the question to address is what levels of exposure to these chemicals are likely to affect human health. This analysis is usually done by official agencies (e.g., the Environmental Protection Agency in the United States), by applying animal and epidemiological studies. From these studies, an *acceptable daily intake* (ADI), or *tolerable daily intake* (TDI) (depending on the jurisdiction), is calculated. These values indicate the maximal daily intake of a chemical that

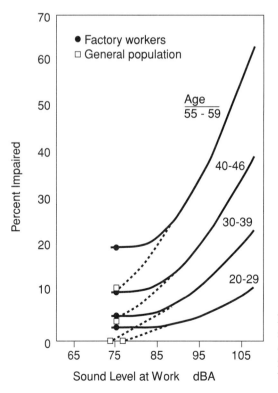

Figure 3.11 Dose–response relationship between occupational sound levels and prevalence of impaired hearing for different age groups. From WHO, 1980a, with permission.

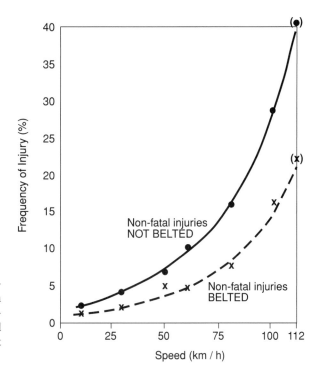

Figure 3.12 Dose–response relationship between speed of a car in a collision and risk of driver injury for seat belt use and non-use. From Beaglehole et al., 1993, with permission.

is not expected to result in adverse health effects after a lifelong exposure. The ADI is usually the NOAEL (or LOAEL) divided by uncertainty factors (UF) (which are discussed below):

$$\text{ADI} = \frac{\text{NOAEL (or LOAEL)}}{\text{UF}}$$

The ADIs can then be used as reference values in establishing guidelines to protect individuals. Note that time and dosimetry factors (such as body weight, surface area, and absorption rate) must be specified for an ADI. For example, an ADI is often prepared for a person of 70 kg who is exposed to a chemical for 3 hr/day. The ADIs and TDIs are often revised over time, as new information is discovered through further studies. Examples of TDIs are given in Table 3.6.

Uncertainty Factors in Establishing Thresholds

Generally it is not possible to specify an exact threshold for any substance, for a variety of reasons: the vulnerability of individuals varies; there is considerable physiological diversity in human populations; measuring techniques have their limitations; study methods are often limited; at very low exposures, the effects may not be easily detectable; and data relating to the upper end of the curve may also be difficult to obtain because massive exposures are relatively rare. Nonetheless, the principal use of dose–response curves is to predict the consequences of very high and very low exposures.

The extrapolation of animal data to humans has a number of fundamental problems. First, the effect on the animal studied may simply not apply to hu-

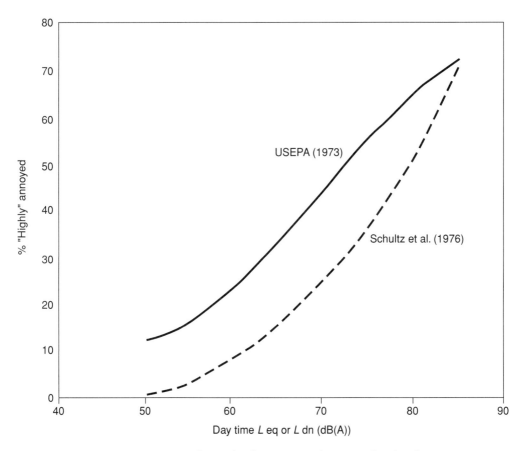

Figure 3.13 Dose–response relationship between outdoor noise level and annoyance. From WHO, 1980a, with permission.

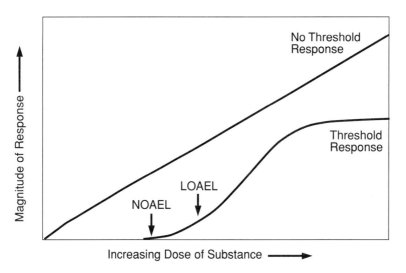

Figure 3.14 No observed adverse effect level (NOAEL): the level of exposure to a chemical at which no adverse effects were observed during studies with animals. Lowest observed adverse effect level (LOAEL): the lowest level of exposure to a chemical at which adverse effects were observed during studies with animals. From HC, 1993, with permission.

TABLE 3.6

TOLERABLE DAILY INTAKES OF ENVIRONMENTAL CHEMICALS

Non-Carcinogen	Tolerable Daily Intake
Copper	0.05–0.5 mg/kg/day
Endrin	1.0 μg/kg/day
Lead in adults	7.14 μg/kg/day
Lead in infants	3.57 μg/kg/day
Mirex	0.028 μg/kg/day
Methyl Hg	0.47 μg/kg/day
Total Hg (methyl Hg+ inorganic Hg)	0.71 μg/kg/day
Tin	2 mg/kg/day

Source: HC, 1993.

mans because of physiological differences between the species (as discussed in Chapter 2). Second, projections from a higher-dose response range to a lower-dose range involve various assumptions that may not prove to be accurate. Third, animal studies are often conducted using routes of administration that do not correspond to the routes of human exposure.

The *safety* (or *uncertainty*) *factor* (UF) reflects the degree of uncertainty that must be incorporated into the extrapolation from experimental data to the human population. When the quality and quantity of dose–response data are high, the safety factor is low. When the data are inadequate or equivocal, the safety factor must be higher. (Safety factors are not relevant to carcinogens, however, as discussed below.) The National Academy of Sciences (NAS) Safe Drinking Water Committee and the EPA in the United States have developed the safety factor guidelines shown in Table 3.7. An example of an application of a safety factor to calculate an ADI is provided in Box 3.4, although in this example the calculation is extended to give information about the accepted dose from water intake, not just intake from all sources combined.

Figure 3.15 is a generalized dose–response curve showing how risks at the lower levels of exposure may be estimated by extrapolating from middle-range observations. The solid line to point A is the dose–response curve, determined

TABLE 3.7

SAFETY OR UNCERTAINTY FACTORS

Factor	Comments
10× factor	Applied to data from valid experimental studies on prolonged human intake. This protects the sensitive members of the population.
100× factor	Applied when experimental results from studies of human intake are not available, or are inadequate but there are valid results from low-dose intake studies on one or more species of experimental animals. This accounts for species-to-species extrapolation.
1000× factor	Applied when there are no low-dose or acute human data and only scanty results on experimental animals. This is applied to account for species to species extrapolation, from high dose to low dose, and from short-term to long-term effects, as well as protecting sensitive members of the population.

BOX 3.4

Calculation of Acceptable Daily Intake

Animal studies of various doses of para-dichlorobenzene have shown hepatic and nephrotoxicity as well as pulmonary damage and other effects. A 1-year gavage (direct exposure into the stomach) study in rabbits using groups of five animals dosed between 0 and 1000 mg of para-dichlorobenzene per kg of body weight per day for 5 days per week resulted in weight loss, tremors, and liver effects. The highest no observed adverse effects level (NOAEL) was 357 mg of para-dichlorobenzene per kg per day. A subchronic study indicated a NOAEL of 150 mg of para-dichlorobenzene per kg of body weight in the rat exposed by gavage, and this number was used for calculating an ADI for humans. The provisional ADI was computed as follows:

[Remember ADI = NOAEL/(safety factor) taking dosimetry factors into account]

$$ADI = (150 \text{ mg/kg of body weight/day}) \times (70 \text{ kg/person})$$
$$\times (5 \text{ days/7 days/week})/(100 \times 10)$$
$$= 7.5 \text{ mg/person/day}.$$

One hundred is the safety factor appropriate for use with a NOAEL from animal studies with no comparable human data; ten is an additional safety factor because the duration of exposure in the experiment was significantly less than a lifetime.

As no data were available on the contributions of food and air to exposure, an arbitrary designation of 20% was chosen as the maximum allocation from drinking water. If the daily water intake per person is assumed to be 2 liters per day, the allocated ADI (AADI) for water is:

$$AADI = ADI \times \text{water allocation}/(2 \text{ liters/day})$$
$$= 7.5 \text{ mg/day} \times 20\%/(2 \text{ liters/day})$$
$$= 0.75 \text{ mg/liter}$$

This number represents the maximum amount of para-dichlorobenzene that an individual can ingest from water in 1 day with relative assurance that the individual will not have any ill health effects. Caution must be made in interpreting this number, because of the multiple assumptions, extrapolations, etc., that have been used to create it.

Source: de Koning, 1987.

by a multiple dosing experiment. Curves AB, AD, and AE are possible dose–response curves at lower doses, with points B, D, and E being the respective threshold for adverse effects in the human population. In setting an ADI concentration (point C), a selected safety or uncertainty factor is applied to the dose at point A. If the curve AB is the true effect curve, then the calculated ADI value will be lower than the threshold dose, thus indicating that the safety factor was appropriate. However, if AD or AE is the true dose–effect curve, then the calculated ADI will be too high and the safety factor too small. In this case, some in-

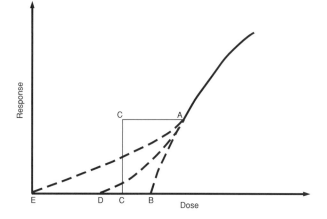

Figure 3.15 Dose–response curves showing different possible estimates at lower dose levels. From de Koning, 1987, with permission.

dividuals in the population will suffer adverse effects. The size of the gap between points C and B is also of interest, because if it is large, expenditure on control methods may be greatly in excess of what is needed.

Once the threshold dose for a toxic substance has been determined for the normal and healthy population, consideration must be given to high-risk groups such as infants, young children, elderly people, pregnant women and their fetuses, the nutritionally deprived, the ill, individuals with genetic disorders, and those exposed to other environmental health hazards. There are many examples of the susceptibility of these high-risk groups. The increased susceptibility of fetuses and infants has been well documented. For example, several Japanese children born to mothers exposed to methylmercury in fish in Minamata suffered congenital malformations even though the mothers showed few or no symptoms of mercury poisoning at all. The fact that nutritional deficiencies increase susceptibility is also well documented. Dietary deficiencies of calcium and iron significantly intensify the toxicity of lead. Individuals who suffer from kidney disease, for example, will experience greater effects from exposure to toxic metabolites that require excretion through the kidneys, and impaired liver function affects the metabolic conversion, particularly detoxification of certain pollutants or their excretion in bile. Individuals suffering from cardiovascular or respiratory disease are at greater risk from the effects of carbon monoxide or sulfur dioxide. It may therefore be necessary to apply an additional safety factor to the dose that is toxic to the general population, in an effort to protect susceptible groups.

Calculating Risks for Non-Threshold Effects

Individuals either get cancer or they do not, and the probability is of an all-or-nothing event. A higher exposure does not result in a worse cancer but in an increase in the likelihood of getting it. Likewise, a lower level of exposure does not mean that the magnitude of the effect is less, so the dose–effect curve is considered irrelevant to assessments involving carcinogens. The dose–response curve, however, is very relevant, and it is generally agreed that the dose–response curve which does not assume a threshold is thus the preferred tool for analyzing risk associated with exposure to carcinogens. The argument against a threshold is that a single point mutation of the DNA can lead to an uncontrolled growth of a somatic cell that eventually produces cancer. It can be argued that different individuals have different thresholds because of differences in DNA repair genes and immune defenses, but these are not easily testable hypotheses.

In the multistage model of carcinogenesis, discussed in Chapter 2, a cell line must pass through several stages before a tumor is irreversibly initiated. The rate at which cell lines pass through these stages is a function of the dose rate. In the multihit model, dose relates to the number of hits to the sensitive tissue required to initiate a cancer. The most important difference between the multistage and the multihit models is that in the multihit models, all hits must result from the dose, whereas in the multistage model, passage through some of the stages can occur spontaneously. The multihit models predict a lower risk at lower doses than that predicted by the multistage model. Aside from the one-hit, the multihit, and the multistage models, there are other models that explain dose–response relationships between carcinogens and cancer. The different models are each associated with different dose–response curves.

Just as one can produce an ADI for threshold agents such as mercury, one can produce a *risk-specific dose* for non-threshold agents, such as radon. In the case of a threshold agent, as described above, the NOAEL can aid the agency responsible for setting the ADI. In the case of a non-threshold agent, at any concentration of the agent cancer will be caused in some individuals in the population. Thus it is usually desirable to reduce the agent to the lowest possible level, realizing that it is impossible to eradicate it entirely. In setting a guideline value, an *acceptable level of risk* (ALR) must be determined. This is essentially a judgment call, which may or may not be made with the input of the people who are concerned in the community. In some countries, one fatality in a million people at risk is considered to be an acceptable level of risk for many situations, but there may be circumstances in which a greater risk, for example, 1 in 100,000, may be considered tolerable if the risk is balanced by a very considerable benefit. It should be noted that an increase in mortality in the general population at such a small rate would be virtually impossible to detect with current epidemiological techniques. One in 10,000 would be more customary for occupational exposures.

HUMAN EXPOSURE ASSESSMENT

Options in Approach

Human exposure is defined as the opportunity for absorption into the body or action on the body as a result of coming into contact with a chemical, biological, or physical agent. The various routes of exposure have already been introduced. The units of exposure to a chemical are usually the concentration multiplied by time (e.g., mg/ml/hr). The term *total exposure* implies that an attempt is being made to take into account all exposures to the contaminant regardless of media or route of exposure. As shown in Figure 3.16, exposures from air, water, food, and soil form the link between hazards and effects.

The critical parameter with respect to health effects is actually the dose, since it directly identifies the amount of the contaminant that has the potential to at-

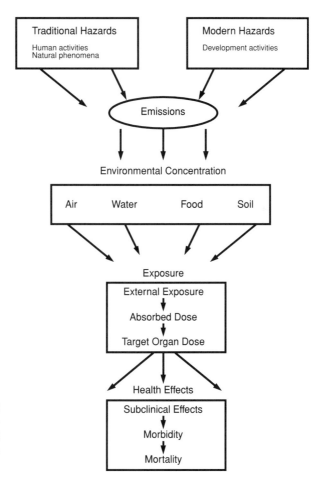

Figure 3.16 Contaminant sources and effects continuum. From Corvalan and Kjellström, 1995, with permission.

tack the target organ. *Internal dose* refers to the amount of the contaminant absorbed in body tissues upon inhalation, ingestion, or absorption. The *biologically effective dose* is the amount of the absorbed or deposited contaminants that contributes to the dose at the target site where the adverse effect occurs. *Total dose* is the term used to indicate the sum of all doses received by a person of a contaminant over a given time interval from interaction with all media.

Because the dose is difficult to measure, the parameter usually considered is the exposure. Therefore, regulators usually establish rules and regulations that are directly linked to reducing exposure, as opposed to dose. Estimates can then be made of the dose, based on the exposure, various assumptions, and animal models. While such estimates often have large uncertainties, it is a more practical parameter than dose. In any case, it has to be clear that measuring exposure, not just environmental concentration, is the critical parameter since it is more directly related to health effects. To put it simply, if someone is not inhaling, ingesting, or absorbing the pollutant, there is no exposure and hence no adverse health effect is possible. In all such investigations the total exposure from all sources must be assessed and not just the concentration in the medium or circumstance of concern. Exposure is usually measured for just one medium at a time. Risk assessment that is intended to optimize mitigation strategies must es-

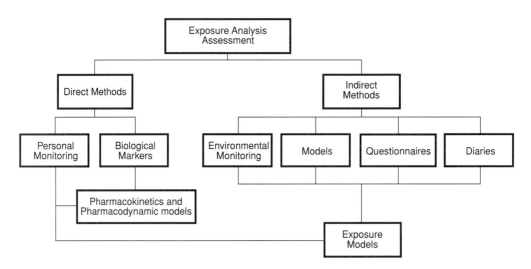

Figure 3.17 Direct and indirect approaches for the analysis of exposures. From NRC, 1991, with permission.

tablish the relative risks associated with absorption from all media and routes of entry in order to gain a clear picture of which is more important.

Monitoring may be *direct* and *indirect,* as indicated in Figure 3.16. Personal environmental monitoring and biological monitoring are considered direct approaches; environmental area monitoring as well as questionnaires, diaries, and mathematical models are considered indirect.

Assessment of exposure can be made in different ways, as illustrated by the various points along the continuum described in Figure 3.17. *Environmental monitoring* measures concentrations of contaminants to which individuals may be exposed. *Biological monitoring* usually measures dose, or more specifically, body burden at a point in time. Each of these can be further subdivided into *area sampling*, which measures concentrations without taking into account the extent of actual exposure, and *personal sampling*, which measures more directly the concentrations to which an individual is exposed throughout a period of time. Similarly, biological monitoring can also be further subdivided to reflect the extent to which the *biological marker* being sampled is a measure of dose, a marker of effect, or a marker of susceptibility.

Personal Exposure Monitoring

Personal air-monitoring devices provide direct measurements of concentrations of air contaminants in the breathing zone of an individual. Generally, samplers worn by subjects record time-integrated concentrations, reading concentrations directly, or they collect time-integrated samples that require lab analysis. Samplers may either be active, requiring a pump to move air, or passive, requiring no pump and collecting the airborne contaminant by diffusion.

For waterborne contaminants, a direct measurement entails sampling from the water source, such as a drinking tap, or from the water actually drunk. To measure food contaminants, duplicate meals are analyzed. In this method, an individual must collect a second portion of everything consumed. This duplicate meal is then homogenized and analyzed for the compounds of interest.

Direct measurements of skin exposure in an occupational environment have been carried out by attaching patches on the skin. After a working day, the patches are removed, extracted, and analyzed. The effectiveness of using gloves to protect skin exposure can be established in a comparable way. Cotton gloves worn underneath latex gloves can be analyzed for specific chemical agents absorbed during handling. The results should indicate whether and to what extent the compound of interest can penetrate the gloves. These results can indicate how frequently gloves should be changed to prevent exposure.

Biological Monitoring of Exposure or Effect

In biological monitoring, the contaminant of interest, its metabolite (see Chapter 2), or the product of interaction between it and some target molecule or cell is measured in the relevant body tissue. If lead is the contaminant of interest, for example, area sampling can be conducted to determine the operations associated with the greatest lead concentration; personal air monitoring for lead exposure may be conducted, blood lead levels may be drawn from exposed workers to measure dose, or a marker of effect such as free erythrocyte protoporphyrin (FEP) may be evaluated. Examples of some biological markers of exposure are shown in Table 3.8.

A *marker of effect* must be a measurable, biochemical, physiological, or other alteration within an organism that, depending on magnitude, is recognized as relating to the potential to cause health impairment or disease (NRC, 1991). Some markers of effect signal preclinical or presymptomatic stages in disease development, whereas others signal adaptive changes that are not themselves pathological. This often presents a difficult clinical situation—for example, with respect to workers' compensation (see Chapter 10). Workers may be told that they have an elevated leveled FEP, but they have no clear symptoms of lead poisoning. In most jurisdictions, this case would not be considered compensatable by a workers' compensation board. Also, these markers may be complicated by various interpretations and confounders. For example, FEP levels may be proportionally elevated because of iron deficiency. Or, although the presence of carboxyhemoglobin (COHb) in blood signals that carbon monoxide exposure is occurring, the source could be the inhalation of carbon monoxide or the metabolism of methylene

TABLE 3.8

EXAMPLES OF USEFUL MARKERS OF EXPOSURE

Substance	*Biological Marker*
Carbon monoxide	COHb in blood
Cadmium	Cadmium in urine
Lead	Lead in blood
Methyl-mercury (in fish)	Mercury in hair
PCP	PCP in urine
Alcoholic beverages	Ethanol in exhaled breath
Organic solvents	Metabolites in urine
VOCs	VOCs in exhaled breath
Tobacco smoke	Cotinine in urine

COHb, carboxyhemoglobin; PCP, pentachlorophenol; VOCs, volatile organics.

chloride. It may also be due to hemolytic anemia with increased breakdown of hemoglobin.

Biological monitoring for susceptibility markers is a highly controversial area. Markers of susceptibility may relate to induced variations in absorption, metabolism, and response to environmental agents. For example, measurement of airway reactivity to inhaled bronchoconstrictors can be used as a marker of susceptibility to asthma.

Recently, the application of markers in a rapidly developing field sometimes called *molecular epidemiology* has attracted much interest. There has been particular enthusiasm for the study of DNA and protein adducts. However, chemical methods to detect and quantify adducts often rely on costly methods that require highly sophisticated and expensive instrumentation (such as gas chromatography and mass spectrometry) operated by highly skilled technologists. Furthermore, most of these methods still have to be validated and cannot be considered routine measurements.

Indirect Approaches to Estimation of Exposure

The indirect approach to estimating an individual's or a population's exposure to a pollutant combines concentration measurements in the environment with information on human activities obtained through the use of questionnaires or diaries (see Fig. 3.17). Exposure assessment surveys, whether they be questionnaires, telephone interviews, or measurements, usually attempt to obtain information in four areas: demographic profile, health status, environmental factors, and time–activity. There are three general approaches for obtaining time–activity information. One is called the *estimation approach*, in which an estimate is made of the amount of time spent by study participants in various activities during the time period of interest. The second approach uses *time activity diaries*, in which participants are asked to describe all of the activities in which they were engaged during the study period. The third approach is the *observational approach*, in which participants are monitored by outside observers. While this adds a degree of completeness and accuracy to the data, many people may refuse to participate in a study in which their activities are being monitored. Using data on concentrations in various environments and human activity data as input variables, *calculation models* can predict exposures at an individual or population level. To estimate exposures via different exposure routes, standard values for the amount of inhaled air and ingestion of drinking water and soil can be used. One set of such standard values is presented in Table 3.9 for various age-groups. The standard value for total soil adhered can be used as a proxy measure for potential dermal exposure.

Estimating Inhalation Exposure

Outdoor measurements have been an integral part of environmental monitoring in many countries for several decades. Indoor air was largely ignored however, until the 1970s and 1980s. Thus, while many air pollutants are at higher concentrations indoors than outside, indoor air quality monitoring procedures are less well developed. This will be discussed further in subsequent chapters. To estimate an inhalation dose, an estimate of the amount of air a person breathes in a day is required. A person's gender, age, and amount of physical activity are major factors affecting the volume of air breathed. Age-specific standard values

TABLE 3.9

RECOMMENDED STANDARD VALUES FOR DAILY INTAKE OF AIR, WATER, AND SOIL

Age (years)	Air Inhalation $(m^3/day)^a$	Water Ingestion^b (liter/day)	Soil Ingestion (mg/day)	Total Soil Adhered (mg/day)
0–<0.5	2	BF: 0/0	35	2200
		NBF: 0.2/0.8		
0.5–<5	5	0.2/0.8	50	3500
5–<12	12	0.3/0.9	35	5800
12–<20	21	0.5/1.3	20	9100
20+	23	0.4/1.5	20	8700

^{a}1000 liters = 1 m³.
^{b}The first value represents straight tap water only; the second includes tap water–based beverages such as tea, coffee, and reconstituted soft drinks. Exclusively breast-fed infants (BF) do not require additional liquids. Estimates for non–breast-fed infants (NBF) are based on volume consumed as drinking water and on consumption of 750 ml/day of formula made from powdered formula and tapwater for total drinking water.
Source: HC, 1992.

are given in Table 3.9. Other factors influencing the volume of air breathed include temperature, altitude body weight, smoking habits, history of heart disease, and possibly background air pollution. The absorbed dose is dependent on the deposition of the chemical in the respiratory tract and the absorption of the deposited chemical into the bloodstream.

Estimating Ingestion Exposure

Water To estimate the exposure to contaminants from drinking water, the amount of water people drink and otherwise consume (for example, by bathing) must be determined. Ingestion of water includes plain water, water in coffee, tea, or other drinks made with tap water, and water in cooked food. If precise values for a community are not available, standard values such as those presented in Table 3.9 can be used. To calculate the water ingestion dose, it is usually assumed that 100% of the contaminated water is absorbed after ingestion, and a similar formula to that shown for inhalation is used.

Soil Soil can be eaten unintentionally when soil sticks to hands or to food. Soil can also be ingested when other objects are put in the mouth or swallowed. All children do this to some extent. The frequency that children swallow and put objects in their mouths varies. Children between the ages of 1 and 3 years, and children with iron deficiency or certain mental disorders develop a habit of swallowing objects more often than other children (known as *pica*). Standard values for the daily ingestion of soil by children who do not swallow objects regularly and by adults are presented in Table 3.9. To calculate the soil ingestion dose, it is assumed that 100% of the contaminant ingested with soil is absorbed. The equation, however, should convert the concentration of the contaminant in the soil (C) from $\mu g/kg$ of soil to $\mu g/kg$ of soil, so that the units for soil concentration are the same as those for soil ingestion.

Food To determine the amount of a contaminant eaten with food, a knowledge of eating habits of the group or population being studied is required, along with the concentration of the contaminant in different kinds of food. Eating habits—the amount of each different kind of food eaten—in a community may differ from the national average or environmental estimates. To measure the amount of contaminant absorbed into the body with food (estimated dose), a separate calculation is carried out for each kind of food or food group eaten. Although this equation looks more complicated, the extra steps are just a repetition of the basic equation used in calculating all other estimated doses (ED).

Estimating Skin Exposure and Doses

The absorption of contaminants through the skin depends on a number of factors, including the following:

- the total surface area of the exposed skin
- the part of the body in contact with the contaminant
- the duration of contact
- the concentration of the chemical on the skin
- the ability of the specific contaminant to move through the skin into the body (this is called the *chemical-specific permeability*)
- the type of substance through which the contaminant comes into contact with the skin (for example, whether the contaminant was dissolved in water or in soil when it came into contact with the person)
- whether the skin is damaged in any way before coming into contact with the contaminant.

The area of the skin that is exposed will be influenced by the activity being performed and the season of the year. To estimate the absorption of a contaminant in water through the skin, a permeability constant (P) should be used. However, such constants have been established for only a few chemicals. Even for chemicals that have been tested, the value of the constant can depend to a very large degree on the design of the experiment used to test the chemical. Box 3.5 summarizes the information needed to calculate estimated daily intake (EDI) via ingestion and skin absorption.

Principles of Population Sampling

In the selection of a population sample for human exposure assessment, a *sampling frame* should be established, which should include (*a*) all the people in the target population, or (*b*) areas and the approximate number of people linked to each area. If the people in the target population are mobile, they may have to be linked to the areas where they eat or sleep. Developed countries usually have a central statistical bureau that maintains registries or conducts a population census, which may form an ideal frame for sampling from the general population. As these listings are rarely complete, sampling frames often need to be conducted in stages, as discussed below, with these data constituting a sampling frame for the initial stages of a multistage sample. In developing countries, where census data are generally not available, special efforts may be needed to estimate the population linked to the areas to construct a sampling frame.

Basic Equations for Calculating Estimated
Daily Intake (EDI) Via Ingestion and Skin Absorption

$$\text{Ingestion EDI} = C \times \text{IgR} \times \text{EF}/\text{BW}$$

$$\text{Skin absorption (water) EDI} = C \times P \times \text{SA} \times \text{ET} \times \text{EF}/\text{BW}$$

$$\text{Skin absorption (soil) EDI} = C \times A \times \text{BF} \times \text{EF}/\text{BW}$$

where C = concentration of the contaminant; IgR = ingestion rate (usually liters/day); P = permeability factor of the skin site; SA = surface area exposed; ET = exposure time; EF = exposure factor; BW = body weight; A = total soil adhered (often need to use standard tables); and BF = bioavailability factors [percent of the contaminant in the soil that is actually free to move out of the soil and through the skin (unitless)].

If the target population consists only of people with specific characteristics, lists of these people may be available. For example, if the target population consists of lactating mothers, clinics in the area may be able to provide lists of mothers who have recently delivered babies. If available information does not provide complete enough coverage of the target population, samples from the lists must be supplemented with samples from other, possibly less efficient, frames that provide more complete coverage of the target population (see UNEP/WHO, 1993).

Figure 3.18 provides a visual representation of *multistage sampling*, in which researchers begin by sampling relatively large units and work their way down to increasingly smaller units. Using estimates of the number of people residing in each area, a sample of the geographic areas is selected. At the next stage, either the sample can be listed or smaller geographic areas can be listed within each area selected at the first stage of sampling. At the final stage of sampling, a list of the people residing in each sample area is prepared, and a sample of the people is selected from the lists. For example, to select a sample of adults living in a large city, researchers might (1) randomly select ten neighborhoods; (2) within each neighbourhood, randomly select two urban blocks; (3) within each block, select ten households; (4) within each of the households, select one adult for the study. Methods for implementing simple random sampling and systematic sampling are discussed in numerous other publications. In *stratified random sampling*, an effective technique used to ensure that subgroups are adequately represented, the subpopulation of special interest (e.g., people between certain ages) is sampled at a higher rate than the remainder of the population to obtain sufficiently precise results for that group. The total estimated dose is calculated by simply adding these EDIs together. Note that the equations are very similar, except that the rate of contact varies depending on the type of exposure.

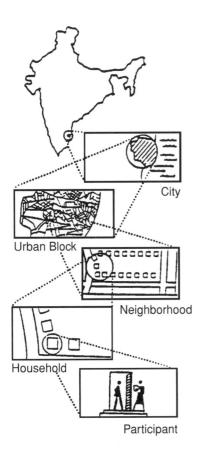

City

Urban Block

Neighborhood

Household

Participant

Figure 3.18 Multistage sampling procedures. From UNEP/WHO, 1992a, with permission.

Errors and Quality Assurance

The potential for errors in environmental exposure assessment is large. Errors may occur with respect to the representativeness of sampling sites, the method of sample collection, the analytic procedure, and data handling.

The *representative error* refers to whether the sample collected represents the average concentration in the media under study. For example, an outdoor monitor on the roof of a multistoried building may not yield the concentration data needed to estimate average community air exposure. Even if sampling is conducted at a reasonable site, there is always a question as to how representative it is of exposure to residents at different times or when the wind blows from different directions. Portable sampling done in various directions and at variable distances from a fixed site can often provide more accurate data.

Sample collection errors (e.g., for water, soil, or food samples) can usually be minimized by simply using containers that are free of the contaminant of interest. Air samples are more difficult to properly collect and there is considerably more controversy over which instrument to use in various situations. Industrial hygienists therefore obtain considerable training in techniques of proper sample collection, and only people trained in these techniques should conduct air sampling.

Analytical errors may arise from the use of improper calibration procedures, variations in temperatures or line voltage in the laboratory, operator mistakes, as well as the intrinsic imprecision and inaccuracy of the analytical method chosen.

Finally, *errors in data preparation* may occur at a number of stages and often relate to the number of individuals involved in obtaining an environmental measurement. These specialists include the field person who collects the sample, the laboratory technician who does the analysis, the computer programmer who enters the data, and the epidemiologist who, often with the help of the statistician, interprets the data.

Quality assurance programs have therefore been developed and much international guidance has been provided on this subject. Effective procedures include the use of standard reference materials when calibrating instruments, monitoring of the line voltage and temperature to keep them constant, and duplicate analyses of some of the collected samples. A number of methods have been employed for quality assurance, such as interlaboratory comparisons, in which different analytical methods are used to analyze the same sample, and various statistical procedures to highlight bad data or extreme values.

Ensuring Adequate Sample Size

Determining an appropriate sample size requires balancing precision and cost. When the cost of a study is high, it may not be possible to obtain a very large sample size. Guidelines for calculating necessary sample sizes for accurate estimates are available in many textbooks and WHO publications, including that by UNEP/WHO (1993). Even if the final sample sizes are determined primarily by cost constraints, rather than for desired precision, it is essential to calculate the precision that is expected for important parameter estimates and the power expected for important hypothesis tests. Studies that do not meet minimum standards for reliability of inferences are not useful—they cannot be interpreted. In general, a sample size of 50 persons is the minimum acceptable for human exposure–monitoring studies, with a range of 250 or more people considered desirable. The problems regarding inferences to the target population must be discussed in the reports of all studies but this is particularly important for studies with small sample sizes. Such problems include (*1*) unreliable point estimates, (*2*) unreliable estimates of precision, and (*3*) lack of normality for interval estimates and hypothesis tests (see UNEP/WHO 1993 for greater detail).

HEALTH RISK CHARACTERIZATION

General Approach

Risk characterization brings together the first three components of the risk assessment process: hazard identification, dose–response assessment, and exposure assessment. The incidence and severity of potential adverse effects are estimated as well. The major assumptions, scientific judgments, and uncertainties are described in detail to fully understand the validity of the estimated risk. Risk characterization (or *risk estimation* as it is also known) may be subdivided into four different steps as indicated in Table 3.10.

The first equation of total exposure combines the concentration of pollutants (by direct measurement through sampling and analysis, modeling, analysis of biological markers, and questionnaires) with the duration of exposure, expressed ac-

TABLE 3.10

CONSECUTIVE STEPS IN HEALTH RISK CHARACTERIZATION

Step	Description
1. Exposure	Pollutant concentration × exposure duration (or it is directly measured by integrated sampling)
2. Dose	Exposure (1) × dosimetry factors (absorption rate, inhalation rate, etc.) divided with body weight or surface area
3. Lifetime individual risk	Dose (2) × risk characterization factor (carcinogenic potency, noncarcinogenic threshold, e.g., NOEL) or severity (e.g., NOAEL), with uncertainty factors
4. Risk to exposed population	Individual risk (3) × number in exposed population (this should take into consideration age, and other susceptibility factors, population activities, etc.)

cording to the health effects of concern. For carcinogenic effects, the total time (hours or days) of exposure during a person's lifetime is the principal concern (exposure every day over a lifetime would be 25,550 days, assuming a 70-year lifetime). For noncarcinogenic effects, short-term exposures at elevated concentrations are targeted, therefore a duration of hours or even minutes may be important. For chronic exposure, an average daily pollutant concentration is usually used with the assumption that it is relatively constant over a lifetime. For children, exposure periods are generally divided into age categories, e.g., 0–6 months, 6 months to 5 years, and 5 years to 12 years, because of their differing body weights.

The second equation combines the exposure information with dosimetry factors in a simple model to estimate the average dose per day over a lifetime. These factors include absorbed rate, average body weight, average lifetime, and others, as relevant. Dose is usually expressed as pollutant mass per kilogram of body weight per day. It should also include exposures from all media (air, water, soil, direct skin contact, etc.), such that the total dose is the sum of all of the individual doses.

The third equation integrates this exposure assessment with the dose–response relationship. As discussed in the section Relationship Between Dose and Health Outcome, it incorporates uncertainty factors (and any other modifying factors that reflect professional judgment regarding scientific uncertainties of the entire database) with the NOAEL. This creates a benchmark against which to evaluate the significance of the dose with respect to its implication for health. The U.S. EPA has estimated potency factors that can be applied for many carcinogens. (Methodologies to estimate the chance of toxic outcomes other than cancer are less developed.) The reference dose, or *recommended maximum concentration* in some jurisdictions, is the NOAEL divided by the uncertainty factors multiplied by any modifying factors of concern. The lifetime individual risk is therefore the product of the dose multiplied by these response factors. For cancer, this is expressed as the lifetime excess risk of cancer for an individual exposed at the given lifetime exposure. For noncarcinogenic agents, it is usually assumed that there is a threshold below which there is no effect. The ratio of the exposure level to the estimated threshold dose gives some indication of the likelihood that adverse health effects will result from exposure to the toxic substance.

To generalize these average exposures and risks to the individual to an entire exposed population (consisting of many individuals, who may be very different from one another), one multiplies the estimate of average or worst lifetime individual risk by the number of individuals in the population (or each subpopulation) exposed. This final figure is the excess risk for a given effect that an exposure produces for an entire population. How this risk should then be interpreted and communicated to the public and the approach used to manage this risk will be discussed further in Chapter 4. First, though, an example is provided of how the above principles can be applied in field studies.

Specific Health Risk Assessments in Field Situations

When risk assessment framework is applied to a new field situation, new or unexpected problems and pitfalls inevitably occur. In some cases it is obvious what risk factors are involved. In others the potential hazards is extremely difficult to recognize. In still other situations the ingested dose may be easily calculated from food contamination levels and average consumption data. In others the situation is very complicated because many different exposure routes are involved and dosimetry factors are not available. In such cases, the use of biomarkers may be the only effective way to come to an acceptably accurate estimate of the total dose.

HEALTH IN ENVIRONMENTAL IMPACT ASSESSMENT

Health risk assessment may also be used to anticipate the potential health effects of projects or activities planned for the future. During the formulation of development policies and the planning of projects, health effects often receive inadequate attention. In many countries where there are requirements and the capacity in place to assess environmental impact, only (or predominantly) impacts on the biophysical environment are assessed routinely. When expected environmental effects of pollution or ecosystem disturbance still conform to the legally established environmental standards, routinely it is then assumed that adverse human health effects are not likely to occur. This assumption is based on the idea that adverse human health effects are always adequately presented by standards designed to protect the environment.

Methods have been developed to identify, assess, and mitigate the environmental and health effects of major industrial, agricultural, and other large developmental projects before they occur. Guidelines on *environmental health impact assessments* (EHIA) have been prepared by several international organizations, including the WHO's regional office for Europe (WHO, 1985, 1986). Several countries have also prepared national guidelines. With the declaration adopted at the 1992 UN Conference on Environment and Development that "human beings were at the centre of concern for sustainable development," it is now widely acknowledged that environmental impact assessments must address health concerns.

In principle, the assessment of adverse health effects follows an approach similar to the risk assessment framework discussed in the previous sections of this chapter. First, potential hazards associated with the project that require further investigation have to be identified. Subsequently, emissions have to be calculated or estimated using technological specifications of the project. From these data, emission concentrations, exposure, and total dose should be calculated with mathematical models that have been developed specifically for these purposes and that take local geographical characteristics and climate factors into account. (The interpretation of the generated data requires specific skills and expert judgments. It may not be easy to determine the importance of, for instance, a 10 dB(A) increase in noise levels for the inhabitants of a particular residential area). The relative importance of some impacts in comparison with other impacts may also have to be considered. Finally, health risks can be characterized as discussed in Table 3.10. At this stage, it should be realized that certain projects may change the nature and demographics of the exposed population and the percentage of vulnerable persons. For example, large projects involving resettlement of populations will increase the percentage of elderly people among the exposed population simply because older individuals are more reluctant to move. Large construction projects, in contrast, may increase the number of young male adults.

Since an *environmental impact assessment* (EIA) is a practical process, it is not generally possible to await results from new research. Consequently, conclusions must generally be based on currently accepted scientific knowledge, while simultaneously conducting research to evaluate future environmental impacts. Usually the only actual measurements that can be performed during the preparation stage of a project and the baseline assessments or measurements taken from pilot projects. Extrapolation of data regarding emissions, exposures, and (if available) health effects from similar projects can be extremely useful. Extrapolation from one situation to another situation where there are different geographical and demographic features as well as exposure characteristics usually requires a number of assumptions, and specific expertise.

The health component of environmental impact assessments should incorporate more than the best scientific information available. It should draw upon community-based information and traditional knowledge of native peoples and others in the community. It should also recognize that many projects have beneficial as well as adverse effects on health and well-being. By creating jobs and providing other economic benefits that contribute to a better standard of living, health may be greatly improved because of the project in question. As noted in Chapter 1, economic well-being has been repeatedly linked with longevity and other indicators of health, because, among other reasons, people with adequate income can afford to eat balanced diets and live healthy lifestyles. Adverse effects on health may be disproportionately experienced by people who do not share in a project's benefits. Thus the health component of the EIA should assess who will benefit and who may experience adverse effects. If potential adverse effects are identified, recommendations for mitigation and follow-up measures should be included in the environmental impact statement (EIS) that the project's proponent is required to do. The EIAs may also contain alternatives to the project, including the potential effects on health of not allowing the project to proceed. Although there may be jurisdictional considerations regarding which government department is responsible for occupational versus public health in some countries, both components are essential to ascertain the potential benefits and adverse effects of a proposal.

The Lower Seyhan Irrigation Project in Turkey

One of the greatest water-related projects in Turkey, known as the Lower Seyhan Irrigation Project, was started in the Cukurova region in the early 1950s. The activities in the project included the construction of a dam on the Seyhan river to store water for hydroelectric and agricultural purposes; the establishment of a spillway for excess water; construction of irrigation canals to distribute the water throughout the plain and for irrigation of fields; and construction of drainage canals for excess water from the fields.

The Cukurova authorities did not consider it a danger when malaria-infected workers arrived from the southeastern part of Turkey (where malaria transmission still occurred). It was thought that the disease was totally under control because of the very low number of malaria cases reported from the entire country. The consequences of the project can be listed as follows:

1. Populations from areas to be covered by water were resettled around newly irrigated areas.
2. Productivity of irrigated lands increased.
3. Insects and different kinds of insecticides were introduced into the area, creating vector resistance to insecticides.
4. Irrigation expanded the number of arable fields, creating an increase in the need for laborers.
5. People moved from poorer parts of the country (most of them came from areas where unnoticed malaria epidemics still occurred) to be seasonal workers in the newly developing areas.
6. Seasonal workers settled along the canals (attracted by vegetation and slopes of less than 1%), where water collections became efficient breeding places for malaria vectors.
7. Malaria parasites were introduced to the local mosquito vector (*An sacharovi*), which has a great capacity for transmitting the disease.
8. Industries increased their work on local products because of the agricultural development.
9. The increase in industrial activity created increased demand for workers.
10. Workers and families gravitated toward industrial activities, resulting in an increase in the population of the Cukurova region.
11. Unhealthy settlements were established around towns for the incoming population.
12. New, high-rise apartment buildings were built to meet the housing needs of the newcomers. The underground floors of these buildings became new breeding places for vectors because of the high level of the water table and deep basement excavation.
13. Malaria parasites were transmitted to nonimmune local people.
14. Finally, there was a resurgence of malaria in the area. During 1970, the number of cases reported in the Cukurova region increased from 49 to 149.

Source: WHO/CEMP, 1992.

Multidisciplinary collaboration is crucial in an EIA. It is important to ensure that the health components at each stage of the assessment are adequately addressed. To be effective, the EIA should occur at the project planning stage. It must be an integral component in the design of a project, rather than something added on after the design is completed. In this way the EIA may suggest alternative project designs with greater health benefits and fewer health risks. For any large project, some description of the baseline environmental health and social conditions is essential. This should include the demographic characteristics of the potentially affected populations, the current health status, the local health care and occupational health services, the characteristics of any incoming groups of people, such as construction workers or miners, the history of the potentially affected populations in relation to development, and any traditional behaviors that may be impacted by the development. An irrigation project in Turkey (described in Box 3.6) illustrates how one project can influence a community's health through various mechanisms.

Increasing public awareness of technological and environmental health risks has been accompanied by increasing public participation in the decision-making framework. As a result, public involvement should be an integral part of any EIA process. Following are advantages of including the general public and other interest groups in the EIA:

- greater awareness of the environmental issues important to the public
- possible identification of alternative actions
- an increase in the acceptability of the project, as the public will better understand the reasons and risks related to the project
- minimizing of conflict and delay

Study Questions

1. Consider all information that is needed to assess human exposure to a specific hazard. Consider how this information could be gathered.

2. What are the advantages and disadvantages of environmental and biological monitoring?

3. Which of the consequences indicated in Box 3.6 are directly or indirectly related to health? Which of these impacts on human health can be expected to be positive or negative? Which of these aspects would have to be taken into account in an EHIA, and what specific information would be needed to assess quantitative health risks prior to the onset of the project? What would be needed to assess quantitative health risks prior to the onset of the project?

4

RISK MANAGEMENT

LEARNING OBJECTIVES

After studying this chapter you will be able to do the following:

- discusss the principles of risk management, including the process for the selection, implementation, and evaluation of appropriate control strategies
- identify the factors affecting risk perception and the principles of risk communication and be able to take these into consideration in risk management
- discuss the advantages and disadvantages of controlling pollutants at each stage: at the source, along the path (the environment), and at the level of the person
- describe the basic requirements of a surveillance system
- outline the approach to managing an environmental emergency
- apply the principles of economic evaluation of environmental health interventions

CHAPTER CONTENTS

Risk management brings together the evaluation and perception of risk to control exposure to hazards (Fig. 4.1). It is partly a scientific, quantitative exercise in which the results of a risk assessment (Chapter 3) are compared to standards, guidelines, or comparable risks. Having made this comparison, and knowing the assumptions, extrapolations, and estimates that go into the two numbers in the comparison (as discussed in Chapter 3), an environmental health professional can determine whether a significant risk is present. But the perception of the risk by the individuals or community facing the risk must also be taken into account. Of course, the manner in which the risk evaluation is communicated will also affect risk perception, as will the effectiveness of communicating the plans for and results of exposure control.

After the risk is evaluated and the exposure is controlled as appropriate, the risk must be monitored to ensure that it remains under control. Although sometimes the problem can be solved, usually the process is an iterative one in which the risk must be reassessed and community perception reevaluated on a continual basis. In reality, this interactive process means that the different steps in risk assessment and management may be carried out simultaneously.

RISK EVALUATION

Comparing Risks to Standards or Guidelines

A health risk may range from minor physiological changes to premature death (see Table 3.5). What is understood to be an important or unacceptable level of risk depends in large part on the concept of health accepted in the community in question. For example, in setting most environmental and occupational standards in North America, authorities have assumed that there is no threat to health as long as the exposure does not induce disturbance of a kind and degree that overloads the normal protective mechanism of the body. In the former Soviet Union, in contrast, maximum permissible concentrations for environmental pollutants were set below the level that causes physiological and other changes of uncertain significance. These standards had the status of guidelines rather than absolute limits, and were not necessarily enforced.

In some jurisdictions *guidelines* are established, which cannot be enforced by law, while in others, *standards* are set, and individuals or companies that exceed

Risk Assessment
1. Hazard identification
2. Dose-response assessment
3. Exposure assessment

4. Risk Characterization

Risk Management
5. Risk evaluation
6. Risk perception and communication
7. Control of exposure
8. Risk Monitoring

Figure 4.1 Risk assessment and management framework.

the standards may suffer the penalties prescribed by legislation. In either case, the general approach for evaluating risk is to compare the estimated exposure to that which is considered acceptable, based on guidance values or standards (e.g., the acceptable daily intakes [ADIs] or risk-specific doses [RsDs] that were calculated in Chapter 3).

The purpose of any risk management effort is to help make decisions to control hazards. While comparison with administratively established standards or guidelines (e.g., ADIs or RsDs) is essential for inspectors and other enforcement officials, it is important for environmental health professionals to gain some perspective on the magnitude of the risk and to be able to convey its meaning to decision makers and to the public. The way in which risks are perceived relates strongly to the manner in which they have been estimated. Risks calculated from historical data tend to be easier to understand. For example, there are plenty of data on automobile accidents, and any risk in one jurisdiction can be compared with data from another (with certain methodological limitations). Data on a given risk in a given jurisdiction can also be compared with data from the same jurisdiction at an earlier date.

However, this historical approach to estimating risks is only applicable in situations in which the hazards causing the risks are known and exposure to them is predictable and the outcomes resulting from exposure can be directly measured in a population and related back to exposure to the hazard. For example, if the aim is to calculate the risk of cancer arising from exposure to cigarette smoke, one would need to know that smoking rates rarely change dramatically from year to year, that smoking a certain amount is associated with a certain level of risk, and that the numbers of people in the population of concern who smoke at various levels can be specified. This calculation can be done only because cancer cases can be identified and counted in the population and it is already well known that cigarette smoking causes cancer.

Comparing Risks When There Are No Historical Data

If there is no historical database for a hazard, so that dose–response information does not exist, the evaluation of the risk is much more complicated. With respect to new technology for which there is no historical database (e.g., a new power plant or industrial facility), one approach is to consider it in separate parts, calculating the risks from each part and adding them together to estimate a risk for the whole. In this approach all possible chains of events from an initiator to a final accident are followed in what is referred to as an *event tree*, with the probability of each event in the tree being estimated from historical data in different situations.

It is particularly helpful to compare risks that are calculated in a similar manner. For example, the risk of traveling by automobile can be compared to traveling by horse or by airplane. Similarly, radiation risk from a medical X-ray can be compared to that of radon gas, to the dose an average resident experienced near Chernobyl, or to the natural radiation dose an individual receives on a long-distance trip by air.

Setting standards regarding water quality, food contamination, and air pollution is discussed in chapters addressing air, water, and food (Chapters 5, 6, and

7). Threshold limit values used in occupational health will be discussed further in the chapter on industry (Chapter 10).

FACTORS AFFECTING THE PERCEPTION AND ACCEPTANCE OF RISK

Risk Perception

Environmental health professionals often discover that the public perception of an environmental health risk differs widely from that of scientists. The level of public *outrage* toward an environmental health hazard plays a major role in the acceptability of the risk associated with this hazard. In past decades, it was often thought that if the public were educated about the risks associated with the hazard, people would find the hazard more acceptable. It is now known that understanding the risk is only one of many dimensions that affect risk perception and acceptance. Moreover, this has been shown to be a fairly minor factor relative to other dimensions. Some of the more important dimensions that affect environmental health risk perception and the strategies for risk management and communication in light of these dimensions are shown in Table 4.1. Aside from these (e.g. voluntarism, attribute of blame, understanding), risks that have delayed health effects and those that affect future generations are accepted less readily than those that are immediately apparent.

Coping Strategies

Many factors influence how people respond to environmental health risks. As discussed above, one person's perception of a risk may be completely different from another person's perception. In addition, individuals have different coping strategies to deal with perceived risk, or stress in general. A distinction can be made between coping strategies that concentrate on either the individual emotional response, called *emotion-focused coping,* or eliminating or reducing the observed hazard, *problem-focused coping*. These strategies may involve both direct action and mental processes.

Most of this text addresses problem-focused responses to risks. Viewing an individual's health problems in terms of emotion-focused coping may lead the environmental health professional to attribute them to the emotional stress of a situation (e.g., Chernobyl; see Chapter 9) or to the person's own actions, inability to cope, or other personal characteristics. This may inadvertently lead to victim blaming, which in turn may obscure the real threat that a risk imposes and in any case does not help the professional address the individual in an effective manner. Nonetheless, it is important for environmental health professionals to have some understanding of coping strategies to manage environmental health risks appropriately.

Cognitive coping strategies are characterized by the use of thought processes aimed at the reduction of experienced stress. These mental strategies take many different forms:

Problem denial. The individual tries to convince himself or herself that the health risk is exaggerated by others or by the media, and that the authorities will exercise their responsibility to protect the community.

Problem amplification. The individual perceives the problem as much larger than it is, usually because of the stress in their lives.

Problem suppression. The individual does not deny the perceived risk, but just tries not to think about it.

Problem redefinition. The individual redefines the problem in such a way that the positive effects (e.g., stimulation of the regional economy, or increased employment) are more important.

Problem acceptance. This strategy aims at regaining emotional stability in a situation in which the individual sees no possibilities to influence change.

Coping strategies may lead to direct action-based strategies. These include the following:

Action aimed at risk reduction. This could be achieved by trying to influence the decision-making process, for example by demonstrating against a given situation or organizing action groups.

Searching for information. This could result in a better understanding of the risk and may be a valuable strategy since unfamiliarity usually relates to overestimation of the risk.

Searching for help. This would include contacting environmental action groups that can give advice or practical assistance in reducing the risk. Working off one's feelings in discussion groups is another active form of coping.

Active search for distraction. Immersing oneself in sports, hobbies, or other activities and avoiding thinking about the problem would characterize this type of action.

Emotional modification. Use of tobacco, alcohol, or drugs can be seen as a form of emotional modification. These coping strategies, however, involve exposure to health hazards and may result in disrupted social structures, violence, and criminal behavior.

Apart from coping strategies, it is likely that an individual's personality and degree of social support will influence the stress response. Evidence indicates that both the health and well-being of individuals with more social support are generally higher than for those individuals without this support. This social support may consist of actual assistance or information provided to resolve problems, or it may include emotional support. Personality characteristics that have been associated with lower stress responses include a general attitude of trying to influence important events in life; a tendency to define sudden changes or threatening situations as a challenge rather than a threat; motivation of being involved in society and having a purpose in life.

Principles of Risk Communication

Risk communication is defined as the purposeful exchange of information about the existence, nature, form, severity, or acceptability of risks. The objectives of risk communication could be either (*a*) to alert the public or decision makers to

TABLE 4.1

DIMENSIONS OF RISK, THEIR EFFECTS ON RISK PERCEPTION, AND RELATED STRATEGIES FOR RISK MANAGEMENT AND COMMUNICATION

Dimension	Conditions Associated with Higher Perceived Risk	Conditions Associated with Lower Perceived Risk	Strategy to Manage
Voluntarism	Involuntary exposures (e.g., air pollution)	Risks taken by choice (e.g., skiing, smoking)	Make the risk more voluntary by empowering community; negotiate conditions of acceptability
Attribution of blame	Risk caused by human failure (e.g., explosion at an industrial plant)	Risk caused by nature (e.g., lightning, aflatoxin in peanut butter)	Don't compare natural risks with anthropogenic risks
Familiarity	Unfamiliar risk (e.g., ozone depletion, hazardous waste treatment facilities)	Familiar risks (e.g., household accidents, radon in basements)	Make a risk familiar by conducting open meetings and tours, displays; keep talking about the risks until they are familiar and better understood
Understanding	Lack of understanding of mechanisms or processes involved (e.g., nuclear power plant accidents)	Understanding of mechanisms or processes involved (e.g., slipping on ice)	Educate, build trust in technical experts
Media attention	Much media attention (e.g., airline crash, industrial accident)	Little media attention (e.g., work injuries)	Recognize the media attention and address it openly
Memorability	Highly publicized events (e.g., Exxon Valdez oil spill)	Nonmemorable outcome	Recognize the image and address it openly
Dread	Risks that evoke fear (e.g., abandoned hazardous waste site)	Risks not dreaded (e.g., food poisoning)	Legitimize the dread and agree with the disgust
Clustering	Fatalities or injuries grouped in time or space (e.g., large industrial explosions)	Fatalities or injuries distributed randomly in time or space (e.g., auto accident deaths)	Take worst-case scenario seriously; give more attention to magnitude than probability

Catastrophic potential	Risks uncertain (e.g., disagreements among scientists about the risks of nuclear power)	Risks relatively well known to scientists (e.g., war, auto accidents)	Acknowledge range of risk to minimize the debate
Extent of personal control	Little personal or community control (e.g., traveling as a passenger in a car or airplane)	Some personal or community control (e.g., driving a car)	Empower community board, community audits
Equity	No direct benefit for those at risk (e.g., living near an abandoned hazardous waste site)	Seemingly equitable distribution of risks and benefits (e.g., vaccinations)	Share the benefits in proportion to risks (ask the community what they want in return)
Moral relevance or clarity of benefits	Benefits from or need for activity generating risk in question (e.g., nuclear power)	Clear benefits (e.g., traveling by car)	Don't be smug about the moral values of a community
Trustworthiness	Lack of trust in institutions responsible for risk management (e.g., regulatory agencies with ties to industry)	Responsible institutions are well treated (e.g., management of recombinant DNA research by universities)	Don't try to convince people that an institution can be trusted; make it accountable
Responsible process	Risks that are denied (e.g., garbage in the river)	Risks that are acknowledged (e.g., child abuse)	Don't be secretive, apologize, or compensate; explain measures taken to prevent adverse health effects
Impact on children	Children specifically at risk (e.g., birth defects)	Risks threaten adults only (e.g., occupational risks)	Characterize risks in terms of the whole family or community

Adapted from various sources, including Sandman, 1986, and Covello, 1989.

TABLE 4.2

THE U.S. ENVIRONMENTAL PROTECTION AGENCY'S
SEVEN CARDINAL RULES OF RISK COMMUNICATION

Accept and involve the public as a legitimate partner.
Plan carefully and evaluate your efforts.
Listen to the public's specific concerns.
Be honest, frank, and open.
Coordinate and collaborate with other credible sources.
Meet the needs of the media.
Speak clearly and with compassion.

Source: Covello and Allen, 1988.

a significant risk of which they may be unaware, or (*b*) to calm concerns about a small risk that the public or decision makers perceive as serious.

With increased public concern over various environmental health risks, increasing demands are placed on environmental health professionals to provide information that explains the nature of risk in clear, comprehensible terms and that conveys credibility and trustworthiness. Increasing attention has been paid to risk communication to respond not only to the public's desire to be informed but also to the need to overcome opposition to decisions and to develop effective alternatives to direct regulatory control. Such alternatives can require greater accountability on the part of individuals, agencies, or private corporations.

It must be stressed that merely disseminating information without relying on communication principles can lead to ineffective messages regarding risk and inadvertently convey ineffective control of a hazard. The U.S. Environmental Protection Agency (EPA) has articulated seven cardinal rules of risk communication (Table 4.2) to prevent such miscommunications. In addition to these rules, it must be emphasized that to provide effective risk communication, the health professional must understand the appropriate technical information that may arise. Because in some countries the public obtains much of the environmental health risk information from the news media, the guidelines for dealing with the media in Box 4.1 are worth considering.

PREVENTION AND CONTROL OF EXPOSURE
TO ENVIRONMENTAL HAZARDS

Framework for Approaching Control Strategies

An essential step in risk management (Fig. 4.1) is the prevention and control of exposures to environmental hazards. In the classic occupational hygiene model of controlling a hazard (as discussed in any industrial hygiene textbook), the ideal situation is to prevent such exposures altogether; this model is known as *control at the source*. Here substitution or enclosure of the hazard as well as other means of control are used. If this cannot be achieved, exposure should be reduced *along the path*—through ventilation, protective barriers, or related measures. As a last resort, exposure should be controlled *at the level of the person*, by means of personal protective equipment, administrative controls, or other primary prevention measures,

BOX 4.1

Tips for Dealing with the Media

1. Don't take the questions personally. If you sound defensive the media will pick that up and push to find out "what you are hiding."
2. Never say "no comment." This is often interpreted by journalists as an admission of guilt. Instead, say why you are unable to comment (e.g., "We are currently investigating the situation and are unable to comment on our findings at this time").
3. Always tell the truth. If there is a problem for which you share in the responsibility (e.g., errors in judgement were made), explain it, but remember to list many positive aspects so that the negative ones will be outweighed (e.g., "We initially had difficulty with our communication procedures, but they have since been corrected and following this fire, the entire emergency plan will be reviewed and improved").
4. Never speculate. Only comment on the facts; the rest is "under investigation," "unconfirmed," or "not known."
5. Don't speak off the record. Unless you have good reasons to believe you can trust the journalist to honor an agreement to allow you to speak off the record, you should consider any comments you make to be fair game in the pursuit of a good story.

OTHER GENERAL TIPS

- Return calls from the media as soon as possible. This gives journalists time to digest the information you give them and build their stories around it, instead of adding it in after most of the story has already been written.
- Come to the interview with two or three key points that you want the journalist to present to the public. Repeat the points several times.
- Assume the journalist has no background in the subject—explain everything.
- Avoid jargon (otherwise they will simplify things for you—possibly incorrectly).
- Come prepared with a written summary of risk information (e.g., outcome diseases, factors, rates, confounders, standards, and guidelines).
- Stay within the limits of your expertise. Refer to others when indicated.
- Do not say more than you want to.
- Do not comment on facts or figures you haven't seen.
- If you don't know, indicate that you want to verify the facts and will get back to them with the information.
- If the questions are becoming repetitive, the health specialist can end the interview by saying "I think we have covered everything. Why don't you call me later if any new questions that occur to you."
- If a reporter is bullying you, remain calm. Asking to have the question repeated gives you time to control the urge to get angry.
- If you are misquoted you have to weigh your injured pride against having the whole issue rehashed. It may be best to just phone the reporter and explain the error. (You may consider sending a polite letter to the reporter so that you have documentation of the corrected version for possible legal purposes.)
- Fight the journalist's tendency to dichotomize risk (i.e., risky? yes/no). Do your best to have them understand the grade of risk.
- At the conclusion of the interview, feel free to ask the journalist about his or her understanding of the issue and what parts of the information you have provided will be used. While journalists are under no obligation to reveal these things, they often will cooperate and it may provide an opportunity to clear up a misunderstanding before it ends up in print.

TABLE 4.3

HIERARCHY OF INDUSTRIAL CONTROLS

Stages

1. CONTROL AT THE SOURCE

Substitution
Engineering controls
General ventilation

2. CONTROL ALONG THE PATH

Exhaust ventilation
Protective barriers

3. CONTROL AT THE LEVEL OF THE PERSON

Personal protective equipment
Training
Administrative controls (e.g., shift rotation)

4. SECONDARY PREVENTION

such as training, or even biological measures, such as immunization. The final measure of controlling a hazard is *secondary prevention*, i.e., early detection of effects of exposure and subsequent remediation. The hierarchy of methods for controlling a hazard is shown in Table 4.3. The same hierarchy of controls can also be used in environmental health hazard control and in setting standards (Fig. 4.2).

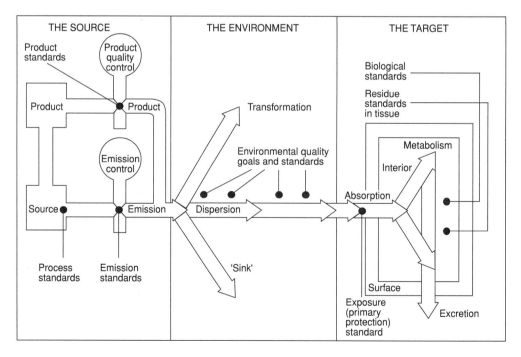

Figure 4.2 Pollutant pathway showing possible points at which standards may be set. From de Koning, 1987, with permission.

It should be noted that control actions may be taken at more than one point. When making decisions regarding the points of intervention and the type or level of control to be used one must take into account the chemical and physical characteristics of the hazard, its transport through the environment, and possible concomitant exposures. Other considerations may include the technology available, the financial resources of both the industry and the government that must enforce the decisions, as well as the legal and cultural traditions of the jurisdictions.

Control at the Source

A hazard may be controlled at the source by eliminating it entirely or by using innovative engineering means to eliminate or minimize exposure to the hazard. A common method of controlling exposures that are not very toxic is *general ventilation* (or *dilution ventilation*) of indoor air, through which large amounts of air are introduced into a workplace (or other hazardous environments) by either natural means, such as opening doors and windows, or the use of fans to move large amounts of air. Rather than removing the contaminants, general ventilation dilutes them in a large volume of air to reach an acceptable concentration of the contaminant. As shown in Figure 4.2, control at the source may be regulated by product standards, process standards, or emission standards.

Product Standards If a substance does not have a known threshold level or has not been adequately tested, it may make sense to redesign the product to minimize the amount of the substance required, or search for a substitute. Governments can ban the use of a substance for specific purposes. Sweden, for example, banned the use of cadmium except in electroplating, pigments, and stabilizers for plastics (and soldering if the product does not come into contact with drinking water or food). Governments may also encourage the use of substitutes by imposing strict labeling requirements.

Process Standards If a pollutant enters the environment during a manufacturing process, governments can encourage the use of other processes for manufacture, through such measures as tax incentives or information exchange programs; legislation is another option. In Japan, for example, the outbreak of Minamata disease prompted the government to require the recycling of all water containing mercury and the replacement of mercury catalysts with other technology.

Emission Standards Emission limits on industrial discharges to air and water, and more recently to soil, have been in place for decades in many jurisdictions. These standards may be expressed in terms of the permissible concentration of a pollutant in units of air emitted or wastewater discharged by a source or in terms of a total load of pollutant per time, unit of production, or unit of energy or materials input. Emission or effluent standards may also be expressed in terms of danger to health or the environment, with a preferred method of control being specified. In this approach, the best available and economically feasible control technology is used.

Standards can also relate to operating practices, including maintenance measures to avoid spills, and measures to promote prompt clean-up, careful storage, and segregation of wastes. They may stipulate rules for cleaning and maintenance of equipment as well as training. Emergency measures may also be required. Many jurisdictions do, in fact, have regulations concerning the packaging, storage, handling, transportation, and disposal of toxic substances.

Control Along the Path

An environmental quality standard (Fig. 4.2) may range from a guideline value designed to provide a degree of health protection, to a regulatory standard with specifications of permissible concentrations of the contaminant, compliance requirements, prescribed sampling method and frequency, and acceptable analytical methods. Calculating acceptable daily intakes (ADIs) for drinking water was discussed in Chapter 3, and the development of threshold limit values (TLVs) will be discussed in Chapter 10.

For chemical hazards, *local exhaust ventilation* is an example of a control that is along the path between the source and the target. Through local exhaust ventilation, airborne contaminants are captured at or near the place where they are generated and removed from the workplace. For some exposures, for example, fumes and gases produced by welding, local exhaust ventilation is much more effective than general ventilation. It is also more economical, as it requires less air to be moved. A local exhaust system usually includes a hood or enclosure, ductwork, an air-cleaning device, and an exhaust fan to draw the contaminated air through the exhaust system and discharge it to the outside. The system must be designed to capture the contaminants before they reach the breathing zone of the workers. Overhead hoods should not be used if their design draws the contaminants through, instead of away from, the workers. Figure 4.3 shows three examples of local exhaust ventilation for welding operations.

For physical hazards such as noise, barriers can be effective, as are acoustic treatment of walls, ceilings, and floor, and increasing the distance between the source and receiver.

Control at the Level of the Target/Person

Particularly in occupational settings, control at the level of the person may also be regulated (the "target"; see Fig. 4.3). *Administrative controls*, which involve reducing the number of exposed workers and the duration of exposure, are fraught with controversy. Clearly, only those workers needed for a job should be in an area that is hazardous. Maintenance workers, electricians, cleaners, or other workers should do their job when the hazardous process is not in operation. Maintenance workers may be more highly exposed to hazards than operational workers since procedures are often not developed for their protection and their work often requires close proximity to hazardous plant processes. Thus, special provisions for the protection of maintenance workers must be included in chemical safety procedures. Although a reduction in the length of time or the frequency of exposure of workers may be achieved by a system of job rotation, it is not acceptable to simply expose more workers less often to unacceptably high levels as an alternative to reducing exposure levels.

Personal protective equipment (PPE) should be used only after substitution and engineering controls have been fully considered and have been implemented as much as is feasible. Personal protective equipment includes face masks, respira-

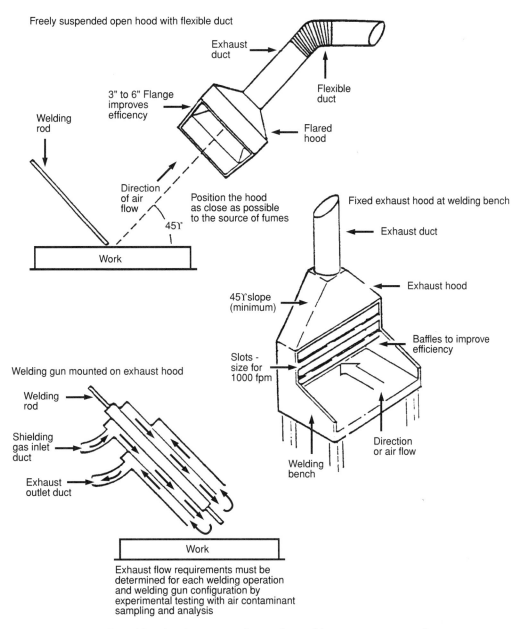

Freely suspended open hood with flexible duct

Exhaust duct

Flexible duct

3" to 6" Flange improves efficency

Flared hood

Welding rod

Direction of air flow

Position the hood as close as possible to the source of fumes

45°

Work

Fixed exhaust hood at welding bench

Exhaust duct

Exhaust hood

45° slope (minimum)

Baffles to improve efficiency

Slots - size for 1000 fpm

Direction or air flow

Welding gun mounted on exhaust hood

Welding bench

Welding rod

Shielding gas inlet duct

Exhaust outlet duct

Work

Exhaust flow requirements must be determined for each welding operation and welding gun configuration by experimental testing with air contaminant sampling and analysis

Figure 4.3 Examples of local exhaust ventilation for welding. Source: Fact Sheet From Hamilton, Ontario, with permission. Canadian Center for Occupational Health and Safety (CCOHS).

tors, gloves, rubber boots, protective clothing, goggles and safety glasses, hard hats, and hearing protection. Table 4.4 summarizes the steps and resources required for a PPE program. Figure 4.4 shows a uranium miner with PPE and monitoring equipment. The International Program on Chemical Safety (IPCS) has provided guidelines for using PPE and for choosing the proper equipment (see *How to Use the IPCS Health and Safety Guides*, UNEP/ILO/WHO, 1993).

Other measures at the level of the target or exposed individual include immunization against infectious hazards. Guidelines regarding which workers

TABLE 4.4

CHECKLIST FOR PERSONAL PROTECTIVE EQUIPMENT PROGRAMS

Correct equipment
Thorough training program
Fit test
Regular equipment maintenance
Secure and clean place of storage for each individual's set of
   equipment

should receive which immunizations are provided by various international agencies and associations. When carrying out such a program it is important to consider several issues, such as whether immunizations should be made mandatory or voluntary, what risks are involved, what the implications are for the individual when immunity fails to develop, or what the consequences are of development of the disease in question.

Health Education as a Risk Management Tool

Many health risks have a behavioral component. For instance, in an occupational setting, protective clothing can be provided that gives adequate protection against exposure but that is not comfortable to work in, thus employees may not want to wear them at all times during working hours. Furthermore, safety guidelines or procedures may not be followed for various reasons, e.g., they are time consuming or considered to be redundant.

When it became generally accepted that diseases should be prevented rather than cured, the importance of health education in the promotion of public health also became obvious. There are a number of instruments that can be used to educate the public, including TV spots, billboards, and local meetings. A frequently occurring misconception, however, is that the transfer of knowledge and relevant information to the population of interest alone will result in behavioral change. To achieve a lasting behavioral change, a number of crucial steps have to be taken:

Problem analysis: characterizing the relationship between the health problem and human behavior.

Behavior determinants: identifying the factors that determine specific behaviors.

Options for changing behavior: assessing the relative importance of such determinants and the extent to which they can be changed

Intervention plan: determining how behavior can be changed most successfully

Intervention implementation: carrying out the intervention to change behavior

Evaluation: ascertaining the effect of the intervention.

When the relationship between the health problem and human behavior is not well established, or when behavior is only of minor influence on the extent of the problem, an intervention plan for changing behavior is not likely to improve public health significantly.

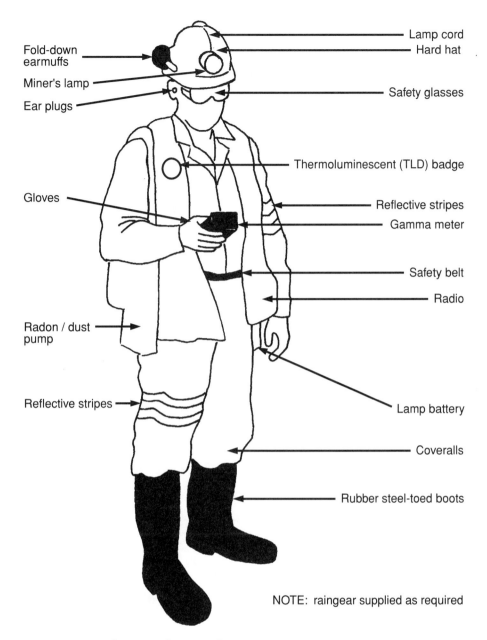

Figure 4.4 Miner with PPE and personal monitoring equipment. From Cameco, 1996, with permission.

The most important types of determinants of behavior include attitude, social influences, perceived behavioral control, skills, and barriers (see Box 4.2 and Fig. 4.5). When trying to change specific behavioral elements, it is essential to understand the reasons behind the undesired behavior. An individual may intend to show the desired behavior but is simply not capable of doing so. For example, someone may want to reduce exposure to organic solvents from paint by using water-based paints, but cannot achieve this goal for various reasons: these

A Theory of Planned Behavior

The main determinants of behavior according to the theory of planned behavior (Ajzen, 1991) are indicated in Figure 4.4. In this model, intentions are assumed to capture the motivational factors that determine the behavior and indicate how hard people are willing to perform the behavior under consideration. The first determinant of an intention is *attitude*, which refers to the degree to which an individual has a favorable or unfavorable evaluation of the behavior. The second determinant refers to the perceived *social pressure* to perform or renounce the behavior. Perceived behavioral *control* is indicated as the third predictor. This factor refers to the perceived difficulty or ease of performing the behavior and is assumed to reflect past experience as well as anticipated impediments and obstacles. However, a strong intention to engage in a behavior does not necessarily imply that one is successful in performing it. Nonmotivational factors such as the availability of resources (money, cooperation, skills) or opportunities determine people's actual control over their behavior.

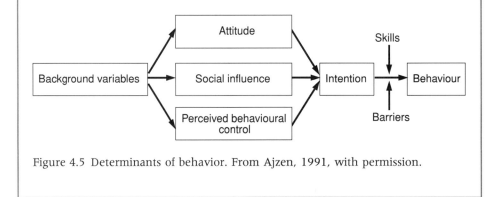

Figure 4.5 Determinants of behavior. From Ajzen, 1991, with permission.

paints are not available in that town (lack of the alternative option), or they are too expensive (financial barrier).

Other conceptual models have also been developed to help health promotion professionals to carry out their duties. One model, which builds upon the Ottawa Charter's definition of health promotion as activities that enable people to increase control over the determinants of their health, is known as the PRECEDE–PROCEED model (Green and Kreuter, 1999). It uses educational approaches to influence the *p*redisposing factors to unhealthy choices through direct communication, the *r*einforcing factors through promoting changes in values that support lifestyle choices, and the *e*nabling factors to permit these changes through training and organization. While the PRECEDE part of the model addresses the predisposing, reinforcing and enabling constructs in *e*ducational and ecological *d*iagnosis and *e*valuation, the PROCEED part addresses the *p*olicy, *r*egulatory, and *o*rganizational *c*onstructs in *e*ducational and *e*nvironmental development. Box 4.3 elaborates on this model and how it relates to the DPSEEA framework used elsewhere in this text.

BOX 4.3

The PRECEDE–PROCEED Model of Health Promotion and its Relation to the DPSEEA Framework

The figure below illustrates the PRECEDE–PROCEED model (Green and Kreuter, 1999), indicating that the place to start is to conduct a social assessment in a community, ascertaining the perspectives of the community members, their hopes, aspirations and concerns. Next, an epidemiological assessment is conducted to ascertain the health problems and risk factors. Phase 3 involves identifying the health-related behavioral as well as physical environmental factors that may be predisposing (e.g., knowledge, attitude, values of the individuals concerned), reinforcing (e.g., attitude and behavior of decision-makers) and enabling factors (e.g., availability of resources and skills) underlying the concerns identified. Phase 4 focuses on assessing the policy and administrative issues that must be addressed, and phases 6 through 9 are the implementation, process evaluation, impact evaluation, and outcome evaluation steps.

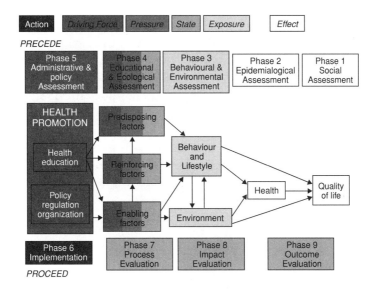

—*adapted from Green and Kreuter 1999*

The shading in the PRECEDE-PROCEED figure corresponds to the shading in the top boxes, which relate to the DPSEEA framework introduced earlier and elaborated upon in Chapter 8. The social and health effects in the Driving Force-Pressure-State-Exposure-Effect-Action model are examined first. The exposure then corresponds to the behavioral and environmental conditions, with pressure relating to the ecological and educational factors. The driving forces are the policy, regulatory, and organizational determinants; and the action and evaluation phase then corresponds to phase 6–9 of the PROCEED model.

The DPSEEA framework grew out of the environmental movement, whereas the PRECEDE–PROCEED model was developed by health promotion experts. The point to note is that there has been a convergence of ideas over the last decade or so, with health promotion specialists and environmental activists both coming to realize the importance of a transdisciplinary and comprehensive approach.

—*contributed by Dr. Jerry Spiegel*

Methods of environmental and exposure monitoring were discussed earlier, as were the pros and cons of biological monitoring and various methods of health surveillance. *Risk monitoring* can be considered a form of auditing the effectiveness of the combination of risk management approaches used. The variables used in risk monitoring are often called *indicators*. Such indicators should be reliable, easy to measure year after year, closely connected to health risks or measurable outcomes, and closely related to the opportunity for exposure to environmental hazards. Also, health outcomes that are used for this purpose should occur within a short time after exposure. Some indicators that have been proposed for use in monitoring environmental health status in populations are the rate of diarrheal diseases (reflecting water quality), the frequency of asthmatic attacks among individuals with known asthma (reflecting air quality), the rate of new cases of leptospirosis (reflecting exposure to rats), the rate of new cases of noise-induced hearing loss (reflecting exposure to noise in the workplace), and the level of lead in blood tests of people living in an area (reflecting exposure to lead in the community).

Some of these indicators, such as diarrheal diseases, are more specifically related to environmental exposures than others. Asthma rates are not as good indicators as one might expect because the connection with environmental exposure is complicated by many other factors that provoke asthmatic attacks, some of which, such as allergen exposure, may be more powerful than air pollution in causing an effect. Likewise, cancer rates do not work very well for ongoing monitoring of exposure to environmental hazards because the effects are delayed by many years. Indicators that are properly chosen to be informative and practical in a given situation provide a picture of how the environmental health risks experienced by a population are changing and how well public health and environmental measures are controlling the risk. They are also useful for comparing the performance of environmental measures in one country or administrative unit to that in another for setting priorities in controlling risk, or for demonstrating the presence of a hazard requiring attention.

Health Surveillance Systems

Periodic health surveillance is conducted by performing a routine standardized set of tests for the early identification of some (often specific) health problems at regular intervals, usually annually. It is often applied to workers who are exposed to a particular hazard to detect occupational disorders early and to prevent them from getting worse. Use of periodic chest X-rays to identify occupational lung diseases, such as silicosis and asbestosis, has played a major role in controlling these diseases. Unfortunately, periodic health surveillance alone cannot prevent occupational diseases and is ineffective for many disorders such as lung cancer and others, for which the conditions shown in Box 4.4 are not met. It is important to stress that screening tests are only part of a surveillance program. To have effective surveillance, the group results must be analyzed and given to the authorities responsible for correcting the problem, and there must be a commitment to act upon these results. An example of an effective surveillance program is shown in Box

BOX 4.4

Principles to Apply in Choosing Screening Tests for
Surveillance Programs

1. The test must be sensitive and specific. *Sensitivity* refers to the proportion of diseased persons in the population who are correctly identified by the test. *Specificity* refers to the proportion of nondiseased individuals who are correctly identified as such by the test. (An insensitive but specific test may yield many
false-negative results (c), whereas a sensitive but nonspecific test may give many
false positives (b). Note that a *positive predictive value* refers to the proportion of
persons who have a positive test and are truly diseased. A *negative predictive value*
refers to the proportion of persons who have a negative test and are not diseased.
These two indices depend on the sensitivity and specificity of the test and the
prevalence of the disease. They are quoted less often than the sensitivity and
specificity of a test, but should be considered when discussing the usefulness of
a screening test.
2. The test must be simple and inexpensive.
3. The test must be safe. The test must have a very high degree of safety as it is
meant to be applied to a large number of normal people who likely have only a
very small risk of the condition in question.
4. The test must be acceptable. The test cannot be inconvenient, time consuming,
uncomfortable, or unpleasant to the subjects being offered the screening.

Source: Fletcher et al., 1982.

4.5. In this case, only when biological monitoring for occupational lead poisoning
through centralized reporting of blood lead results was combined with industrial
hygiene controls and enforcement of lead in air criteria did a sustained decrease
in occupational lead poisoning occur (Yassi et al., 1991, 1996).

Environmental Health Indicators

In the process of monitoring risk management, it is particularly important to establish and use appropriate environmental health indicators. There have been
significant efforts in the international arena to establish a common set of indicators with which to evaluate environmental health policy. For example, experts
came together for this very purpose in March 1993 at The Consultation on Environment and Health Indicators for Use with a Health and Geographic Information System (HEGIS) for Europe, where they defined key environmental, socioeconomic, and health indicators for use in the European region. The potential
environmental indicators are shown in Table 4.5. General health descriptors for
which data already exist at a sufficient level of detail and reliability were restricted to measures of mortality and morbidity. Some potential health indicators
considered are shown in Table 4.6 (see Corvalan and Kjellström, 1995 or Briggs
et al., 1996, or WRI, 1998 for full discussion).

BOX 4.5

Example of an Effective Occupational Lead Poisoning Surveillance Program

An analysis was conducted of 16,199 blood lead samples from employees of nine high-risk workplaces in Manitoba, 1979–94, as part of an integrated regulated occupational surveillance system. Adjusted median blood lead levels were analyzed, as was the proportion of levels above the regulatory target over the years. Trends in individual workers and in each of the targeted firms were also examined.

It was found that a 1979 government regulation specifying the maximum allowable lead in blood as 3.38 μmol/liter (70 μg/dl) was followed by a drop in blood lead concentrations; the 1983 order to reduce maximum allowable blood lead concentrations to below 2.90 μmol/liter (60 μg/dl) was not followed by such a decrease. Longitudinal analysis by individual worker suggested that companies were complying by using administrative control—i.e., removing workers to lower-lead areas until blood lead levels had fallen, then returning them to high-lead areas. In 1987 a further order was issued that required removal of workers from a site when their blood lead level was 2.40 μmol/liter (50 μg/dl) and limited environmental exposure to 50 μg/m^3. This new integrated approach succeeded in bringing about a significant reduction in blood lead concentrations overall as well as in most of the high-risk companies. Moreover, this seems to have been accomplished in most companies without their having to rely on worker rotation.

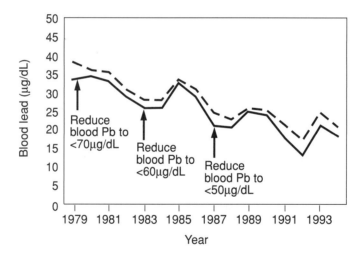

The study concluded that while having an appropriately stringent blood lead target is essential, focusing upon blood lead as the sole criterion for compliance is ineffective. Regulations must specifically require environmental monitoring and exposure controls, with biological surveillance serving to ensure effectiveness of these measures. The analysis that was conducted illustrates the usefulness of a comprehensive, centralized surveillance system linked to inspections and enforcement, as it was invaluable in targeting preventive measures and ensuring the effectiveness of regulatory efforts.

Source: Yassi et al., 1991, 1996.

TABLE 4.5

POTENTIAL ENVIRONMENTAL INDICATORS FOR HEALTH RISK ASSESSMENT

Substance	Indicator and Medium	Proxy/Surrogate
AIR QUALITY INDICATORS		
SO_2	Concentration in air	Exceeding WHO or national guidelines
		Emission
		Use of coal for domestic heating/cooking
NO_2	Concentration in air	Exceeding WHO or national guidelines
		Emissions
		Use of gas for domestic heating/cooking
		Traffic density
Particulates	$TSP/PM_{10}PM_{2.5}$	Exceeding WHO or national guidelines
	Concentration in air	Black smoke
		Emissions of TSP
		Use of coal
Ozone	Concentration in air	
CO	Concentration in air	Emissions
		Traffic density, city gas usage
WATER QUALITY INDICATORS		
Drinking-water quality	Hardness, water color, taste, pH	Water treatment
	Conductivity/TSS	
	VOC, TOC	
	Nitrates, nitrites, phosphates	
MULTIMEDIA AND OTHER INDICATORS		
VOCs	Concentration of specific VOCs in air and water	Emissions
		Petrol usage
PAHs	Concentration of benzo(a)pyrene in air and food	Small-scale wood and coal burning
		Traffic density
Metals and trace elements	Concentration of Cd, Pb, As, Hg in human tissue	Concentration in air, water, soil, food
		Emissions
	Concentration of Al in drinking water	
Persistent organic chemicals	Concentration of PCBs, dioxin, etc., in human tissue	Concentration in air, food, water
		Emissions
		Production/consumption
Pesticides	Concentration in food	Pesticides use
	Concentration in soil, water	Sales
	Concentration in human tissue	Land use
Nitrates	Concentration of nitrate, nitrite, phosphate, etc., in surface water	Fertilizer usage
		Additive use
	Concentration in groundwater, food	

(Continued)

TABLE 4.5

POTENTIAL ENVIRONMENTAL INDICATORS FOR HEALTH RISK ASSESSMENT
(*continued*)

Substance	Indicator and Medium	Proxy/Surrogate
Pathogens and allergens	Foodborne pathogens	Concentration
	Waterborne pathogens	Land use/vegetation
	Airborne allergens (e.g., pollen)	Humidity
	Indoor allergens	Housing quality
		Water treatment
		Wastewater treatment
		Food hygiene
Radiation	Activity of radon in household air	Geology
	Solar radiation	
	Radiation equivalent of food	Sunshine/cloudiness
Exposure to tobacco smoke	Cotinine in urine	Particle concentration in indoor air
		Mutagenicity of air
		Tobacco consumption
		Smoke controls in public buildings, etc.
Nuisances	Nuisance caused by odors	Complaints, waste treatment
	Noise levels in home	Complaints, noise emissions
	Traffic noise	Traffic density

PAH, polycyclic aromatic hydrocarbons; PCB, polychlorinated biphenyl; TOC, total organic carbon; TSP, total suspended particulates; TSS, total suspended solids; VOC, volatile organic compounds.

The linkage between environmental indicators and health indicators is key to accurate monitoring of environmental or occupational health risks (Briggs et al., 1996; Corvalan et al., 1997). To visualize these linkages, Corvalan and Kjellström (1995) developed the driving force–pressure–state–exposure–effect–action (DPSEEA) framework (Fig. 4.6) as an adaptation of the pressure–state–response (PSR) framework used by the Organization for Economic Cooperation and Development (OECD) and the United Nations in the development of indicators for sustainable development monitoring. The environmental indicators listed in Table 4.5 are primarily state indicators and some of the proxy/surrogate indicators are pressure or driving-force indicators. Figure 4.5 highlights the importance of exposure in environmental health risk monitoring and the need to include action indicators in monitoring risk management implementation. A recent example of use of the DPSEEA framework by a community to assist in developing indicators to evaluate interventions aimed at improving health in an urban ecosystem is provided by Yassi et al. (1999).

SPECIAL PROBLEMS IN MANAGING ENVIRONMENTAL HEALTH RISKS

Approach to Environmental Health Concerns of Individuals

Occupational and environmental medicine is the medical specialty dedicated to identifying, evaluating, treating, and preventing occupational disorders and, by ex-

TABLE 4.6

POTENTIAL HEALTH INDICATORS FOR ENVIRONMENTAL ASSESSMENT

General Indicators	Mortality	Morbidity
Perceived health	Life expectancy at birth	Asthma
Body mass index	All causes of death	Chronic obstructive diseases
Healthy life expectancy	(age and gender standardized)	Lung cancer
Birth weight	Premature death (0–64)	Leukemia
	Cause-specific deaths	Stomach cancer
		Mesothelioma
		Skin cancer
		Allergies/hypersensitivity
		Cardiovascular diseases
		Infectious diseases
		Congenital abnormalities
		Chronic liver diseases
		Occupational diseases
		Spontaneous abortions
		Acute poisonings

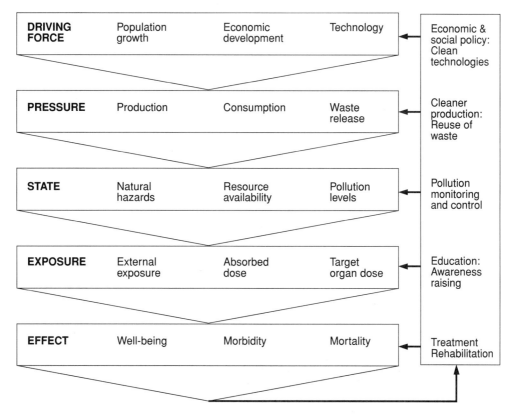

Figure 4.6 Framework for environmental health indicators. Modified from Corvalan and Kjellström, 1995, with permission.

tension, to the evaluation of disorders suspected of arising from environmental factors. Thus persons who believe they have developed a health problem caused by the environment should consult a specialist in occupational and environmental medicine, if possible.

Although the general field of occupational and environmental medicine has a history that goes back to the writings of ancient times, the specialty started in 1700, when an Italian physician named Bernardino Ramazzini wrote the first comprehensive treatise on the subject. In recent years the scope of occupational medicine practice has expanded to include environmentally related disease as well as disorders that are clearly work related. Except where the provision of specialized medical services is required by law, as in France, occupational medicine is a small specialty worldwide and its practitioners tend to work for governments, universities, or large companies. However, any physician can apply the essential principles of occupational and environmental medicine. It is also possible for physicians and other health professionals outside the specialty to play an important role in managing risk.

The first step in addressing a potential environmental health concern in an individual is to identify whether one truly exists. The process here involves (1) diagnosing the disease, which, in turn is based on symptom history and pattern, physical examination, and laboratory investigations; (2) evaluating exposures; and (3) determining, usually through literature review, whether the exposure could have caused the diseases in question. Recognition of occupational injuries is usually obvious. Recognition of occupational and environmental diseases, however, can be very difficult. Many occupational and environmental diseases look like diseases from other causes and can be identified only by taking a careful occupational and environmental history. This is part of the physician's interview when he or she asks patients what they have done for a living and to what they have been exposed in their work and community. The occupational history gives many clues that the physician can follow in determining whether a patient's problem is work related.

Environmental diseases are often more subtle, but many cases do arise from specific events, such as a pesticide spraying incident or an industrial accident in the community. In environmental medicine, it is often difficult to know whether an illness actually exists; patients are often referred for evaluation because their physicians are not sure what the health effects of an exposure might be, and they need reassurance of their diagnosis.

Diagnosis is usually less of a problem in occupational diseases than establishing whether a condition is work related. For example, it may be difficult to prove that a cancer was associated with exposure to asbestos 20 years before. Carpal tunnel syndrome, which is a painful neurological disorder caused by compression of a nerve in the wrist, can be caused by many factors unrelated to work, such as pregnancy and some diseases, but it can also be work related in people whose work involves repeated motion of the wrists. Environmental diseases are often more difficult to pin down with certainty. Some conditions, such as cancer, and certain types of lung disease may result from exposures that took place years before.

The second step in addressing an environmental health concern is usually treatment. There is usually no special treatment for an occupational or environmental disorder that is much different from the treatment of the same disorder from any other cause. Removal from exposure is the most important aspect of treatment.

The third step is rehabilitation, the process of overcoming and accommodating the results of the injury or illness. Usually, the healing process and therapy will restore much of the function that has been lost temporarily after an injury, but there may still be some permanent impairment. In occupational and environmental disease, it is more common for the condition to present itself at a late stage and for there to be limited potential for rehabilitation. As statistics overwhelmingly illustrate, the longer the worker is away from work following, for example, a back injury, the less the chance of successful reintegration into the workplace. Thus early intervention and early return to work using modified work programs are essential. Similarly, the prognosis for recovery from a disease such as occupational asthma is increased dramatically by early recognition and vocational rehabilitation (i.e., removing the worker from exposure to an alternate suitable job).

Impairment assessment is the physician's measurement of the degree to which the patient has lost function as a result of the disorder. For example, reduced strength or loss of motion resulting from an occupational injury can be measured, as can a patient's reduced capacity to breathe and perform physical activity because of lung disease. Unfortunately, pain cannot be measured objectively, and this leads to many problems in impairment assessment. This assessment is important in determining whether a worker can go back to work and the degree of permanent disability that has resulted. Permanent disability is reflected in the benefits given to a worker under workers' compensation and may figure into the award given to a person who has sued in an environmental case.

In practice, there are almost always several members of the team involved in assessing and managing an environmental health problem, whether for a population or for individuals. Box 4.6 gives an example of a multidisciplinary environmental health team assessing and managing a common workplace health risk.

Managing an Environmental Health Emergency

A true environmental health emergency is best managed by a specialist with training in toxicology, epidemiology, and public health. Such specialists are in short supply, however, and may not be on the scene when an incident occurs. Almost any health practitioner may be presented with a problem related to hazardous exposures. In rural or remote areas, practitioners may have to serve, in cooperation with public safety engineers and technicians, as consultants on environmental health hazards without preparation.

In discussing the role of the environmental health professional in managing an environmental health emergency, we must consider four main areas: (*1*) what the practitioner does in an emergency, (*2*) how the practitioner deals with cases of suspected toxicity, (*3*) how the practitioner deals with the "worried well" who fear toxicity but are probably affected, and (*4*) how the practitioner deals with workers involved in clean-up operations. A careful methodological approach to managing an emergency is just as important as having a detailed knowledge of the hazards involved. Three commonsense steps are generally followed. The first

BOX 4.6

A Health Surveillance Program to Monitor the Risk of Noise-Induced Hearing Loss

Noise control and hearing conservation provide an example of how occupational health standards, periodic health surveillance, hazard control, personal protection, occupational medicine, and company policies are interlinked to control an occupational health problem. Authors of the WHO Environmental Health Criteria on Noise (WHO, 1980a) concluded that, although noise-induced hearing loss occurs at 75 dB, many countries have adopted an occupational exposure level of 90 dB averaged over an 8-hr working shift; it is considered too expensive to require reductions to lower exposures. Factories and other workplaces that have noise levels approaching 90 dB are required to carry out noise surveys; the noise is measured with sound level meters and dosimeters (which average the noise over a work shift). If the noise level averages 85 dB or more, the employer must put a hearing conservation program into place, but as WHO investigators (1980a) point out, it would be better to establish such programs at 75 dB.

Hearing conservation measures include controlling sources of noise (through use of acoustic tiles, soundproof containers, sound-absorbing mounts for vibrating equipment, and whatever else is necessary), making available to workers an assortment of personal hearing protection (ear plugs, ear muffs), and providing annual audiometric screening examinations. Using a device called an audiometer, a technician tests the ability of workers to hear tones played at different frequencies; the loudness required for the worker to first hear the tone is recorded as the threshold of hearing. When workers lose hearing at a particular tone, it is called a *permanent threshold shift*.

Noise-induced hearing loss starts with a specific loss at the frequency 4000 Hz and gets worse thereafter. This is unfortunate, because this same frequency is the mid-range of human speech, which means that workers who develop noise-induced hearing loss find it difficult to understand speech and to follow a conversation. An early sign of hearing loss is prolonged ringing in the worker's ears or a temporary threshold shift in the ability to hear, which goes away after a few hours.

When these signs are present or a permanent threshold shift is first noticed, the occupational physician must determine whether the cause is truly noise exposure, whether the noise was associated with work (some workers listen to loud music, have hobbies such as shooting guns, or have had their hearing impaired from gunfire in military service), and how great the impairment is. If a new case of noise-induced hearing loss is identified, the system of protecting workers from hearing loss has somehow failed and that part of the workplace where impairment occurs requires attention to improve noise control.

All parts of this hearing conservation program must work together, including the record-keeping, the prevention of noise-induced hearing loss, and identification of new cases as early as possible while there is still time to prevent severe hearing loss. This is also an example of how screening programs and other procedures applied to groups of workers end up benefiting individuals and identifying individual needs.

step is to evaluate the problem; the second is to contain it; and the third and main step in which the environmental health professional (or other practitioner) is involved is management of the health effects (Guidotti, 1986).

Step 1: Evaluate The Problem The major role of the health practitioner at this step is as an advisor and resource for technical information. To perform this role, the health professional needs the most accurate possible information on the following:

What hazardous substances are involved?

What are their toxic and safety hazards?

How many people have been exposed and how many may be exposed in the near future?

Among these people, are there any who may be at exceptionally high risk?

This information may change constantly during a real episode. In a typical incident, there are innumerable false reports, doubts, and updates. The practitioner involved must be prepared to be flexible.

Correct identification of the substances involved is essential. Labels on drums may be misleading because drums are often recycled. Samples should be taken by an environmental health specialist or industrial hygienist who wears suitable personal protective equipment. Unless there is a compelling reason to act, such as during a fire or a rapid leak, it is usually wise to let the material rest where it is until the material is identified and suitable precautions can be taken. If an emergency forces action before the material is identified, the only prudent move is to assume the worst unless one has evidence that the material is not highly toxic. Unidentified materials usually turn out to be fairly benign. Until they are identified, however, they often cause great anxiety by requiring the use of full protective gear by emergency response personnel. Once the identity of a material is known, the hazard potential must be determined. There are a number of sources of information on the toxicology and safety hazard of common industrial and commercial chemicals.

Users of hazardous materials are required by law in many jurisdictions to keep on file a Material Safety Data Sheet (MSDS) prepared by the manufacturer (see Chapter 3). The MSDSs usually give reasonable information on the safety hazard of chemical formulations, but they are almost always incomplete in their descriptions of the compound's toxic effects and are usually weak or missing information on chronic effects. Many chemical formulations are proprietary mixtures, thus their formulations are considered trade secrets and the MSDS may not identify specific chemicals or their proportions. The MSDSs in the files of many companies are also often incomplete, and not all pertinent MSDSs may be available on short notice.

Other sources of information, such as medical libraries, are familiar to physicians for clinical information. Law libraries also often have information on toxicology. Both usually carry the standard reference works in toxicology and can order computerized literature searches for users. Many familiar medical texts have pertinent information on toxic exposures. Poison Control Centers can be excellent sources of information and advice. Box 4.7 lists reference materials available from agencies in the International Program on Chemical Safety (IPCS) that provide information on specific environmental hazards.

The next part of the evaluation of a hazard presented by an incident is to find out what is happening to the toxic material at the site. Once spilled, the waste seeps into the ground, through the soil, and often into groundwater. The possible migration of the waste materials is an important issue to address in the initial assessment. A clear idea of how the chemical will spread is very important in determining who is likely to become exposed to. For example:

If the incident is a gas leak, how many homes are downwind?

If the incident involves a liquid waste seeping into the ground, how many families draw their water from local wells?

If the liquid waste is flowing downhill as surface runoff, perhaps into a storm drain or stream, where does the water go?

How many children in the area might play in or explore the site?

Will the prevailing winds carry a plume away from or toward residents?

If groundwater is contaminated, is drinking water or irrigation water likely to be fouled?

If it rains or if snow melts, will surface run carry the waste off-site?

If drinking-water supplies are contaminated, must water be supplied to residents?

Not everyone in the community will actually be exposed, of course, and for purposes of planning a medical response, it is important to consider the characteristics of the persons who may actually come into contact with the material. Children may develop skin rashes from direct contact: fumes may be merely annoying to the young and healthy, but could be troublesome or life threatening to the elderly, those who have cardiovascular or pulmonary diseases, to infants, or to asthmatics. Pregnant women require special attention to protect mother and foetus. Knowledge of the community at risk allows health authorities to warn susceptible individuals to take protective measures or to leave the area.

Step 2: Contain the Problem The next step in managing an environmental health emergency is to establish control over the situation to minimize the potential of exposure. This requires teamwork among police, fire, and public health authorities and obviously varies with the nature of the incident. The physician still serves as an advisor in this step. In more complex situations, coordination among and with local authorities is essential. Fire departments are usually best equipped to handle safety hazards but often need advice and assistance in dealing with toxic materials. The most difficult situations, such as fires involving multiple toxic substances, known and unknown, pose serious threats to public safety personnel and may require on-site medical presence.

In extreme situations, evacuation may be unavoidable. The mental health consequences of evacuation are great and this extreme step should never be taken without good reason. Large-scale population evacuations carry a high cost in stress and safety, as well as the potential for violence.

An important aspect of containing the problem is to prevent public overreaction. An incident like this provokes rumors and misinformation that must be set straight to avoid panic or misguided interference in public safety measures. Early establishment of a rumor control committee, a hotline, and good working relations with the media can be very valuable. It is particularly important to funnel all public information, whenever possible, through a single spokesperson. Otherwise, slight differences of opinion, interpretation, and understanding may look like confusion, uncertainty, and rivalry among responsible authorities.

Step 3: Manage the Health Effects Most practitioners feel uncertain and overwhelmed when called on to deal with complex toxic exposures. Although these cases are admittedly complex, there are certain guidelines that can be followed. There are two separate problems that the health practitioner faces: evaluation of persons who probably were exposed and evaluation of the "worried well" who are concerned about the possibility of exposure and need to be reassured. Medical emergencies involving hazardous substances are less common than situations in which people believe themselves to have been exposed to a toxic substance and seek medical evaluation. When the substance is known, an appropriate medical evaluation can be derived. When the substance is not known or involves a complex mixture, the appropriate medical evaluation may be difficult to determine.

Many incidents involve multiple exposures or substances that have multiple effects. It is good practice to provide a basic comprehensive evaluation in all cases. When an individual presents with a specific clinical complaint, it is important not to focus the evaluation too narrowly because important findings may be missed. A basic battery of tests may be recommended, but information collected may not always be useful and careful thought must be put to ease of interpretation before tests are ordered.

An important role for the environmental health practitioner is the protection of workers engaged in cleanup and control activities at the site. The practitioner should inquire about the availability of suitable protective gear, decontamination procedures, and the presence of security and emergency services. One should emphasize to the workers the importance of not smoking and eating on the site, of checking oxygen levels before entering any confined space, using the buddy system (always working with a companion with access to rescue equipment), and leaving contaminated clothes at the site. It is important to stress that managing an environmental emergency is a multidisciplinary activity that requires clear lines of authority, excellent communication with decision makers and the public, and a strong sense of well-coordinated teamwork.

COST-EFFECTIVENESS AND COST-BENEFIT ANALYSIS OF INTERVENTIONS

The use of *benefit-cost analysis* (BCA) in managing environmental health risks has expanded rapidly in recent years. Basically, in this analytical technique the present value of benefits is compared with the present value of the costs to determine the net present value of the management option under review. *Cost-effectiveness analysis* (CEA) is similar to BCA in its treatment of costs, however, the consequences of interventions (i.e., results, impacts, effects, outcomes) are not valued. Instead, the purpose of this analysis is merely to determine the costs in relation to the benefit achieved, measured in terms of natural units, e.g., additional years of life, case of disease incidence, etc.

BCA & CEA provide practical techniques for determining whether resources are being allocated efficiently in achieving objectives. In this regard they provide powerful tools for planning & evaluating alternative programs related to environmental health risks.

In BCA the value of the benefits is compared with the value of the costs, with each of these measurements entailing three steps: (*1*) *identification* of the type of effects, (*2*) *quantification* in concrete terms, and (*3*) *valuation*. First, all items of cost must be identified, uninhibited by potential measurement difficulties. The costs to be considered include the initial design and implementation of the program, as well as the annual cost of enforcing and maintaining it. Producer costs must be also identified, including, for example, the private sector's real resource costs of complying with the regulations and the extent to which this will likely be passed on to the consumer.

The second step is to determine how much each item will cost, and in which year. It is important to include the degree of uncertainty associated with crude measurements of cost estimates, which is best conducted in a sensitivity analysis.

In the third part of the BCA, valuation, these costs over time must be converted into common values. Similarly, benefits as well as any potential ripple effects must be identified. Direct benefits may include lives saved on a statistical basis, life-years gained, reduction in morbidity or mortality, and savings in the cost of health care and social services because the population is healthier. Direct economic benefits, such as increases in productive output, should also be included, as well as the less direct health benefits, such as increased aesthetic value of a cleaner environment, reduction in pain, fear, and anxiety, increased freedom from nuisance, and sense of fairness. The step of measuring these benefits is considerably complex, as measurement of health effects associated with environmental hazards is a subject of considerable uncertainty. Epidemiological studies are relatively insensitive in detecting small effects and there are discrepancies between toxicological studies and human observations. The degree of uncertainty must therefore also be taken into consideration in the overall analysis.

Finally, in order to be compared for policy purposes the value of health improvements converted into a common currency (such as U.S. dollars, yen, or Deutsch marks in a particular year) or scale (such as lives or DALYs). The period in which these improvements will occur is also specified (such as 5, 10, or 20 years). The steps involved in conducting BCA and CEA studies are summarized in Table 4.7.

Many valuation methods are described in the environmental health literature. These include the *cost-of-illness* approach, which estimates direct and indirect costs associated with the avoidance of disease damages together with costs associated with any behaviors taken to avoid exposure to risk; and *contingent valuation* methods, which measure individuals' willingness-to-pay preferences in monetary terms according to how they view changes in utility associated with risk changes. This can be established by asking strategically designed questions about how much individuals would be willing to pay for a certain reduction in the risk of a certain health problem, or by comparing people's relative ranking

TABLE 4.7

SUMMARY OF STEPS INVOLVED IN CONDUCTING BENEFIT-COST AND COST-EFFECTIVENESS ANALYSES

1. Define the study scope and objectives.
2. Define and measure the outcomes or effects of each option under analysis.
3. Identify, measure, and value all costs.
4. Identify, measure, and value all benefits.
5. Compare the costs with benefits, along with sensitivity tests of the magnitude of the costs and benefits where uncertainty may exist regarding measures of outcome or its value.
6. Define the implications of the results for presentation to decision makers.

BOX 4.8

Case Study—Pollution in Japan: Prevention Would Have Been Better and Cheaper Than Cure

In the 1950s and 1960s Japan experienced a period of rapid industrialization and economic growth, but little attention was paid to the environmental consequences. The result was high levels of pollutants in the air, water, and soil in some areas and several infamous outbreaks of diseases. Strong corrective action was taken in the 1970s and 1980s to redress the most severe problems. Three conclusions emerge from the examples given below: allowing the release of toxic substances into the environment can lead to serious health consequences and economic losses; preventing the problem, as Japan is doing now, is less costly than cleaning it up; and taking corrective action now is less costly than allowing problems to persist.

CASE 1: SULFUR DIOXIDE IN THE AIR

Between 1956 and 1973 one of Japan's largest petrochemical complexes was constructed at Yokkaichi City. By 1960 air pollution was causing local concern, and by 1963 1-hr average sulfur dioxide levels exceeded 2800 $\mu g/m^3$, far above the WHO's suggested maximum of 350 $\mu g/m^3$. In 1967 local residents successfully sued six companies, claiming medical costs and compensation for lost income. Seven percent of the total population of the district was certified to have been medically affected by ambient air pollution. Increasingly stringent pollution measures were introduced in 1970, and by 1976 sulfur dioxide levels were in compliance with local standards.

Air pollution control costs since 1971, including technical installations and their operation, monitoring, and creation of environmental buffer zones, have been $114 million a year. Without this investment, however, medical expenses and compensation would have been more than $160 million a year.

CASE 2: MERCURY IN THE WATER

At the turn of the century, Minamata was a scenic coastal town of 12,000 people who made their living from wood products, oranges, and fish. In 1908 a fertilizer plant was established that eventually became the Chisso Corporation, one of Japan's largest manufacturers of chemicals. By the 1920s compensation for damage to fisheries had already become an issue, and in 1956 patients with a severe neurological affliction, later to be called *Minamata disease*, were observed.

In 1968, following extensive research, the disease was linked to the ingestion of seafood containing high concentrations of methylmercury, a compound discharged into Minamata Bay by the Chisso Corporation as a by-product of the manufacture of acetaldehyde. The discharge of methylmercury peaked in 1959; it ended in 1968 when the company ceased production of acetaldehyde, but by then the floor of the bay and its aquatic life had become heavily contaminated. Starting in 1974, 1.5 million cubic meters of polluted sediment were dredged and removed.

By 1991, 2248 people (1004 of whom had died) had been certified as suffering from Minamata disease and were eligible for compensation. An additional 2000 people were pursuing claims for compensation. Had the discharge of mercury continued, the estimated annual costs of the damage, including patient treatment and compensation, sediment dredging, and losses to fisheries, would have been $97 million a year. If acetaldehyde production had continued, pollution abatement through in-plant waste recycling would have cost only $1 million a year.

(*continued*)

CASE 3: CADMIUM IN THE SOIL

In the late 1940s a disease characterized by extreme generalized pain, kidney damage, and loss of bone strength appeared in the Jinzu River Basin. The disease, which primarily afflicted women, was called *itai-itai* ("It hurts, it hurts!") after the cries of the sufferers. After two decades of research in 1968 the conclusion was drawn that the cause was chronic cadmium poisoning, which was traced to the effluent from the Mitsui Mining and Smelting Company located in the upper reaches of the basin. The route for the cadmium poisoning was from river water to irrigation water to soil to rice. By 1991, 129 people had been certified as *itai-itai* sufferers, and 116 of them had died.

A major program of soil restoration was initiated in 1979. By 1992, 36% of the contaminated area of 1500 hectares had been treated. Had the further release of cadmium not been prevented, the annual costs from medical compensation, agricultural losses, and soil restoration would have been $19 million a year. The costs of prevention were $5 million a year.

Source: World Bank, 1993.

of different health states where known probabilities can be used to assess the relative willingness to pay for improved health risks. (Details of these methodologies are beyond the scope of this basic text.) Similar techniques may be applied to determine preferences among different health states so that quality-adjusted life-years can be used as a common denominator to compare the benefits of different risk reduction interventions.

The scope of the study is also important to define. Typically BCA studies are microeconomic in focus and assume prices where quantities of other goods or services remain unchanged as a consequence of the project or policy intervention. Generally, for occupational health and safety interventions or relatively localized air or water pollution interventions, this assumption is reasonable. However, in the case of assessing the environmental health impacts of rapid population growth, ozone depletion, and related global warming, the BCA framework may be difficult to apply. Box 4.8 presents three cases in Japan that illustrate how prevention would have been cheaper than the costs involved in treating and compensating those affected by pollution.

Increasing numbers of articles and textbooks are addressing BCA and CEA in environmental health decision making. Principal issues in the use of economic analyses in the environmental health field include the definition of options, the perspective of the analysis, valuation, issues of benefit cost distribution, and the scope of the study. Each of these will be addressed briefly below.

With respect to defining the options, it is generally accepted that a BCA or CEA is not complete until an assessment is conducted for more than one option or alternative. In the environmental health area, this may entail alternative approaches, e.g., using alternative technology, regulation capacity, or information monitoring. The following example of residential radon exposures illustrates how BCA can be applied by environmental health authorities to determine the economic implications of taking steps to reduce residential exposure to radon gas.

Case Study: The Value of Reducing Residential Radon Exposure in Canada

When exposure to radon gas in homes was initially considered a potential environmental health hazard in the 1970s, it was estimated that the cost of reducing risks would be exorbitant. Subsequent examination has changed that view. This case study provides a summary of how to assess the value of an environmental health intervention. Discussed below are the points that should be understood to conduct such an assessment.

The Potential Health Risk In the case of radon, risk assessment evidence on the health risks are well documented—by case studies, animal tests, and epidemiological investigations. As early as 1556, excess deaths attributed to an unusual and fatal chest disease were noted among Central European miners. Over the years, as knowledge expanded, such disease became clearly linked to exposure to radon and its radioactive decay products. Over 20 case–control studies of occupational cohorts have confirmed the association between exposure and lung cancer. The International Agency for Research on Cancer (IARC) confirmed radon as a lung carcinogen in 1988 (see Chapters 2 and 9 for discussion of radiation and its health effects).

In 1988, a blue ribbon panel of experts organized by the (U.S.) National Research Council's Committee on Biological Effects of Ionizing Radiation (BEIR-IV) developed a consensus position on a dose–response model, with implications that residential exposure could constitute a serious hazard. Epidemiological studies, however, have not produced conclusive results. Nevertheless, while consensus on this issue has not been reached, the suspicions about a connection between radon and lung cancer have more evidence to back them up than other recognized hazards have.

The Potential for Exposure Radon is a naturally occurring inert gas formed by the radioactive decay of radium-226, which itself is a product of the decay of uranium-238. It is present at varying levels of concentration in all rock, soil, and water. While present in ambient air at low levels, concentrations can be considerably higher in closed structures (such as houses) if the gas is allowed to infiltrate. Testing has confirmed that the distribution of radon in homes within a region tends to be log-normal (that is, most homes have low levels, whereas a small number produce high readings). The levels observed, particularly at the higher end, correspond to a range of exposures where a health effect would be expected, especially considering the large numbers of people who are potentially exposed.

The Cost of Prevention Although radon occurs naturally, the level to which humans is exposed is influenced by the technologies used in housing construction and operation. Research has confirmed the effectiveness of various methods to reduce exposure in new and existing homes—from better construction techniques to active ventilation systems for blocking the entry of soil gas into a home. The costs, originally estimated from experimental work in the 1970s at approximately $7500 (Canadian) per home, have been revised downward substantially.

Evaluating Possible Interventions With information about the levels of radon exposure and the costs of mitigating exposure, it is possible to carry out an economic evaluation of various intervention options, following the steps identified in Table 4.7. This analysis can provide decision makers with information about the efficiency of alternate ways to use scarce resources. Preliminary analysis along these lines has been carried out in Canada and the United States, as discussed below. The following steps are widely accepted as a guide to conducting either a BCA or CEA.

Step 1. Define the Study Scope and Objectives A Canadian study (Letourneau et al. 1992), considered five different program options to reduce radon exposure

- change building codes
- test and mitigate (if needed) all existing homes
- test and mitigate (if needed) all existing homes and adopt building code change
- test and mitigate (if needed) at point of sale
- test and mitigate (if needed) at point of sale and change building codes.

Evaluation of these options provides a basis for

- estimating the relative benefits of different residential radon risk reduction options
- identifying the conditions (e.g., implications of acting at different exposure levels that would result in the greatest benefit in relation to the costs.

Step 2. Select the Most Appropriate Outcome Measurement Because lung cancer is the health outcome of concern, measures for determining cost-effectiveness would include such things as cost per cancer case averted, cost per life saved, and cost per additional life-year, or cost per radiation exposure reduction. These measurements provide a way to summarize how much money would have to be spent for each unit of benefit produced. This avoids ethical issues and other controversies that must be encountered in estimating the value of each unit of benefit (in other words, placing a dollar value on a life).

Step 3. Identify, Measure, and Value all Costs Costs were explicitly identified for each program option under review, based on current practices and technologies (notably at levels well below those that had been originally estimated from experimental remediation research). For example, the cost of a screening test was set at $35, the cost of sub-slab depressurization for an existing home at $1500, etc. As costs in the options under review are incurred over a 10-year period, these must be discounted (at a designated interest rate) to allow options to be estimated at present values.

Step 4. Identify, Measure, and Value all Benefits Benefits were based on estimates of the effectiveness of the mitigation in reducing exposure (measured in working level months [WLM] of radiation exposure) and then estimating the health benefit from the dose–response relationship produced by the BEIR-IV review (approximately 3.5 lung cancer cases per 10,000 WLMs of exposure). As this is the sole measure of benefit, any questioning of the health effects of residential radon exposure has tremendous implications for the economic analysis. Nevertheless, the use of the BEIR-IV model (later confirmed by the BEIV-VI review [NRC, 1999]) is quite in keeping with the general protocol for considering risk management options. (Other health and economic benefits from reducing the level of soil gas infiltration in a home [e.g., mildew, moulds] have not been included in the analysis, but can be assumed to exist.)

Step 5. Compare Costs with Benefits (and Apply Sensitivity Tests) Results of the Canadian study are provided in Table 4.8. At a national level (based on the results of national testing conducted in 19 different cities to determine levels of exposure), the greatest cost-effectiveness ($33,000 per WLM reduced) was determined to be associated with the option of testing at point of sale and mitigating if concentrations exceed the Canadian "action level" guideline of 800 Becquerels/m^3.

Comparison of the right column with the left column shows that lowering the action level (to 150 Bq/m^3, which is in effect in the United States) for these options nationally would make the cost-effectiveness more attractive—for example, the cost-effectiveness ratio would be reduced to $15,000 per WLM reduction. (Sensitivity tests conducted to consider the implications of varying the interest rate used to discount future costs indicated that the adoption of a 10% discount rate would lower the cost-effectiveness ratio further—to $9000 per WLM reduced.)

Comparison of estimates for a program to reduce radon risk in cities with high and low mean levels of exposure showed that there can be dramatic differences in the cost-effectiveness of preventing lung cancer cases. The two cities chosen for comparison are a city with high exposure (Winnipeg) and one with lower exposure (Vancouver). Analysis of BEIR-IV and others of the dose–response data showed that for every exposure reduction of one WLM, four cancer cases could be avoided. It would cost $8000 to avert one case of radon-induced lung cancer in Winnipeg, but over $50,000,000 in Vancouver; Vancouver has high screening (testing) costs and very little mitigation, whereas in Winnipeg, a smaller city with high exposures, there are much smaller screening costs and considerably more mitigation.

TABLE 4.8

COST-EFFECTIVENESS RATIOS FOR RADON MITIGATION OPTIONS IN CANADA

National Application of Various Options	Cost-Effectiveness Ratio ($1000/WLM Reduced)	
	@800 Bq/m^3	@150 Bq/m^3
Mitigate existing homes	54	25
Change building codes	75	—
Retrofit to changed building codes	74	64
Screen point of sale and mitigate	33	15
Screen point of sale and mitigate, and change building code	74	65

WLM, working level months, a unit of radiation exposure.

Step 6. Define Implications of Results for Decision Makers From the perspective of cost-effectiveness alone, mitigation of residential radon exposure appears to be an attractive option (as $8000 is not a high price to pay to avoid a case of lung cancer). However, the implications of the options under review would entail a large total expenditure of funds (another important policy consideration) to achieve the benefit that could be realized. The total cost of the most attractive option nationally (point of sale testing and mitigation) would be $350 million, based on the number of houses that would be tested. This would increase to $1220 million if the action level of 150 Bq/m^3 were adopted, as more houses would require mitigation.

The most practical implication of the analysis is that it would make the most economic sense to target intervention (screening test and mitigation if necessary) in areas of high-exposure risk, where the cost-effectiveness ratio of $8000 per lung cancer case avoided would be of considerable interest, but $50 million may be excessive. Thus, this CEA revealed that the screening/mitigation intervention option is less cost-effective in areas of low radon concentrations, where the bulk of total population exposure comes from homes with levels below the action level, but is very cost-effective in smaller population groups where the exposures are higher.

Study Questions

1. The construction of a depot for chemical waste is planned near a residential area. Several residents perceive this new situation as threatening to their health and that of their families. Give examples of possible coping strategies that can be characterized as emotion focused or problem focused.

2. Consider the advantages and disadvantages of a "best practical means" approach as compared to an emission or effluent standard. Which best preserves environmental quality in nonpolluted areas? Which best encourages the development of new abatement technology? Which is most related to actual health effects?

3. Think of an example of the use of immunization in an occupational health context and consider the advantages and disadvantages of this practice. Should this immunization be mandatory? Why or why not?

4. Consider whether you agree with the statement that personal protective equipment should be a last resort. Why or why not? Under what circumstances?

5. Consider to what extent the control measures at the person, indicated for the occupational environment, could also be effective to control for ambient exposures. Indicate if you regard such control options desirable for the general public.

5

AIR

LEARNING OBJECTIVES

After studying this chapter you will be able to do the following:
- describe the importance of air quality as a determinant of health
- describe the nature and extent of air pollution–related diseases
- list the major sources of air pollution
- describe how air quality criteria are developed
- discuss the various approaches to prevention of air-related environmental health problems

CHAPTER CONTENTS

OVERVIEW OF AIR POLLUTION

Air pollution is the result of emission into the air of hazardous substances at a rate that exceeds the capacity of natural processes in the atmosphere (e.g., rain and wind) to convert, deposit, or dilute them. Microbiological air pollution is mainly a problem of indoor air and will be addressed in Chapter 8. Radioactive compounds in air will be discussed in Chapter 9. Here we will focus on chemical pollutants in the air.

    Air pollution is a problem of obvious importance in many places that affects human, plant, and animal health. For example, there is good evidence that the health of about 1 billion urban dwellers is compromised daily because of high levels of ambient air sulfur dioxide concentrations (see the section Control of Ambient Air Pollution, below; WHO, 1997). Air pollution affects health most clearly when compounds accumulate to relatively high concentrations, producing an adverse effect on the body, e.g., bronchoconstriction or other asthmatic symptoms. Recent studies have shown that even low levels of exposure to fine particles can produce illness and deaths in a community. Often, this effect is not visible against the greater number of cases of illness or deaths caused by other factors, such as hot weather. Air pollution can also affect the properties of materials (such as rubber), visibility, and the quality of life in general.

Although people have caused air pollution ever since they learned how to use fire, anthropogenic air pollution has increased rapidly since industrialization began. In addition to the common air pollutants, many volatile organic compounds, inorganic compounds, and trace metals are emitted into the atmosphere by human activities. Worldwide, almost 100 million tons of sulfur oxides (SO_x), 68 million tons of nitrogen oxides (NO_x), 57 million tons of suspended particulate matter (SPM), and 177 million tons of carbon monoxide (CO) were released into the atmosphere in 1990 as a result of human activities. The Organization for Economic Cooperation and Development (OECD) countries accounted for about 40% of the SO_x, 52% of the NO_x, 71% of the CO, and 23% of the SPM, as shown in Figure 5.1 (UNEP, 1992a). The reductions in some of the emissions noted in the figure were likely due to regulation, education, changes in technology, and a rise in fuel prices in OECD countries.

The accumulation of chemically active compounds in the atmosphere is greatly affected by land features and atmospheric movements. Valleys, nearby mountain ranges, and the lack of open space (parks, forests, wilderness areas, bodies of water) strongly increase the severity of air pollution in a locale. These features hold the air mass like a container and prevent dilution and mixing. Stagnant air masses may receive emissions for days on end. When conditions are right, usually in the

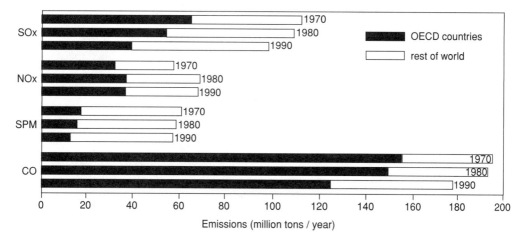

Figure 5.1 Anthropogenic emissions of air pollutants. From UNEP, 1992a, with permission.

morning or when there is descent of air from higher altitudes, a special atmospheric condition is created that is called *an inversion*. In an inversion, the temperature rises with increasing altitude rather than falling, which is normally the case. An inversion layer is a mass of air with an inverted temperature gradient (warmer above, cooler below). The motion of air in an inversion layer is suppressed and it limits the mixing and dilution of air pollution. Inversions are very common, especially in valleys and coastlines. The worst episodes of air pollution usually occur when inversions stay in place for days on end and the atmosphere underneath receives air pollution day after day with no mixing or wind to dilute it.

Air pollution is a very complicated physical and chemical system. It can be thought of as gases and particles that are dissolved or suspended in air respectively. Many air pollutants interact with one another to produce their effects. The severity of air pollution changes with the season, with daylight, with industrial activity, with changes in traffic, with the prevailing winds, and with precipitation (rain or snow), among many relevant factors. The composition of air pollution, therefore, is not constant from day to day or even week to week, but tends to cycle. Average levels go up and down fairly consistently depending on the time of year, but the actual levels are highly variable from one day to the next.

Aerosols

Small solid or liquid particles (fine drops or droplets) that are suspended in air form a mixture called *aerosols*. Forming are complex systems in air pollution. Aerosols often consist of a mixture of solid-phase particles, combined solid- and liquid-phase particles, and sometimes liquid droplets suspended in air. Even aerosols that are predominantly solid may contain absorbed water. On the coast, some aerosols are formed by salt water droplets.

Dust consists of particles in the solid phase. The term is usually used for the particles themselves or the accumulation of particles after they have settled or have been deposited. When they are up in the air, the particles are called *suspended particulate matter*. This term is usually reserved for particles that are created by dry processes and are chemically and physically unchanged from the original material except for their size. *Smoke* consists of particles in both the solid and sometimes liquid phase and the associated gases that result from combustion. Smoke is very complicated chemically and varies in composition depending on what has been burned. Tobacco smoke and air pollution are both examples of smoke and both undergo chemical transformations over time as they age. *Ash* is the solid phase of smoke, particularly after it settles into a fine dust.

The most important characteristics of aerosols that determine their behavior are size and composition. Size affects how the particle will travel in air and composition determines what will happen when it settles or lands on something. The range in size of common particles associated with different constituents of air pollution and occupational exposures is shown in Figure 5.2.

The individual particles in aerosols may be relatively uniform in size, or *monodispersed*, or highly variable in size, or *polydispersed*. In nature, all aerosols are polydispersed. Monodispersed aerosols are most commonly created for research and for certain medications where it is important for the droplet or par-

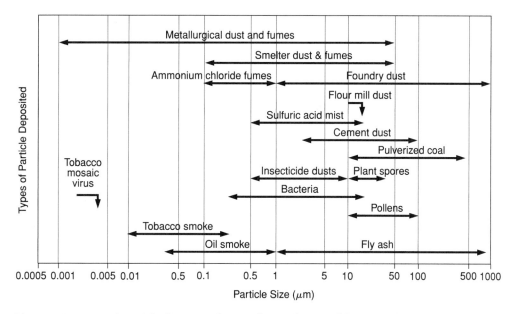

Figure 5.2 Range of particle diameters from airborne dusts and fumes. Adapted from Levy and Wegman, 1988, with permission.

ticle to land at a certain place in the respiratory tract, as in asthma inhalers. Aerosols in air pollution are all polydispersed. *Fumes* are polydispersed fine aerosols consisting of solid particles that often aggregate together, so that many little particulates may form one big particle. Some gases, such as sulfate and nitrate, also may precipitate and then aggregate to form solid particles. Air pollution includes solid-phase particles and even droplets in a range of sizes, some of which will behave one way while others behave differently. Larger particles are kept up in the air by winds and local air movement and have a tendency to settle out by the effect of gravity if the air is very quiet. The smaller particles are kept up in the air by the movement of molecules in air (which is heat), a phenomenon called *Brownian movement*.

The size of particles in aerosol governs where the particles will tend to go in the respiratory tract and that, in turn, determines some of the effects on the lung. Size is also related to mass; the smaller the particle, the less the mass. In all polydispersed aerosols, the greatest number of particles will be small but together they will account for only a small fraction of the total mass; the larger particles will be many fewer but will carry most of the mass. This is important because some particles, such as those containing lead or mercury, will not necessarily damage the lung but the mass of their toxic material may be absorbed and have an effect elsewhere in the body.

Particles are generated with different size distribution depending on the source. The composition of particles will depend on the local sources. Particles from different sources may have different size distributions. Large particles are most often the result of blowing dust or soot as the result of open combustion and some are formed by aggregation of smaller particles. Large particles are mostly solid but may contain adsorbed gases or be liquid on the surface. Smaller, and especially fine particles are mostly caused by certain types of combustion, associated with diesel exhausts, power plants, and other forms of rapid, hot combustion. Small particles of around 10 μm may also be formed by the aggregation of fine particles, around 2.5 μm. Fine particles generally consist of a matrix of carbonaceous compound, and dissolved or absorbed or solid-phase sulfate, nitrate, and trace metals and some water. The effects of small particles on the body are different from those produced by larger particles and are considered more toxic. The composition of an aerosol determines the chemical reactivity of its particles and their density.

From the human health perspective, however, the most important aspect of particle size relates to how a particle behaves in the respiratory tract. In discussions of health a special measure of size, the *aerodynamic diameter*, is used, which is different from the actual measurement of the particle and reflects the behavior of a particle more accurately than a physical measurement would. The aerodynamic diameter of a particle is defined as the diameter of a sphere with a density of 1. This means that if the particle in question had the density of water they would both settle at the same velocity. This measure allows one to compare particles that are different in shape, density, or mass. For example, a piece of fluff (e.g., cotton) has a relatively large surface but a low density and will therefore be easily suspended or carried away by the wind. Thus it has a small aerodynamic diameter whereas its geometric diameter is relatively large. From this point on in the text, the size of particles will be expressed in terms of the aerodynamic diameter measured in micrometers. Larger particles have more mass and thus more inertia; they are less likely to make it through the twists and turns of the human respiratory tract.

The effect of particles on the body reflects the efficiency with which they penetrate all the way to and within the lung and their chemical reactivity and toxicity once they arrive. Larger particles carry much more substance but are much less likely to have an effect on the body because they do not penetrate into the lower respiratory tract (below the first division of the windpipe, or trachea). The largest particles, visible to the naked eye as specks of dust, are mostly filtered out in the nose. Particles above 100 μm may be sources of irritation to the mucous membranes of the eyes, nose, and throat but they do not get much further. Those particles below this cutoff make up the *inhalable fraction* because they can be inhaled into the respiratory tract. Particles larger than about 20 μm generally do not enter the lower respiratory tract, below the throat (trachea). Those particles below 20 μm comprise the *thoracic fraction* because a high proportion can penetrate into the lungs. Particles below 10 μm enter the airways with greatest efficiency and may be deposited in the alveoli, or airspaces, that are the deepest structures of the lungs. Particles between 10 μm and 2.5 μm are called coarse particles. Particles below 2.5 μm are deposited in the alveoli with very high efficiency and are called "fine particles." Particles below 0.1 μm are called "ultrafine particles." Air pollution is predominantly in the coarse and fine range. Notwithstanding the efficiency of penetration, ultrafine particles, smaller than about 0.1 μm, tend to remain suspended in air and be breathed out again unless they carry an electrostatic charge. Thus, as a practical matter, the greatest penetration and retention of particles is in the range 10.0 to 0.1 μm, which is

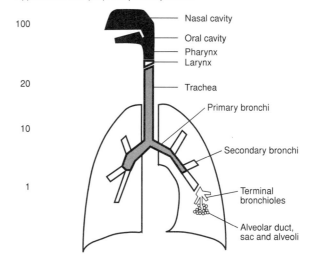

Approximate size (um) of deposited particles

100 — Nasal cavity
— Oral cavity
— Pharynx
— Larynx

20 — Trachea

— Primary bronchi

10

— Secondary bronchi

1 — Terminal bronchioles

Figure 5.3 Deposition of dust particles by size. From Newman, 1992, with permission.

— Alveolar duct, sac and alveoli

called the *respirable range*. This is because particles in this range can be inhaled all the way to the deepest structures of the lung. These patterns of deposition are shown graphically in Figure 5.3.

Once in the lung, particles may have different effects, depending on their size. Particles predominantly in the size range between 10 and 20 μm are more likely to have effects on the airways. A large proportion of particles below 10 μm but above 0.1 μm may be retained in the lungs. When they accumulate in large numbers and the lung responds to their presence, they may cause a type of disease called *pneumoconiosis*; this is seen following high exposures, usually over several years, in occupational settings. Pneumoconiosis is not a consequence of ambient air pollution where the effects tend to be on airways rather than alveoli.

In air quality studies, the total aerosol suspended in air once was measured as *total suspended particles* (TSP) or an optical measurement known as "British Smoke." This measurement reflects the perception of smoke in the air and diminished visibility. These measurements are comparatively easy compared to measurements of coarse and fine particles. PM_{10} and $PM_{2.5}$ have become the preferred measurements of particulate air pollution. Ultrafine particles are very difficult to measure.

Although disregarded for purposes of measuring the size of the particle, shape is important in determining the effects of a particle. The human body handles longer and thinner particles, called *fibers*, somewhat differently from particles that are more rounded in shape because fibers are more difficult to remove from the lungs by natural protective mechanisms. The very long and thin shape of fibres of asbestos are particularly damaging to the lung and can cause lung cancer and mesothelioma of the pleura. Fibers are described by the ratio of their length to their width. A particle at least five times longer than it is wide is considered to be a particle.

Liquid constituents of air pollution exist as aerosols, either as liquid-phase particles, which are *droplets*, or in association with solid-phase particles. Liquids that are constituents of air pollution are always aqueous, or water-based, because droplets of more volatile organic compounds evaporate to the gaseous phase very quickly. A cloud or dense collection of droplets is called a *mist*.

Small solid-phase particles also contain a small amount of absorbed water. Both liquid- and gas-phase constituents of air pollution are often attracted to and ride on the surface of solid particles; this is called *adsorption* (not to be confused with *absorption*, in which the liquid or gas is actually taken into the particle).

The humidity in the atmosphere is an important determinate of the water content of particles; the lower the humidity, the faster the water evaporates. A particle may be reduced to a solid phase, which is called a *droplet nuclei*. Droplet nuclei are small and easily inhaled and are particularly important in the spread of some infectious diseases such as tuberculosis, when they come from an infected person who coughs. Dry particles may also take on water when they are released into a humid atmosphere. Small particles typically absorb large amounts of water if it is available in the atmosphere; these are said to be *hygroscopic*. Through this absorption mass is added to the particle and its capacity to carry other dissolved constituents may be increased. Air pollution from the same types of sources may therefore be different in humid climates and dry climates.

There are processes in the atmosphere through which liquid is converted to gas and back again or liquid is converted to solid. Volatile liquids may evaporate to become gases. The evaporated compound in the gas phase is called a *vapor* and behaves like a gas in air pollution. Droplets may also form from condensation of vapor in a saturated atmosphere. Fog is a familiar example of an aerosol of liquid water droplets that forms from condensation in an atmosphere saturated with water vapor. Droplets may also form from ocean spray. Droplets often form by condensation of liquid around a small solid particle. In coastal areas, the droplets of seawater may evaporate to form solid-phase particulates that contain salt (this is an important source of PM_{10} near oceans).

Precipitation, in the form of rain and snow, reduces air pollution by dissolving soluble gases and by attracting and holding small airborne particles, bringing them down to the ground. The air may then be much cleaner, but the constituents of air pollution in the rainwater or snow may present a serious problem (acid rain; see Chapter 11, Acid Precipitation). Acid-forming compounds, such as sulfates and oxides of nitrogen, reduce the pH in exposed lakes and soils (surface water acidification), which if it exceeds the buffering capacity of the water may lead to fish deaths and other ecological damage.

Gases

Air pollution can also consist of gaseous constituents, the properties of greatest importance being *solubility* in water and *chemical reactivity*. At concentrations found in air pollution, solubility is a major determining factor of the health effects of gases. Relatively soluble constituents of air pollution include nitrogen oxides or sulfur dioxide, which may be ionized in water and which in the atmosphere may coalesce to form ultrafine particles and fine particles. In addition, a number of gases occurring more commonly as occupational exposures are water-soluble, including hydrochloric acid vapor and ammonia. Other gases, such as ozone, hydrogen sulfide, and organic compounds are less soluble.

Solubility for gases is much like size for particles; it is a characteristic that determines the efficiency with which they penetrate deeply into the respiratory tract. A gas that is soluble in water will be dissolved in the water coating the mucous membrane of the lungs and upper respiratory tract and will be removed from air passing more deeply. A gas that is insoluble in water will not be so removed and will penetrate to the alveoli, the deepest structures of the lung, more efficiently.

Gases that are reactive, such as ozone, tend to have their major effects on the airways rather than the alveoli, even if they are relatively insoluble, except at very high concentrations. They may irritate the walls of the airway and cause bronchitis or induce asthmatic attacks, for example. Occupational exposures to toxic gases or uncontrolled releases during an industrial emergency may expose workers or local residents to much higher concentrations than they would experience in ambient air pollution. In such cases, the effects are correspondingly severe and may result in serious toxic effects at the alveolar level, such as pulmonary edema, a condition in which the damage to the lungs allows accumulation of fluid in the lungs in a manner similar to drowning. In this situation, the solubility of the gas is critically important as a determinant of toxicity.

As mentioned above, many gases, including ozone and sulfur dioxide, adsorb onto the surface of particulates and penetrate deeply into the respiratory tract in this way. When this happens, the effects may be different and greater than exposure to either the particulate or the gas alone. The solubility of a gas becomes much less important as a determinant of its toxicity when it is adsorbed onto a particle in the respirable range. Under these circumstances, it may penetrate much more deeply than it would as a simple gas.

Inhalation

Inhalation of toxicants often constitutes the most rapid avenue of entry into the body because of the intimate association of air passages in the lungs with the circulatory system. On inhalation, soluble gases tend to dissolve into the water surface of the pulmonary tract; insoluble gases generally penetrate to the alveolar level. Because the alveoli bring the blood into very close and direct proximity to air, gases may pass directly across the alveolar membrane and into the bloodstream very efficiently. Particles, once deposited in the alveoli, may dissolve and release their constituent compounds. The degree to which they enter the blood, are circulated, and delivered to the body's tissues depends on the concentration inhaled, duration of exposure, solubility in blood and tissue, reactivity of the compound, and the respiratory rate. (The respiratory rate determines how much air is breathed in and therefore the total amount taken into the body.) Unlike many toxic substances that are ingested and therefore passed through the liver and metabolized, inhaled compounds are not significantly metabolized prior to circulation throughout the body. They may therefore have a direct and immediate effect, not unlike direct injection into the bloodstream. To understand the health problems associated with airborne contaminants it is essential to have at least a basic understanding of the structure and function of the respiratory tract.

Anything that decreases the partial pressure of oxygen in the alveoli reduces the oxygen available for exchange and thus deprives the body of oxygen. At high altitude, the partial atmospheric pressure is lower than at sea level and the corresponding pressure of oxygen in alveoli air also decreases, reducing the saturation of blood with oxygen. When the oxygen in air is displaced by another gas, so that there is not enough to support life, or when a person is prevented from breathing, it is called *asphyxiation*. Substances that dilute or displace the oxygen in air without any other effect are simple asphyxiants. Examples include carbon dioxide, nitrous oxide, nitrogen, or hydrocarbons, such as natural gas. Compounds that block the transfer of oxygen to the tissues or the utilization of oxygen once it reaches the tissues are called *chemical asphyxiants*. The two most common examples of such inhibitors of oxygen uptake or utilization are carbon monoxide (CO), which blocks the site on hemoglobin that binds and transports oxygen, and hydrogen cyanide (HCN), which (in the form of cyanide) blocks the pathway by which the tissues utilize oxygen. Carbon monoxide is particularly common as a hazard resulting from incomplete combustion of fuels (such as in automobile exhaust or open-flame heaters): It is especially dangerous because it has no odor and thus gives no warning of exposure.

Chemical agents that irritate the lung may also impair oxygen uptake by other means. Irritants may inflame the respiratory tract, causing bronchitis or provoking an asthmatic attack or causing the lungs to be filled with fluid (pulmonary edema), a process much like drowning.

COMMON HEALTH EFFECTS OF AMBIENT AIR POLLUTION

Respiratory symptoms are the most common adverse health effects from air pollution (Table 5.1). Common symptoms include cough (which may produce sputum), nose and throat irritation, and mild shortness of breath. These respiratory symptoms are often associated with eye irritation and a sense of fatigue. Exacerbation of allergic symptoms is typical. Athletes often report that their performance is off and that they become tired more rapidly when exercising during periods of high pollution levels. Asthmatics and patients with chronic obstructive pulmonary disease (COPD) often experience worsening of their symptoms during air pollution episodes. Recent studies suggest a close association between frequency and severity of asthma attacks and atmospheric oxidant and sulfate levels. People with bronchitis may also experience more coughing due to increased irritation of the bronchial mucosa. Acute upper and lower respiratory tract infections also appear to occur more frequently in residents of areas with higher pollution levels. Fever is not a feature of air pollution exposure alone and suggests a possible infection.

Direct cardiovascular effects of air pollution are associated primarily with CO, which is known to reduce oxygen delivery to the myocardium and suspected to aggravate the process of atherosclerosis. These effects may occur in normal individuals who have no unusual susceptibility, but they are particularly severe among people with existing heart disease.

Respiratory effects of air pollution, particularly in people who suffer from chronic bronchitis, may place an additional strain on the heart as well. Air pollution is associated with increased risk of death from heart disease and lung disease, even at levels below those known to be acutely toxic to the lungs or heart. It is thought that the compromise in lung function places an additional burden

TABLE 5.1

COMMON CONDITIONS TO WHICH AIR POLLUTION EXPOSURE MAY CONTRIBUTE

Disease or Condition	How Air Pollution May Affect Condition	Associated Factors/Comments
Acute bronchitis	Direct irritative effects of SO_2, soot, and petrochemical pollution	Cigarette smoking may have a more than additive interaction
Acute respiratory infections	Increased risk in young children	Poverty, malnutrition, exposure to infectious agents
Asthma	Aggravation from respiratory irritation, possibly on reflex basis	Usually preexisting respiratory allergy or airway hyperactivity
Chronic bronchitis	Aggravation (increase in frequency or severity) of cough or sputum associated with any sort of pollution	Cigarette smoking, occupation
Deaths	Fine particulate increases mortality in heart and lung disease; mechanism is unknown	Preexisting heart or lung disease
Eye irritation	Specific effect of photochemical oxidants, possibly aldehydes, or peroxyacetyl nitrates; particulate matter (fly ash) acts as a foreign body	Susceptibility differs
Headache	Carbon monoxide sufficient to lead to more than 10% carboxyhemoglobin	Smoking may also increase carboxyhemoglobin, but not enough to lead to headache
Lead toxicity	Adds to body burden	Close proximity to lead source; exposure at home

on the heart, which cannot tolerate this. The stimulation of nerve reflexes connecting the heart and the lung may cause additional problems in a diseased heart.

Mucosal irritation in the form of acute or chronic bronchitis, nasal tickle, or conjunctivitis is characteristic of high levels of air pollution, although individuals vary considerably in their susceptibility to such effects. Eye irritation is particularly severe in the setting of high levels of particulates (which need to be in the respirable range described and may be quite large soot particles) or of high concentrations of photochemical oxidants and especially aldehydes.

The link between cancer associated with the organic contents of air pollution has always been a concern but an association has not been proven for ambient urban air pollution, of the types described. There is little evidence to suggest that community air pollution is a significant cause of cancer except in unusual and extreme cases. Examples of cancer associated with community air pollution include point-source emissions from some poorly controlled smelters that release arsenic, which can cause lung cancer. There are also important examples of indoor air pollution in homes (radon) and workplaces (asbestos) that are linked to lung cancer. Tobacco smoking is more carcinogenic than arsenic, radon, or as-bestos in the air, multiplying the lung cancer risk from these toxins.

Central nervous system effects, and possibly learning disabilities in children, may result from accumulated body burdens of lead. Air pollution contributes a large fraction of exposure in many countries because of lead additives in gasoline. Even in countries where lead has been removed from gasoline the lead remains in the environment as one source of exposure.

There are several documented occurences in which severe mortality from many causes is associated with short-term exposure to fine particles. Air pollution has been associated in several severe episodes of high mortality, usually among persons with pulmonary or cardiovascular disorders. Recent studies have shown an association between particulates in urban air pollution and mortality from a wide variety of causes, not just lung diseases. This finding was unexpected, as the levels studied were much lower than those that had been previously linked to increased mortality. The reason for the newer findings is probably that the methods of statistically analyzing large populations are much better and the methods of measuring exposures, such as $PM_{2.5}$, are much more refined than those used earlier.

HEALTH EFFECTS OF SPECIFIC AIR POLLUTANTS

Some of the more common ambient air pollutants, their sources, and their health effects are summarized in Table 5.2 and are described further below. It is important to understand that these pollutants are seasonal in their pattern. Both ozone and sulfates, together with ultrafine particulates, tend to occur together during the summer months in most developed areas. Ozone, oxides of nitrogen, aldehydes, and CO tend to occur together in association with traffic, especially in sunny regions. Some pollutants, such as radon, are only hazards indoors or in a confined area, usually a workplace such as a mine. Others are present both indoors and outdoors, with varying relative concentrations.

Ozone

Ozone is a highly reactive compound that irritates airways in the lungs and interferes with host defense mechanisms in the body. It also has an unusual effect on breathing patterns as the result of changes in the reflex breathing mechanism.

In the lower atmosphere, oxygen, with light from the sun as a source of energy, reacts with nitrogen compounds and volatile hydrocarbons to create ozone. This occurs especially in stagnant weather conditions and inversions under conditions of sunshine, where there is ample time for the photochemical reactions to take place. Ozone is chemically unstable and will react with a variety of substances. (The effects of ozone depletion in the upper atmosphere are discussed in Chapter 11.) Ozone appears to trigger a reflex response in the lungs that alters breathing patterns. People without asthma cannot inhale as deeply and will have small changes in airflow.

Studies using pulmonary function testing have found that healthy persons can experience adverse effects from ozone exposure. This is especially true when they have an increased respiratory rate, for example when they are involved in

TABLE 5.2

SELECTED URBAN AIRBORNE POLLUTANTS, SOURCES, AND HEALTH EFFECTS

Pollutant	Source[a]	Health Effects
Acetic Acid	Biomass fuel combustion, construction materials	Mucous membrane irrigation
Aldehydes	Biomass and fossil fuel combustion, cigarette smoke	Eye irritation, upper respiratory tract irritation
Carbon monoxide	Biomass and fossil fuel combustion, cigarette smoke, traffic	Headache, nausea, dizziness, breathlessness, fatigue, low birth weight, visual disturbances, mental confusion, angina, coma, death
Formaldehyde	Biomass fuel combustion, construction and furnishing materials, cigarette smoke	Eye and respiratory tract irritation and allergies, possible cancers
Lead (and other heavy metals)	Leaded gasoline, smelting	Neuropsychological effects, central nervous system damage, learning disabilities
Microorganisms	Furnishings, humans, animals	Infectious disease, allergies
Nitrogen oxides	Biomass and fossil fuel combustion, cigarette smoke, traffic	Eye irritation, respiratory tract infection (children are especially vulnerable), exacerbation of asthma, irritation of bronchi
Ozone	Traffic, hydrocarbon release, fossil fuel combustion (sending pollutant)	Eye irritation, respiratory tract irritation, reduced exercise capacity, exacerbation of respiratory disease
Particulates	Biomass and fossil fuel combustion, furnishing and construction materials, cigarette smoke, industry, traffic	Eye irritation, respiratory tract infections, allergies, exacerbation of respiratory and cardiovascular disease
Phenols	Biomass fuel combustion, household chemicals	Mucous membrane irritation
Polycyclic aromatic hydrocarbons	Fossil fuel combustion, traffic, acute incineration	Includes carcinogens
Radon	Underlying rock and soil	Carcinogen
Sulfur oxides	Biomass and fossil fuel combustion, industrial emissions	Respiratory tract irritation, impaired pulmonary function, exacerbation of cardiopulmonary diseases
Sulfuric acid (formed by sulfur oxides in air)	Biomass and fossil fuel combustion, industrial emissions	Respiratory tract infection, bronchospasm
Volatile organic hydrocarbons	Biomass and fossil fuel combustion in traffic, furnishing and construction materials, household chemicals	Headache, dizziness, upper respiratory tract irritation, nausea, includes carcinogens

[a]May be a source of emissions (most), source of release (e.g., radon), or source of emissions that give rise to secondary pollutants (e.g., ozone, aldehydes).

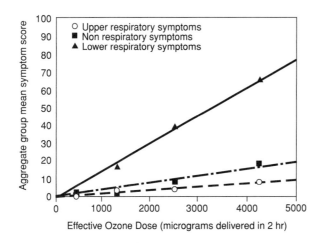

Figure 5.4 Effect of ozone on respiratory symptoms. From Kleinman et al., 1989, with permission.

outdoor physically strenuous activities. A dose–response curve for the symptoms associated with ozone is presented in Figure 5.4. Symptoms include upper respiratory symptoms (nasal discharge, throat irritation), lower respiratory symptoms (cough, wheeze, chest pain), and nonrespiratory symptoms (headache, fatigue).

Kleinman et al. (1989) produced a dose–effect curve indicating how pulmonary function tests vary with dose of O_3 (see Fig. 5.5). Over a short period the effects of ozone are cumulative. After several days, however, people become tolerant to ozone and have fewer symptoms. Their breathing becomes more normal, but persons with asthma may still develop airflow obstruction. Within a brief period, the inflammation produced by the irritant effect of ozone results in a reduction of airflow and a worsening of asthma. Ozone also appears to make persons whose asthma is triggered by allergies more susceptible to the allergen. Ozone may provoke asthmatic attacks in people who already have asthma, although ozone does not appear to cause the disease in the first place. The attacks tend to occur 1 or 2 days after the ozone concentration is at its highest, not during the peak.

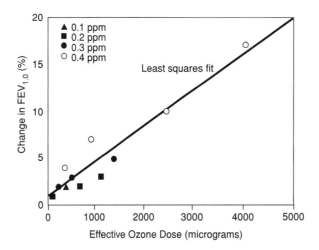

Figure 5.5 Effect of ozone on pulmonary function. From Kleinman et al., 1989), with permission.

BOX 5.1

London Fog

On December 5, 1952, a phenomenon known as a temperature inversion occurred in the atmosphere in London, England. This resulted in a dense fog forming in the center of the city. (During a temperature inversion very little air movement occurs, and air, including the particulate matter and other pollutants it contains, gets trapped in a given location. Suspended matter in the air can provide nuclei on which particles of moisture and other pollutants, such as acids, are deposited.)

During this time, the temperature hovered around 0°C. The burning of fossil fuels (coal) in open hearth fires in homes, in the industrial generation of electricity, and the emissions from transportation vehicles contributed to the atmospheric pollution. Measurements for total suspended particulate matter (TSPM) and sulfur dioxide were routinely made in both central and peripheral London during this time. During December 6–8, 1952, daily averages from all monitoring points increased about fivefold to 1.6 mg/m^3. Peak values were 3 to 10 times the normal values, and were highest in central London. In comparison, the mean December 1957 concentration for TSPM was in the range of 0.12 to 0.44 mg/m^3.

The demand for hospital beds increased on December 8, and the central London hospitals issued an Emergency Bed Warning that they had sufficient beds for fewer than 85% of applicants. The mortality rate in certain parts of London increased dramatically during this time (see Fig. 5.6). The major causes of death were a variety of respiratory-related illnesses, cardiac illness, and ill-defined illnesses. At least a few deaths were caused by injuries and a few people drowned when they could not see and fell into the Thames River. In addition, many animals (e.g., cattle) had to be slaughtered because of illness during this time, likely because of the fog.

Based on the epidemiological data collected during the London smog episodes, it was felt at the time that the increased number of deaths in London during the fog was more closely related to the particulate matter in the air, rather than the SO$_2$. A reanalysis later, though, suggested that the acid aerosols (e.g., sulfur dioxide) were the major factor in causing the increased mortality.

Adapted by A. Morham; from Kjellström and Hicks, 1991.

Sulfur Dioxide

Sulfur dioxide (SO$_2$) has been a serious problem in air pollution since the earliest days of industrialization. It has been the major problem in reducing (see section Industrial Air Pollution, below) or acidifying air pollution during the period of rapid economic growth in many countries. It was one of the major components of the so-called London Fog, which had serious direct health effects, as illustrated in Box 5.1 and Figure 5.6.

Soon after the London Fog incident experimental studies of the effects of sulfur dioxide on humans showed that, at least in acute exposures, concentrations of up to 8 ppm caused respiratory changes that were dose dependent. Later studies revealed that the main effect of sulfur dioxide is bronchoconstriction (closing

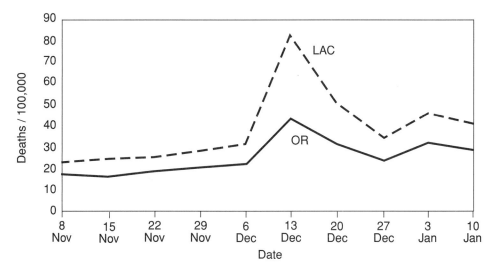

Figure 5.6 Weekly death rates in London Administration County (LAC) and the outer ring (OR) 1 November 1952–10 January 1953. From WHO, 1998b, with permission.

of the airways causing increased resistance to breathing), which is dose dependent, rapid, and tends to peak at 10 min (Folinsbee, 1992). Persons with asthma are particularly susceptible and in fact asthmatics suffer more from the effects of sulfur dioxide than does the general public. Persons with asthma who exercise will typically experience symptoms at 0.5 ppm (1.4 mg/m³), depending on the individual.

Sulfate, a major sulfur-containing ion in water, is a major constituent of air pollution capable of forming acid. Sulfate itself appears to trigger bronchoconstriction in persons with vulnerable airways and it is a major constituent of ultrafine particulates. There are other acid ingredients in air pollution, such as nitric acid, but less is know about them. Through their emission into the air by industry and motor vehicles, these acids cause a phenomenon known as *acid rain*. This is discussed further in Chapter 11.

Because of the small size of acid-forming aerosols such as sulfur dioxide, sulfates, and nitrogen dioxide and their tendency to ride along on particles, these aerosols can deposit deeply in the distal lung and air space. Combined with ozone they appear to provoke airways responses in an additive or synergistic manner. They have also been implicated in causing mortality in association with ultrafine particulates.

Oxides of Nitrogen

As mentioned above, nitrogen compounds, especially nitrogen dioxide, are involved in the formation of ozone at ground level. The oxides of nitrogen also produce adverse health effects and are important air pollutants in their own right.

Nitric oxide (NO) is produced by combustion. Nitrogen dioxide (NO₂), which has greater health effects, is a secondary pollutant created by the oxidation of NO under conditions of sunlight, or it may be formed directly by higher-temperature combustion in power plants or indoors from gas stoves. The direct

TABLE 5.3

POTENTIAL HUMAN EFFECTS OF NITROGEN DIOXIDE

Health Effect	Mechanism
Increased incidence of respiratory infections	Reduced effectiveness of lung defenses
Increased severity of respiratory infections	Reduced effectiveness of lung defenses
Respiratory symptoms	Airways injury and bronchospasm
Reduced lung function	Airways and possibly alveolar injury
Worsening of the clinical status of persons with asthma, chronic obstructive pulmonary diseases or other chronic respiratory conditions	Airways injury and reduced effectiveness of host defences

Source: Samet and Utell, 1990.

effects of NO include increased incidence of infectious lower respiratory disease in children (including long-term exposure as in houses with gas stoves) and increased asthmatic problems. Extensive studies of the oxides of nitrogen have shown that they impair host defenses in the respiratory tract, increasing the incidence and severity of bacterial infections after exposure. They have a marked effect in reducing the capacity of the lung to clear particles and bacteria. Nitric dioxide provokes bronchoconstriction and asthma in much the same way as ozone but it is less potent than ozone in causing asthmatic effects.

Despite decades of research, the full effects of NO_2 are not known. Known human health effects are summarized in Table 5.3. Other effects are known but difficult to evaluate. For example, NO has a major effect on blood distribution in the lungs. In animals, it has been shown that exposure to NO_2 makes cancerous metastases from the lung much more likely to appear elsewhere in the body, although NO_2 itself does not cause cancer. Nitric dioxide is also a significant contributor to acid precipitation (see Chapter 11).

Particles

Particulate matter in the air (aerosols) is associated with an elevated risk of mortality and morbidity (including cough and bronchitis), especially among populations such as asthmatics and the elderly. As indicated earlier, they are released from fireplaces, wood and coal stoves, tobacco smoke, diesel and automotive exhaust, and other sources of combustion.

In recent years we have learned a great deal about the health effects of particles. As noted above, fine particulates in urban air pollution, below 2.5 μm in diameter, differ in their chemical composition from larger particles. Larger particulates that are included in PM_{10} (particulates 10 μm and smaller) consist mostly of carbon-containing material and are produced from combustion; some fraction of these is produced by wind blowing soil into the air. These larger particulates do not seem to have as much effect on human health as the smaller particulates. Particulates in the fraction $PM_{2.5}$ (2.5 μm and below) contain a proportionately larger amount of water and acid-forming chemicals such as sulfate and nitrate, as well as trace metals. These smaller particulates penetrate easily and completely into buildings and are relatively evenly dispersed throughout urban regions where they are produced. Unlike other air contaminants that vary in concentration from place to place within an area, $PM_{2.5}$ tends to be rather uniformly distributed.

The health effects of $PM_{2.5}$ CO, sulfate, and ozone cannot be easily separated because they tend to occur together in urban air pollution. Recent research strongly suggests that at least $PM_{2.5}$ and sulfate, and probably ozone as well, are associated with an increase in deaths in affected cities. The higher the air pollution levels for these specific contaminants, the more excess deaths seem to occur on any given day, above the levels that would be expected for the weather and the time of year. Likewise, depending on the time of the year and the weather, there are more hospital admissions for various conditions when these contaminants are high. Ozone in particular is linked with episodes of asthma, but all three elements seem to be associated with higher rates of deaths from and complaints about lung disease and heart disease. It is not yet known which is the predominant factor in the cause of these health effects; some combination of each may be responsible for some effects.

At the much higher concentrations of CO, sulfate, and ozone encountered in many developing countries, the health effect is likely to be proportionately greater. There are many factors that complicate such studies in developing countries. The very high rates of respiratory disease during the winter among even nonsmokers in some northern Chinese cities, for example, have been attributed to air pollution, and although this is likely to be true, cigarette smoking, indoor air pollution from coal-fired stoves, crowded conditions, and the risk of viral infections may also be important factors.

Carbon Monoxide

Carbon monoxide is produced primarily by the incomplete burning of fossil fuels—for example, by cars and other gasoline-powered engines and by charcoal or oil heaters. As it is odorless, colorless, and slightly heavier than air, it tends to collect in confined spaces and affects people without warning. The written history of CO goes back centuries, as Roman records discuss deaths associated with fires in enclosed spaces.

Basically, as CO concentrations go up, the oxygen-carrying capacity of the blood goes down, because oxygen molecules are literally being replaced by CO molecules and the ability of hemoglobin (carboxy-hemoglobin [COHb]) to bind oxygen depends on O_2 binding at neighboring sites. The CO molecule's bond to hemoglobin is 200–300 times stronger than the hemoglobin-oxygen bond, so CO

TABLE 5.4

PREDICTED CARBOXYHEMOGLOBIN LEVELS FOR SUBJECTS ENGAGED IN DIFFERENT TYPES OF WORK

Carbon Monoxide Concentration		Exposure Time	Predicted COHb Level for those Engaged in		
(ppm)	(mg/m³)		Sedentary Work	Light Work	Heavy Work
100	115	15 min	1.2	2.0	2.8
50	57	30 min	1.1	1.9	2.6
25	29	1 hr	1.1	1.7	2.2
10	11.5	8 hr	1.5	1.7	1.7

Source: WHO, 1987a.

TABLE 5.5

HUMAN HEALTH EFFECTS ASSOCIATED WITH LOW-LEVEL CARBON MONOXIDE EXPOSURE: LOWEST OBSERVED ADVERSE EFFECT LEVELS

Carboxyhemoglobin Concentration (%)	Effects
2.3–4.3	Statistically significant decrease (3%–7%) in the relation between work time and exhaustion in exercising young, healthy men
2.9–4.5	Statistically significant decrease in exercise capacity (i.e., shortened duration of exercise before onset of pain) in patients with angina and increase in duration of angina attacks
5–5.5	Statistically significant decrease in maximal oxygen consumption and exercise time in young, healthy men during strenuous exercise
<5	No statistically significant vigilance decrements after exposure to carbon monoxide
5–7.6	Statistically significant impairment of vigilance tasks in healthy experimental subjects
5–17	Statistically significant diminution of visual perception, manual dexterity, ability to learn, or performance in complex sensorimotor tasks (e.g., driving)
7–20	Statistically significant decrease in maximal oxygen consumption during strenuous exercise in young, healthy men

Source: WHO, 1987a.

is not cleared easily from the circulatory system. Exposure to short periods of high-concentration CO is just as bad as long periods of low concentrations. Carbon monoxide is also a messenger molecule in the human nervous system and some of its effects may be direct.

Normal amounts of CO in the blood are in the range of 1%. Smokers can have higher concentrations, around 3%–5%, and if one were to exercise at rush hour in heavy traffic (at 10–15 ppm), levels of 3%–4% could be expected. Different predicted COHb levels for subjects engaged in different types of work are shown in Table 5.4. Different lowest observed adverse effect levels (LOAELs) are shown in Table 5.5. Exercise tolerance does not seem to be decreased until after a level of about 5% is reached in healthy subjects. People at increased risk include those with heart and lung problems. Follinsbee (1992) found that "for every 1% increase in COHb there was a 4% decrease in time to ischaemic changes." At low levels of CO exposure, symptoms include fatigue, headaches, and dizziness, but higher concentrations of around 3%–5% can lead to impaired vision, disturbed coordination, nausea, and eventually death. To prevent COHb levels from exceeding a 2.5% to 3% level in the nonsmoker, the following guidelines have been proposed: a maximum permitted exposure of 100 mg/m^3 for <15 min; 60 mg/m^3 (50 ppm) for <30 min; 30 mg/m^3 (25 ppm) for <60 min, and 10 mg/m^3 (9 ppm) for 8 hr (WHO, 1987a).

Volatile Organic Compounds

Volatile organic compounds (VOC) include benzene, chloroform, methanol, carbon tetrachloride, and formaldehyde, among hundreds of other compounds. Gasoline is a mixture of many such compounds. In the past two decades some 261 VOCs have been detected in ambient air. While most of these chemicals occur in the environment at very low levels, some are highly reactive. Like nitrogen compounds, they cause indirect effects (such as helping to create ozone) as well as having direct human physiological effects. They may originate from household products such as painting supplies, dry cleaning establishments, refineries, gasoline stations, and many other sources. They can cause irritation to the respiratory tract (from increased rhinitis, or runny nose, to asthma) as well as headaches and other nonspecific complaints. At high concentrations, VOCs have markedly toxic effects, some of which vary by compound, but which include neurological effects in all cases. Direct toxicity from VOCs is primarily an indoor air pollution problem and an occupational hazard, as levels indoors and in the workplace can reach many times that of outdoor levels.

Trace Metals

The trace metals include cadmium, mercury, zinc, copper, lead, and a dozen others. These are called *trace elements* because they are present in the environment or body only in small amounts. Human activity has led to the increase in release of these elements into the environment. Trace metals may have direct health effects on the nervous and respiratory systems, such as liver and skin.

Lead is the best studied of these trace metals. It is known to be a highly toxic substance that particularly causes nerve damage. In children, this can result in learning disabilities and neurobehavioral problems. An estimated 80%–90% of lead in ambient air is thought to be derived from the combustion of leaded petrol. Because of its effects on the behavior and learning abilities of children even at low levels of exposure, efforts throughout the world are being directed at removing lead from gasoline and consumer products such as house paint. The WHO guidelines value for long-term exposure to lead in the air is 0.5–1.0 $\mu g/m^3$/year (WHO, 1987a). Lead is discussed further in Chapter 10 as an occupational hazard.

Other trace metals that occur in air pollution include mercury, vanadium, and iron; all at very low concentrations.

INDUSTRIAL AIR POLLUTION

Types of Industrial Air Pollutants

Industrial air pollution occurs as the result of the release of pollutants (called *emissions*) into the atmosphere. The pollutants mix in air and are diluted but may travel long distances on slow, steady winds if an industrial chimney is tall enough to propel them high into the atmosphere. A fundamental problem of air pollution science is the difficulty of measuring pollutant concentrations accurately.

There are three general types of industrial air pollution as defined by their different chemical characteristics, distribution, and sources (outlined in Table 5.6). *Reducing air pollution* is caused by the emission of SO_2 and particulates, substances that are chemical reducing agents in the atmosphere. Emissions of SO_2 are caused by burning fossil fuels containing sulfur; emissions of particulates occur most heavily when combustion is inefficient. Reducing air pollution is produced primarily by fossil fuel power plants, industrial furnaces, steel mills, and large diesel-powered vehicles.

TABLE 5.6

TYPES OF AIR POLLUTION BY CHEMICAL CHARACTERISTICS AND SOURCE

Type	Composition	Source
Reducing	Sulfur dioxide, particulates	Stationary combustion sources, such as fossil fuel power plants, industrial furnaces, home heating units
Photochemical	Hydrocarbons and nitric oxide emitted by the internal combustion engine undergo complex photochemical reactions in the presence of sunlight, resulting in an atmosphere with significant concentrations of ozone, nitrogen dioxide, aldehydes, and organic nitrates	Mobile emissions sources such as cars, fossil fuel powerplants, petrochemical plants, and oil refineries
Point source	Specific to source of emission, e.g., lead near a smelter	Specific industries; industrial or transportation accidents

Photochemical air pollution, much newer in human history, results from complicated chemical reactions in the atmosphere that are driven by the energy in sunlight. In photochemical smog, emissions rich in oxides of nitrogen and hydrocarbons undergo reactions to produce ozone, specific compounds of nitrogen, and aldehydes—all of which are highly reactive and chemically oxidizing. This type of smog is caused primarily by automobile traffic, to which are added emissions from stationary sources, such as hydrocarbons from gasoline and dry cleaning solvents and oxides of nitrogen from power plants. Many cities have been able to bring reducing air pollution under control. However, as automotive traffic has increased worldwide, photochemical smog became a problem. This type of air pollution may occur in settings that do not have a concentration of industry, if there is enough motor vehicle traffic. It is most common, and usually most severe, where the sunlight is strong and temperatures are warm because these conditions favor the chemical reactions that are characteristic of this form of air pollution. Because these characteristic chemical reactions takes time, photochemical air pollution is often worse downwind of the source and several hours after peak emissions.

A third type of industrial air pollution is *point-source emissions*, which affects the immediate vicinity of the plant but does not usually involve atmospheric reactions to any great extent. Examples include lead in the vicinity of a smelter, hydrogen sulfide from a sour gas plant, pesticides from agricultural application, and concentrated fumes from a spill or tank rupture. Such emissions are frequently the result of accidents, particularly those related to transporting hazardous substances by truck or train.

Air Pollution from Industrial Accidents

Industrial activities or accidents may release a relatively large quantity of a specific type of air pollution that becomes a local problem. Severe episodes that have been well-documented include one in Belgium in 1930 (Meuse Valley), one in the United States in 1948 (Donora, Pennsylvania), one in Mexico in 1950 (Poza Rica), two in England in 1952 and 1962 (both in London; see Box 5.1), and one in India in 1984 (Bhopal). The Bhopal incident is presented in Box 5.2.

Air Pollution in the Workplace

Airborne hazards are common problems in occupational health; these are discussed more fully in Chapter 10. Several diseases are known to be caused by inhalation of substances found in particular occupations. For each category of disease noted previously in Common Health Effects of Ambient Air Pollution, there are long lists of workplaces where such diseases have been documented to be excessive because of inadequate air quality controls. The incidence and prevalence of these conditions have changed over time. For example, the fibrotic lung diseases (pneumocomosis that causes scarring of the lungs), which used to be quite prevalent, still occur in developing countries where exposure controls are inadequate. This category of diseases includes silicosis, asbestosis, coal miners' pneumoconiosis, and others. Occupational lung cancer is well documented, as are COPDs and chronic bronchitis occurring in association with workplace exposures. Occupational asthma is now increasingly common, with the list of substances known to be capable of causing asthma growing rapidly. Chapter 10 profiles the common occupational lung diseases.

For many people, the distinction between the work environment, the home, and the general environment is an artificial distinction, as discussed in Chapter 1. Exposure control in the community should always be linked to exposure control inside the plant, and the fact that exposures are usually much higher inside the plant should always be taken into account in prioritizing prevention activities.

AIR POLLUTION AND THE COMMUNITY

Magnitude and Sources of Ambient Air Pollution

Industrial development has been associated with the emission to air of large quantities of gaseous and particulate emissions from both industrial production and burning of fossil fuels for energy and transportation. When technology was introduced to control air pollution by reducing emissions of particles, the problem was much improved but it was found that the gaseous emissions continued and the fine particles that are still generated caused problems of their own. Current efforts to control both particulate and gaseous emissions have been generally successful in much of the developed world, but air pollution remains a health risk even under these relatively favorable conditions.

In rapidly developing societies, resources are rarely invested in air pollution control, initially because other economic and social issues took priority. The rapid expansion of industry in these countries has occurred at the same time as increasing automotive traffic, increasing demands for power for the home, and concentration of the population in large urban areas called *megacities*. The result has been some of the worst air pollution problems in the world, at levels much higher than those usually observed in countries where development has already occurred.

Exposure to air pollution is part of urban living throughout the world. Over the past 20 years there has been a shift in the type of air pollution affecting developed countries, as the traditional pollutants from stationary sources (such as SO_2 and suspended particulate matter [SPM]) have been effectively controlled by the implementation and enforcement of legislation in many developed countries. Also, a change from domestic coal burning to electricity and natural gas for heating and cooking purposes has lead to a lower level of emissions of SO_2 and SPM with a concomitant improvement in air quality. However, further economic development (and increasing personal wealth) has resulted in increases in industrial emissions and especially in motor vehicle traffic. This in turn has led to increases in pollutants associated with motor vehicle transport, most notably NO_x, CO, and hydrocarbons, as well as ozone and other photochemical oxidants and lead in many jurisdictions. Attempts to control emissions, primarily through the introduction of catalytic converters and more fuel-efficient engines, have largely been outstripped by growth in motor vehicle traffic (see Mage and Zali, 1992). Meanwhile, in many developing countries, rapid urbanization has resulted in a duplication of many of the problems faced by developed countries. In certain countries, heavy reliance on coal and oil for fuel means that urban SO_2 and SPM levels remain high. In addition, rapid economic development has meant that emissions from industry and motor vehicles are increasingly causing air quality problems (Table 5.7). These issues are discussed further in Chapters 8 and 9.

TABLE 5.7

RELATIVE CONTRIBUTION OF DIFFERENT EMISSIONS AND RESPECTIVE
POLLUTANTS IN SÃO PAULO, BRAZIL

	Particulate Matter (%)	Sulfur Oxides (%)	Carbon Monoxide (%)	Nitrogen Oxides (%)
Vehicles	40	64	94	92
Industry	10	36	3	7
Other	50	0	3	1

Source: Stephens et al., 1995.

Urban air pollution at extremely high levels is implicated in acute and chronic lung diseases, heart disease, and neurological damage. In the past decade, some of the highest air pollution levels (for SO_2) have been found in cities in developing countries (seven of the world's ten worse cities were in developing countries). Today, the worst megacities for SO_2 pollution are in developing countries. More than a billion people live in urban areas with unacceptable air quality conditions. Some of the most severe situations of air pollution are in these megacities, such as Mexico City and São Paulo (Brazil).

Ambient Air Quality Standards and Guidelines

Some air pollution problems, such as foul odors, can be dealt with as a public nuisance. Industrial and urban air pollution is more complicated, and effective control requires (*a*) identifying and measuring the pollutants that are most responsible for the problem and (*b*) reducing or preventing their emission at the source. Control of air pollution requires the identification and control of individual sources of emissions to air to prevent the accumulation of air pollution in a certain region, or airshed. An *airshed* is a space, such as a valley, basin, or plain, within which air mixes relatively freely but beyond which movement is relatively slower, and typically depends on winds. To improve air quality within an airshed it is necessary to control all the sources within the airshed.

To set targets for the control of air pollution, it is necessary to set standards or guidelines. The word *standard* implies a set of laws or regulations that limit allowable emissions or that do not permit degradation (deterioration) of air quality beyond a certain limit. The word *guidelines* implies a set of recommended levels against which to compare air quality from one region to another over time. Table 5.8 presents the standards developed by the U.S. Environmental Protection Agency (USEPA) for the United States. Table 5.9 presents the revised air quality guidelines for Europe recommended by the WHO for "classical" air pollutants. Two additional lists exist for specific air toxics, one for carcinogens and one for chemicals that are not carcinogenic (WHO, 1998).

Standards may take two forms: ambient air quality standards and emissions standards. *Ambient air quality* is the general quality of outdoor air in the region. Guidelines are usually for ambient air quality only. *Emissions standards* set the amount of pollution that is allowed to come from a particular source (see Chapter 4). Ambient air quality standards or guidelines are levels of general air quality

TABLE 5.8
AIR QUALITY STANDARDS, UNITED STATES, 1989

Pollutant	Primary Standards	Average Time	Health Effects
Carbon Monoxide	9 ppm (10 mg/m^3) 35 ppm (40 mg/m^3)	8 hr 1 hr	Aggravation of coronary artery disease
Lead	1.5 μg/m^3	Quarterly average	Development effects on children
NO$_2$	0.053 ppm (100 μg/m^3)	Annual (arithmetic mean)	Increased respiratory infections, risk of acute lung disease
Ozone	0.12 ppm (235 μg/m^3)	1 hr	Decrements in lung function, possibly chronic lung disease
PM$_{10}$	150 μg/m^3 50 μg/m^3	24 hr Annual (arithmetic mean)	Chronic respiratory disease, altered lung function in children, increased mortality
SO$_2$	0.14 ppm (365 μg/m^3) 0.03 ppm (80 μg/m^3)	24 hr Annual (arithmetic mean)	Exacerbation of asthma

in the region that the jurisdiction responsible cannot allow to be exceeded. Sometimes the penalty for this is withholding of funds from the national government or some administrative penalty. Ambient air quality is monitored in various places within the region; an *exceedance* occurs when the level of a particular pollutant is exceeded. The number of exceedances, the average levels of air pollution, and the peak levels during 1 hr may all be used as indicators in air quality standards or guidelines. Ambient air quality standards may include a *nondegradation policy*, which

TABLE 5.9
WHO AIR QUALITY GUIDELINES FOR EUROPE, REVISED 1999

Compound	Guideline Value		Averaging Time
Carbon monoxide[b]	100 mg/m^3	(90 ppm)[b]	15 min
	60 mg/m^3	(50 ppm)[b]	30 min
	30 mg/m^3	(25 ppm)	1 hr
	10 mg/m^3	(10 ppm)	8 hr
Lead[c]	0.5 μg/m^3	n.a.	1 year
Ozone	120 μg/m^3	(0.06 ppm)	8 hr
Particulate matter[a]	n.a.	n.a.[a]	n.a.
Nitrogen dioxide	200 μg/m^3	(0.11 ppm)	1 hr
	40 μg/m^3	(0.021 ppm)	Annual
Sulfur dioxide	500 μg/m^3	(0.175 ppm)	10 min
	125 μg/m^3	(0.044 ppm)	24 hr
	50 μg/m^3	(0.017 ppm)	Annual

[a]No guideline values were set for particulate matter because there is no evident threshold for effects on morbidity and mortality. Authorities are referred to risk estimates for particulate concentrations on the WHO website.
[b]The guideline is to prevent COHb levels in the blood from exceeding 2.5%. The values above are mathematical estimates of CO concentrations and averaging times at which these concentrations should be achieved.
[c]Critical level of lead in blood: <100 to 150 μg/litre.
n.a. = not applicable.
Source: WHO, 1999.

means that not only should air pollution not exceed certain levels but it cannot be permitted, on average, to get worse over time even within the allowable levels.

Control of Ambient Air Pollution

Control of emissions at each source is the key to managing air quality, but transportation policy, energy policy (such as the choice of fuels), and siting of facilities that may emit pollution all play a critical role. A major element in the success of air pollution control is the degree of authority that can be exerted by the government agency that has this responsibility. The ability to close or shut down a plant is the ultimate tool for enforcement agencies, but the ability to fine, bring lawsuits, and prosecute offenders is just as important. Often just the threat of such action motivates the management of a plant to cooperate and correct the problem.

Emissions standards (rules about how much pollution a particular source may emit to the atmosphere) require periodic inspection and regular monitoring to be effective. These are generally easier to enforce for stationary sources, where equipment can be set up on a permanent basis and the pollution control apparatus can be inspected directly. The source or facility may require a permit from the government to operate or may be required to register and to provide regular reports on the pollution it has generated.

Generally, emissions standards for individual factories, power plants, or other stationary sources allocate an allowable level of emissions based on their past performance and share of contribution to the regional airshed. They must not exceed this allowable level of emissions or they will receive a citation and must pay a fine. (In practice, the fine must be high enough to deter violations and not be just another cost of doing business.) If they are repeat violators, their permit to operate can be suspended if the law allows.

In some jurisdictions, the entire plant is considered a single source for purposes of regulation; if engineers can reduce emissions in one part of the plant, they are allowed to build new facilities that increase emissions in another part or to build a new addition to the plant that may generate new emissions. The overall level of emissions from the entire plant must not increase, however. This is called the *bubble concept,* because the plant is thought of as being enclosed in a bubble and the air quality in the bubble cannot be allowed to deteriorate.

Mobile sources are more difficult to monitor, however, and many jurisdictions require regular vehicle inspections to ensure that emissions from each truck or automobile are within acceptable limits (see Mage and Zali, 1992). Box 5.3 summarizes some strategies to address motor vehicle air pollution.

To effectively manage air quality in an urban region, an administrative mechanism must be set up that includes trained inspectors and technical staff who can operate the complicated equipment needed for air quality monitoring and who can interpret the results. A permitting or registration system is needed for enforcing emissions standards. Public education should be very much a part of the duties of the staff, as should enforcement and monitoring. Many air quality agencies are operated separately from public health agencies, which are often attached to the environmental departments of government. Ideally, these agencies have the authority to meet with plant owners or managers before facilities are even built to avoid problems before they occur.

Motor Vehicle Air Pollution: Control Strategies

Studies of human exposures to air pollutants from motor vehicles have revealed the following:

- Concentrations of some air pollutants inside motor vehicles and along roadsides are typically higher than those recorded simultaneously at fixed-site monitors.
- Exposures tend to be higher inside automobiles than in buses and other vehicles used in public transit.
- Priority lanes used to afford speed advantages to buses and car pools tend to reduce air pollutant exposures.
- Concentrations of air pollutants in enclosed settings are similar to outdoor concentrations in the absence of indoor sources, but tend to lag behind the peak concentrations observed outdoors. (A notable exception is commercial buildings attached to inadequately ventilated parking garages.)
- Concentrations of motor vehicle air pollutants decline with greater distance from the road, suggesting that passengers and vehicles are at greatest risk, followed by pedestrians and street merchants along roadsides, and then the general urban population.

Motor vehicle emissions may be reduced by (1) controlling vehicle performance, and (2) altering fuel composition. With respect to vehicle performance, this can be controlled by ensuring that vehicles are designed and built to meet standards. It is also necessary that they be properly maintained. Proper maintenance, in turn, can be promoted by providing incentives to car owners to obtain proper maintenance and by using marketplace incentives. Requiring maintenance through a mandatory inspection and maintenance program is considered by many to be the most effective incentive for car owners.

Control of fuel composition is a direct means of controlling emissions, e.g., reducing the lead content in leaded gasoline or reducing sulfur content to control sulfate emissions. Studies suggest that gasoline hydrocarbon emissions decrease significantly with lower fuel sulfur. Control of gasoline volatility is another strategy for reducing vehicle evaporative and refueling emissions, especially in areas with warmer climates. Some additives have been effective in lowering hydrocarbon emissions and carbon monoxide.

Reduction of emissions per vehicle mile traveled can be very effective in controlling emissions. Strategies for emission reduction include car pooling, increased use of mass transit, parking restrictions, and gas rationing. Policies would therefore be needed to create more efficient public transportation systems; increase the load factor of existing vehicles; shift time of peak traffic (e.g., staggering work hours); improve circulation through use of synchronized signals, and reduce travel demand, e.g., by redistribution of urban activities. Chapter 8 presents some examples of successes regarding bicycle use.

Source: Mage and Zali, 1992.

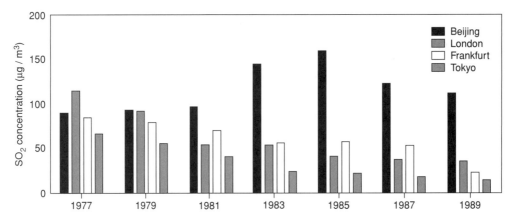

Figure 5.7 Trends in sulfur dioxide concentrations in selected cities around the world. From UNEP, 1992a, with permission.

Due to growing public concern, many nations initiated air quality monitoring in the 1960s. In 1973, the WHO set up a global program to assist countries in operational air pollution monitoring. This project, which became a part of UNEP's Global Environmental Monitoring System in 1976, covers some 50 countries, and data from this project suggest that nearly 900 million people living in urban areas around the world are exposed to unhealthy levels of SO_2 and more than one billion people are exposed to excessive levels of particulate matter (see Figure 5.7 for trends in SO_2 concentrations in selected cities around the world).

Indoor Air Pollution

Indoor air pollution has been identified as one of the foremost global environmental problems (World Bank, 1993). This source probably exposes more people worldwide to important air pollutants than pollution in outdoor air, as discussed in Chapter 9. Whereas outdoor air in such cities as Delhi, India, or Xi'an, China contains a daily average of 500 $\mu g/m^3$ of SPM, smoke inside houses in Nepal and Papua New Guinea contains a daily average of 10,000 $\mu g/m^3$ or more. An SPM level of 50–100 $\mu g/m^3$ may cause adverse health effects (WHO, 1987a). Rural people in developing countries may receive as much as two-thirds of the global exposure to particulates. Women and young children suffer the greatest exposure.

Inefficient and smoky fuels burned for cooking and heating are a source of serious air pollution in many traditional and developing societies. The use of such fuels causes problems both indoors and outdoors. In homes where open fires burn, especially when the climate is cold, the pollution from the fires accumulates and exposes the inhabitants, especially women, to the risks associated with smoke inhalation. The result can be serious lung disease and an increased risk of cancer, as occurs in some parts of China among women who tend fires in homes heated with coal.

The quality of air indoors is a problem in many buildings in developed countries because they were built to be airtight and energy efficient. Chemicals from burning fuels, smoking, and other sources in the building accumulate and create pollution. The most important indoor air contaminants in developed countries are tobacco smoke, radon decay products, formaldehyde, asbestos fibers, combustion products (such as NO_x, SO_x, CO, CO_2, and polycyclic aromatic hydrocarbons), and other chemicals used in the household. Tobacco smoke is a primary contributor to respirable particle exposures indoors. In the United States, concentrations of about 50 $\mu g/m^3$ in houses with smokers and about 500 $\mu g/m^3$ in smoky bars have been recorded (Brooks et al., 1995). Several microbiological air contaminants also cause indoor air pollution, including molds and fungi, viruses, bacteria, algae, pollen, spores, and their derivatives. In airtight buildings especially (e.g., buildings that are energy efficient, but with poor ventilation), indoor air pollutants can accumulate, causing "sick building" syndrome. This is discussed further in Chapter 8.

Indoor air pollution contributes to acute respiratory infections in young children, exacerbation of asthma, chronic lung disease and cancer in adults, and adverse pregnancy outcomes for women exposed during pregnancy. Acute respiratory infections, principally pneumonia, are the chief killers of young children, causing a loss of 119 million disability-adjusted life years (DALYS) per year, or 10% of the total burden of disease in developing countries (World Bank, 1993). The World Bank estimates that smoky indoor air, largely from biomass fuel for cooking or heating, contribute to the acute respiratory infections that kill 4 million people a year, again mostly children under age 5.

Study Questions

1. Draw a diagram showing how the physical forms are related and how substances may change from one form to another.

2. Describe the specific composition of particulates and gaseous constituents of (*1*) wood smoke, (*2*) cigarette smoke, (*3*) automobile exhaust, and (*4*) emissions from a coal-fired power plant. Which has the most matter? Which is predominantly gas? Which is most complicated chemically? Which is likely to be most dangerous?

3. Is air pollution a problem in your area? What are the main sources? What control measures are being used to reduce air pollution at the source? along the path? at the level of the person?

4. How have criteria for developing air quality been developed? What are the scientific and nonscientific issues in setting standards for air quality?

5. Air quality management may involve controlling sources of emissions from industry, transportation, and homes. What effect on air quality may be expected from a national transportation policy that favors automotive transportation over mass transit? What may be expected from a national energy policy that favors the burning of fossil fuels over hydroelectric or nuclear energy? Does the economic base and structure of the community have any implications for air quality in the region? What role does city and regional planning play in influencing air quality? Use your home community as an example of these issues, then compare the situation in another city, town, or village in your country. A number

of initiatives and suggestions for better management of air resources have been discussed in this chapter. Try to develop other initiatives that could be used to promote air quality conservation—these could be economic, social, legal, or physical in nature. (Chapter 8 will return to the issue of air quality as it relates to urbanization; Chapter 9 will discuss it with respect to energy policy; and Chapter 10 will discuss it with respect to industry.)

6. Is indoor air pollution a problem in your home? What are the main sources? How do you maintain air quality?

6

WATER AND SANITATION

LEARNING OBJECTIVES

After studying this chapter you will be able to do the following:

- discuss the importance of clean water as a determinant of health and discuss the nature and extent of waterborne diseases
- list the major sources of water contamination
- discuss how drinking-water criteria are developed
- outline the various approaches to prevention of water-related environmental health problems and the debates associated with implementation strategies

WHY WATER IS ESSENTIAL

Water (or liquids based on water) is essential for basic survival (see Chapter 1). When a person has nothing else to drink, even poor-quality water must be consumed to stave off death through dehydration. The relief may only be temporary since contaminated water can spread disease and cause poisoning. People and animals drink water but they also bathe in it and depend on it to grow crops. Every person on earth requires about 2 liters of clean drinking water each day, which amounts to 12 million m³/day for the world's population. Animal consumption is considerably larger, but animals do not require the same quality of water needed for human consumption. Most of the world's fresh water is used for irrigation: 70% of fresh water is used daily. As the world population increases, the demand for drinking water and irrigation will grow. Water is also used in the generation of hydroelectric and thermoelectric power. Dammed reservoirs provide the gravity-driven force that turns turbines to produce electricity (energize dynamos). Water also acts as a coolant for nuclear and coal/oil power stations. Industry uses significant amounts of water, particularly in the production of paper, petroleum, chemicals, and primary metals. Attempts have been made in these industries to cut back on water consumption through reuse of water, as well as through new processing methods. Water is used for the transportation of goods and people, as a means of recreation through swimming and boating, and as a natural habitat for many forms of fish and wildlife. Seawater is also used to produce salt. The quality requirements for different water uses vary and the impact on water quality varies with the type of use (see Box 6.1).

This chapter will emphasize the health hazards related to contaminated drinking water and lack of proper sanitation. Lack of good-quality water is a key problem in economic development in many parts of the world. In dry parts of the world, lack of water sources is complicated by the poor quality of what is available. The term *water privation diseases* comprises those health problems that occur because of lack of water.

WATER QUALITY, SANITATION, AND HEALTH

Communicable Diseases Associated with Water

Bacteria, viruses, and parasites can spread by water and cause disease. These agents of disease are called *pathogens.* Most of these diseases are considered communicable because they can spread from one person to another via contaminated water or other vectors. The water is a vehicle for spread of the pathogens and other environmental health hazards. The most common diseases of this type are diarrheal diseases, such as cholera, typhoid, paratyphoid, salmonella, giardiasis, and cryptosporidiosis (Box 6.2; see Chapter 2). The minimal infectious dose (the number of bacteria required to make a person ill) is much lower for cholera than for the other diseases, so cholera can spread even via water that looks reasonably clean. The feces of an ill person with cholera or carrier contain large numbers of pathogenic organisms and the contamination of drinking water by feces creates the opportunity for spread of the disease to another person. Many of the communicable diseases that spread via water can also spread via food (see Chapter 7). Successful prevention would have to address both exposure routes. A person does not even need to drink the water to get diseases associated with it. In schistosomiasis, a parasitic tropical disease, for instance, the parasite enters the human body through the skin and causes disease after being transported inside the body to the target organs—the gut and the urinary bladder (Box 6.2).

Water Use and Water Quality

Uses affecting water quality:

- Municipal   sewage discharge, storm water run-off
- Agricultural   manure disposal, agrochemicals, drainage water discharge
- Industrial   wastewater effluents, cooling water discharge, acid mine drainage

Uses limited by water quality:

- Municipal   drinking, domestic and public uses
- Agricultural   domestic farm supply, livestock watering, irrigation
- Industrial   food and other processing, boiler feeding, cooling, mining
- Recreational   swimming and other water-contact sports, aesthetic enjoyment, fishing
- Aquatic life   aquatic and wildlife, fish, swamp and wetland habitat, aquaculture

Uses less or not at all affected by water quality, and with usually less impact on water quality:

- Commercial   hydropower generation, navigation
- Recreational   boating, landscape watering

Source: WHO/UNEP, 1989.

A flowing body of water partially cleans itself. Dissolved oxygen, clay and soil particles, and living organisms in the water all play an important role in the process. Flowing water can dilute, oxidize, and remove pathogens as long as its capacity is not exceeded and sufficient time elapses before water is withdrawn downstream for human use. When the population density of a given area places intense pressure on water resources, this self-purifying capability of water is exceeded. Bodies of water that have their natural flowing properties removed, as, for example, through damming, are much less able to cleanse themselves.

According to *Agenda 21*, the United Nations Program of Action from the Rio Conference in 1992 (UN, 1993), 80% of all diseases and over one-third of deaths in developing countries are caused by consumption of contaminated water. As much as one-tenth of every person's productive time is sacrificed to water-related diseases (UN, 1993). An estimated 1.4 billion people still do not have access to safe drinking water and 2.9 billion do not have access to adequate sanitation (UN 1997), and according to the World Resources Institute (WRI, 1998) this inadequate access to water and sanitation contribute to 2.5 million childhood deaths each year from diarrhea. Most pathogens come from animal or human feces, a result of insanitary excreta disposal. Inadequate water supply plays an equally important role in the spread of disease. Most diseases that are waterborne may also be transmitted by person-to-person contact, aerosols, and food intake; thus, a reservoir of the bacteria is maintained in the people carrying the disease and a sick individual may contaminate water or food supplies and thus continue disease transmission (WHO, 1993a). Some people get infected but do not get the disease symptoms. These people may become carriers of the disease. One of the most famous carriers, known as "Typhoid Mary," lived in New York (Federspiel, 1983). An Irish immigrant who was infected with typhoid around 1900 but did not become ill herself. Instead she became a carrier of the disease because the bacteria lodged permanently in her gallbladder and constantly passed into her gastrointestinal tract. Mary, a kind and well-liked woman, repeatedly took jobs as a food preparer because she did not believe that she could spread disease. By the time she was put in permanent custody by public health authorities in 1915, she had infected at least 47 people and three had died. At the time, it has been estimated that there were at least 200 such carriers in New York City alone!

Most diseases associated with water are caused by pathogens. These diseases are traditionally classified according to the nature of the pathogen. However, such a classification is not very useful for prevention. As explained in *Our Planet, Our Health* (WHO, 1992a), a more useful way of classifying these diseases is according to the various aspects of the environment that human intervention can alter, hence this classification will be used here.

Waterborne Diseases These arise from the contamination of water by human or animal feces or urine infected by pathogenic viruses or bacteria, which are directly transmitted when the water is drunk or used in the preparation of food. Cholera (see Box 6.3), typhoid, and cryptosporidiosis are typical examples of waterborne diseases.

Water-Privation Diseases This category of diseases is affected more by the quantity of water rather than by quality. These diseases spread through direct contact with infected people or materials contaminated with the infectious agent. Infrequent washing and inadequate personal hygiene are the main factors in these types of diseases, such as certain types of diarrheal diseases, helminths, and skin and eye infections.

Water-Based Diseases In these diseases, water provides the habitat for intermediate host organisms in which some parasites pass part of their life cycle. These parasites are later the cause of disease in people as their infective larval forms in fresh water find their way back to humans, either by boring through wet skin or by being ingested with water plants, minute water crustacea, or raw or inadequately cooked fish. Schistosomiasis is an example of a water-based disease.

Water-Related Diseases Water may provide a habitat for insect vectors of water-related diseases. Mosquitoes breed in water and the adult mosquitoes may transmit parasite diseases, such as malaria, and virus infections, such as dengue, yellow fever, and Japanese encephalitis.

Water-Dispersed Infections The disease categories listed above are primarily problems in developing countries. A fifth category of diseases associated with water is emerging in developed countries—infections whose pathogens can proliferate in freshwater and enter the body through the respiratory tract. Some freshwater amoebae that are not usually pathogenic can proliferate in warm water, and if they enter the host in large numbers, they can invade the body along the olfactory tracts and cause fatal meningitis. These bacteria can be dispersed as aerosols from air-conditioning systems; an example of this type of disease is Legionella (WHO, 1992a).

BOX 6.3

Latin American Cholera Epidemic

Cholera is one of humankind's oldest diseases and one of the best-known water-borne diseases. Drinking water that has been contaminated at the source or during storage is the most common source of infection. Any foods that have been taken from contaminated water (fish, shellfish) or washed with it (fruit, vegetables) are also important sources of infection. Severe diarrhea and vomiting are the main symptoms of cholera. The diarrhea is so severe and rapid that patients suffer severe loss of liquid. The main treatment is therefore intravenous or oral liquid rehydration, which prevents the patient from becoming fatally dehydrated. About 90% of cholera cases are mild and difficult to distinguish clinically from other types of acute diarrhea.

The first cholera epidemic in Latin America since the turn of the century began in Peru and quickly spread to a number of neighboring Latin American countries, spreading as far north as the United States. Peru was hardest hit by the disease with a total of close to 300,000 cases reported by January 1992. The spread of disease during the initial period, by February 1992, and by March 1993, is shown in Figure 6.1.

In assessing what had led to the devastating cholera outbreak in Peru, a number of factors were identified: (*a*) urban water supplies were operated on an intermittent basis and thus subject to contamination from leaks, back siphoning, and

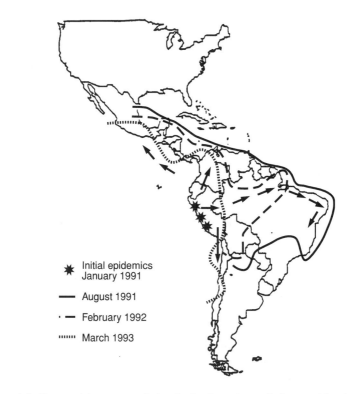

★ Initial epidemics
January 1991

— August 1991

· — February 1992

···· March 1993

Figure 6.1 Geographic extent of the Latin American cholera epidemic over time. From Hug and Colwell, 1996, with permission. *(continued)*

(continued)
cross connections; (b) most households had inadequate hygiene practices related to water storage; (c) in periurban areas most households were not connected to the piped water or sewage systems; (d) organized garbage and solid waste storage, collection, and disposal were nonexistent in the periurban areas and inadequate in many of areas of the central city; and (e) among the poor, fundamental health and sanitation practices were often not applied. A WHO document released following the outbreak outlined a number of guidelines for controlling cholera. These include providing a safe water supply, properly disposing of human waste and educating communities about how to prepare safe water at home (WHO, 1993b).

Chemical and Radioactive Constituents of Water

Some chemical substances dissolved in water as a result of natural processes may be essential ingredients of dietary intake, and some may be dangerous to health when they occur above certain concentrations. Others have both properties simultaneously. To assess the health impact of all of these substances, the Global Environment Monitoring System (GEMS), discussed further in Drinking-Water Supply and Monitoring (below), classifies chemicals in drinking water into three typical categories:

1. Substances (various metals, nitrates, cyanides) that exert an acute and/or chronic toxicity when consumed. As the concentration of these substances in the drinking water increases, so does the severity of the health problem; below a certain threshold concentration, however, there are no observable health effects.

2. Genotoxic substances (synthetic organics, many chlorinated microorganics, some pesticides, and arsenic) that cause adverse health effects such as carcinogenicity, mutagenicity, and birth defects. There is no threshold level for these substances that would be considered safe, since any amount ingested contributes to an increase in risk.

3. Essential elements (fluoride, iodine, selenium) that are a mandatory part of dietary intake to sustain human health. Deficiencies or high concentrations of these elements cause a variety of adverse health effects (WHO/UNEP, 1989).

Some chemicals present in water are of particular importance with regard to their effect on human health. These include arsenic, fluoride, iodine, and nitrates.

Arsenic Arsenic is naturally present in all lead, copper, and gold ores. Groundwater enriched through the weathering of arsenic-bearing minerals is generally the most important source of arsenic in drinking water. There are several geological areas in Asia, North America, and Latin America where dermatological effects were the first manifestation of groundwater enrichment of arsenic. At chronic poisoning levels, various effects are observed, such as vascular disease, liver disease, skin lesions, skin cancer, and neurological disorders.

Fluoride Fluoride is naturally present in some foods as well as in water, but for the most part, it is the amount provided by drinking water that determines the daily intake. Since fluoride is an important component in bone and tooth structure, it is considered an essential element. It is also a toxic chemical. Only a relatively narrow range of fluoride concentrations in drinking water provides optimal conditions. Too-low levels of fluoride increase the incidence of dental caries whereas elevated levels cause mottling of the teeth as well as skeletal fluorosis. Fluoride is added to drinking water in some countries to improve dental health.

Iodine Water is one of the main sources of dietary intake of iodine. In areas where there is very low concentration of groundwater iodine, resident populations suffer from iodine deficiencies resulting in an enlargement of the thyroid gland (goiter) and, in severe cases, mental retardation and cretinism.

Nitrates Excessive and widespread application of nitrogenous fertilizers and manure spraying are the main sources of elevated nitrate concentrations in groundwater. High levels of nitrates in drinking water are of concern because they may lead to serious, even fatal consequences in infants below 6 months of age. Nitrates are reduced to nitrites and, once absorbed, combine with hemoglobin to form methaemoglobin, which is unable to bind with oxygen and therefore transport it from the lungs to the tissues (WHO/UNEP, 1989). The nitrate concentration in selected river systems is shown in Figure 6.2 (WHO, 1992a). With time there is an apparent increase in concentration in many of these rivers.

Other Aspects of Water Quality

Color The color of drinking water is usually due to the presence of colored organic matter associated with the humus fraction of soil. Color is influenced by the presence of iron (usually rusty brown) and other metals—this may be caused

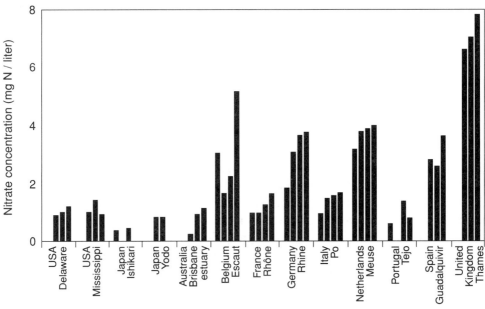

Figure 6.2 Nitrate concentrations in selected rivers: 1970, 1975, 1980, and late 1980s. From WHO, 1992a, with permission.

by natural impurities or may be a signal of corrosion products. It may also result from the contamination of the source with industrial effluents, which could indicate a hazardous situation.

Taste and Odor Taste and odor originate from natural and biological sources, from contamination by chemicals, or as a side effect of water disinfection. Taste and odor may develop during storage and/or distribution. Any deviations in taste and odor may indicate some sort of pollution or malfunction with the storage or distribution systems.

Temperature The temperature at which water is consumed is very much a matter of personal preference. Generally, cool water is more palatable than warm water. High-temperature water enhances the growth of microorganisms and may increase taste, odor, color and corrosion problems.

Turbidity Turbidity in water is caused by particulate matter that may be present as a consequence of inadequate treatment or the presence of inorganic particulate matter in some groundwater. High turbidity levels can protect microorganisms from the effects of disinfection and can stimulate bacterial growth.

Although deviations in the physical characteristics of drinking water may be harmless, any significant changes over time should be investigated, as these may indicate potentially hazardous situations.

ADEQUACY OF FRESHWATER SUPPLY TO MEET THE WORLD'S NEEDS

Adequacy of Supply

Freshwater quality and quantity are inextricably linked. There is sufficient freshwater worldwide to meet human demands at present and in the foreseeable future, but because of uneven distribution of groundwater, surface water, and rainfall, many arid and semi-arid parts of the world lack reliable sources. Of all the world's water, 97% is in oceans or lakes. Of the remaining 2.53%, by far the largest part, 69%, is in the form of snow and ice. The available liquid fresh surface water upon which most communities depend accounts for only 0.008 (2.53% × 0.34) (see Fig. 6.3).

Sources of freshwater include rivers, lakes, and groundwater. The last three centuries have witnessed a significant growth in the volume of water being withdrawn from these sources, an increase of more than 35 times compared to a sevenfold increase of the population. In recent decades, there has been a further increase in water withdrawal, with the highest rates of growth occurring in developing countries. The main increase in water withdrawal is for agricultural purposes (see Fig. 6.4).

Access to water is at least as important a problem for health as water contamination. Water is distributed very unevenly around the world and those areas with less access have had much greater problems with hygiene and quality of water. The tropics and the mid-level of the Northern Hemisphere has much more potential freshwater available than other parts of the world.

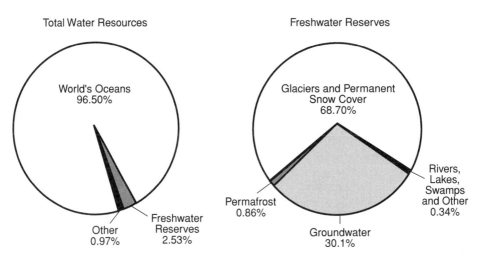

Figure 6.3 Global total water and freshwater reserves. From Shiklomanov, 1993, with permission.

Countries are not simply water-rich or water-poor; there is wide variation within many countries. Calculations based on the level of precipitation per unit of area, for example, are very misleading. Users of water upstream may affect the quality of water available to users downstream. Many countries draw water for sources that come from the territory of other countries, e.g., as Egypt does with the Nile, and The Netherlands does with the Rhine. In the case of Egypt, river inflow provides 50 times more water than does rainfall. The intensity with which local river runoff is used may be a more revealing indicator of water scarcity.

Global Trends

The issue of water scarcity carries many political, legal, and economic implications. Many of the important water basins of the world are shared by more than one country, as in the Great Lakes of Africa and the Aral Sea. The Aral is badly depleted and contaminated on both the Kazakhstan and Uzbekistan sides. It draws

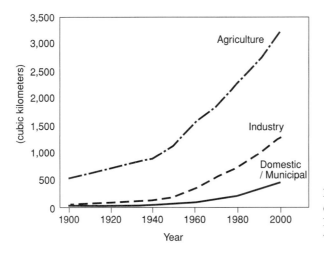

Figure 6.4 Global water withdrawal by sector, 1900–2000. From Shiklomanov, 1993, with permission.

its water from Turkmenistan, Tajikistan, and Kyrgistan and was heavily affected during the days of the Soviet Union by economic decision to benefit Russia. The significance that countries attach to their water resources is reflected in the existence of over 2000 treaties relating to water basins, such as the Great Lakes Compact between Canada and the United States. The first modern treaty on joint environmental management was conducted over the Baltic. In many areas of the world, agreements on sharing water resources are inadequate or do not exist. An example is the Nile Waters Agreement of 1959, an Egyptian and Sudanese attempt to distribute the flow of that river that did not take into account the requirements and demands of upstream countries like Ethiopia. Turkey's construction of a system of dams on the Euphrates River is expected to reduce inflow of water to Iraq to as little as 10% of normal flow (WRI, 1994).

Conflict over shared water resources is a reality in many parts of the world. Attempts in Ethiopia to enhance the flow of the White Nile by building a canal to bypass the Sued (a large swamp in Southern Sudan) was one factor that began the civil war in The Sudan. Dispute over control of the headwater of the Jordan River (a basin shared by Syria, Jordan, Lebanon, and Israel) and the possibility that the river might be diverted into the Israeli National Water Carrier helped to spark the 1967 Arab–Israeli war. Danger of conflict continues due to the competing demands for surface and groundwater in the Jordan River basin. Water sharing agreements are expected to be a key issue in any future Middle East peace agreement. When Solvakia and Hungary had a dispute over damming the Danube River, the matter went to the International Court of Justice.

One area that has been seriously affected by water use for irrigation is the Aral Sea river basin. The large-scale cotton-growing projects established in the 1950s eventually used such large quantities of the water in the rivers Amu-Darja and Sur-Darja that the influx of water into the sea was less than the evaporation. The size of the Aral Sea has therefore gradually shrunk and this has seriously affected the living environment, the economy, and the health of the region around this landlocked sea.

Many international development projects have inadvertently affected water resources and have thereby had a negative impact on both the environment and the health of the communities they were trying to assist. This has occurred even though the projects were intended to enhance socioeconomic conditions and the quality of life. Large dams and water reservoirs that were built in Asia and Africa for irrigation or hydropower in the 1960s and 1970s have led to disastrous consequences, with increases in the cases of schistosomiasis, malaria, and Japanese encephalitis. Such projects have even led to the introduction of new diseases in an area, as in the case of intestinal schistosomiasis introduced into the Senegal River delta following the construction of the Diama dam.

Determining Quality of Fresh Water

The quality and quantity of water tend to be closely linked. Where water is scarce, the quality often tends to be poor and the effects of pollution have an even greater impact because there are no alternatives. Over centuries and particularly over the last few decades, the natural quality of water in rivers, lakes, and aquifers has been altered by the impact of various human activities and water uses. Most pollution problems involving water have evolved gradually over time before they became apparent and measurable. The four most important sources of water pollution worldwide are sewage, industrial effluents, storm and urban runoff, and agricultural runoff.

In many developing countries the problem of water pollution has become similar to that in developed countries. In the past, pollution in developing countries resulted primarily from domestic sewage. While sewage remains a source of pollution, the increasing use of pesticides for agriculture and the production of toxic wastes from industry have increased the complexity of water contamination issues. Currently, in some developing countries water pollution is due to domestic sewerage systems or specific pollutants from industry and it is significantly worse than in industrialized countries where there has been a longer history of pollution control activities. Any efforts at the international level to distribute water equitably need to be matched by efforts to combat the pollution of the various water bodies.

Indirect pollution of water from air is also an important factor in water pollution. *Acidification* is due to long-distance air pollution from industry and motor vehicle traffic (see Box 6.4). *Eutrophication* is due to overloading by nutrients (e.g., nitrates and phosphates) from agricultural fertilizers.

Sudden growth of microorganisms in water is called a *bloom*. Blooms of Cyanobacteria (blue-green algae) occur in lakes and reservoirs used for potable supply and can produce different types of toxins. Adverse health effects are known to be caused by these toxins in drinking water and especially in watering holes for livestock. The increased incidence of toxic algae blooms is sometimes the result of pollution, particularly sewage and agricultural runoff, although such blooms can occur naturally in shallow, nutrient-rich bodies of water. There are insufficient data at the present time to form recommended guidelines, but there is a clear need to protect impounded surface-water source from discharges of nutrient-rich effluents.

The problem of maintaining good water quality is particularly acute in urban areas in developing countries. This effort is hampered by two factors: failure to enforce pollution controls at the main point sources and inadequacy of sanitation systems and of garbage collection and disposal. Box 6.5 gives some examples of water pollution in different cities in the developing world.

DRINKING-WATER QUALITY CRITERIA

The WHO *Guidelines for Drinking Water Quality* (WHO, 1993d) are comprehensive in scope and intended to be used as a basis for the development of national standards. Through use of the WHO Guidelines, each country can develop its own standards based on a risk-benefit approach. Standards that are too stringent may have the effect of reducing or limiting available water supplies in some parts of the world. The Guidelines are therefore designed to be realistic, adaptable, and advisory. The overriding priorities in the Guidelines are (in priority order):

1. An adequate supply of water
2. An adequate supply of microbiologically safe water
3. An adequate supply of microbiologically safe water that meets the guidelines for chemical parameters.

Water Pollution Related to Development

ACIDIFICATION

Acidification of surface and some groundwater is a slow process that is principally caused by increased atmospheric deposition of inorganic acids. Atmospheric deposition in the form of acid rain occurs worldwide through the chemical reaction of rainwater with sulfur and nitrogen oxides, ions from coal/oil burning, and motor vehicle traffic pollution to air. Increased acidic deposition in some susceptible areas has reduced the pH of lakes so that they no longer support fish or animal life. In addition, the release of metals into lakes and streams from acidified soils presents possible risks to human health and to fish in the lakes.

EUTROPHICATION

Eutrophication can be a natural phenomenon in lakes over long periods of time through which organic material gradually accumulates in the lake basin during the geological history of the lake. Added nutrients such as phosphorus and nitrogen serve to accelerate eutrophication and make it abnormal and destructive to the lake. Increased concentration of these nutrients has been attributed to the discharge of wastewater into lakes, the use of fertilizers, and changes in land use that increase runoff. Eutrophication is an established problem in many lakes and reservoirs in highly populated industrialized countries and is probably the most pervasive water quality problem on a global scale. One of the results of eutrophication is algal bloom, which produces large increases in algae in the water of the lake, some of them producing toxins. Eventually the lake suffering from eutrophication will get clogged up with weeds and become a swamp or peatmarsh.

DIRECT DISCHARGE

Direct discharge of pollutants into water is usually controlled by regulations, although it certainly still occurs. Effluent from a plant may carry waste and the byproducts of industrial processes. Runoff from the plant site may carry chemical contaminant, including oil, into drains and then into waterways. Holding ponds are often used to impound the discharge and to partly decontaminate it before release. Thermal pollution is a special type of discharge in which warm water heats the piercing waters and may cause a situation similar to eutrophication. It is often a problem downstream from power plants.

Source: UNEP, 1993.

Many organisms present in drinking-water supplies have no real health significance but may affect the appearance, taste, and/or odor of the water. These organisms may also be important indicators of defective water treatment and distribution systems.

Frequent monitoring for fecal indicator organisms is an old method of assessing water quality but remains the most sensitive way of assessing the hygienic quality of water. Fecal bacteria that have been chosen as indicator organisms are present in high numbers in the feces of humans and warm-blooded animals and are readily detectable by simple methods. They do not grow in water itself. The major indicator organisms of fecal pollution are *Escherichia coli*, thermotolerant and other coliform bacteria, the fecal streptococci and sulfite-reducing clostridia. No water intended for human consumption should contain

TABLE 6.1

BACTERIOLOGICAL QUALITY OF DRINKING WATER (WHO GUIDELINES)

Organisms	Guideline
ALL WATER INTENDED FOR DRINKING	
E. coli or thermotolerant coliform bacteria	Must not be detectable in any 100 ml sample
TREATED WATER ENTERING DISTRIBUTION SYSTEM	
E. coli or thermotolerant coliform bacteria	Must not be detectable in any 100 ml sample
Total coliform bacteria	Must not be detectable in any 100 ml sample
TREATED WATER IN DISTRIBUTION SYSTEM	
E. coli or thermotolerant coliform bacteria	Must not be detectable in any 100 ml sample
Total coliform bacteria	Must not be detectable in any 100 ml sample. In the case of large supplies where sufficient samples are examined, must not be present in 95% of samples taken throughout any 12-month period

Source: WHO, 1993d.

E. coli in any 100 ml sample. taken. Treated water should not contain total coliform bacteria in any 100 ml sample (Table 6.1). The indicators may or may not be associated with the disease themselves. For example, most *E. coli* do not cause human disease, although some do. The presence of *E. coli,* however, is a reliable indicator of potential contamination by pathogens.

Monitoring Contaminants

It is not practical or necessary to monitor water for all possible chemical contaminants and pathogens. While it is possible to detect the presence of many pathogens in water, the methods of isolation and enumeration are often complex and time consuming. Therefore, rather than monitoring water for every possible pathogen, the more logical approach is to detect organisms normally present in the feces of humans and other warm-blooded animals as indicators of fecal pollution (see Table 6.1). The strategy that works is one that (*a*) identifies episodes of contamination that might carry a significant risk and (*b*) closely monitors a few specific contaminants (such as arsenic) that could cause serious trouble.

The WHO has identified contaminants that are potentially hazardous to human health and those detected relatively frequently and in relatively high concentrations in drinking water. Certain indicator organisms and some 128 chemical contaminants can now be assessed through comparison with guideline values. *The Guidelines for Drinking Water Quality* (WHO, 1993d) apply the following principles:

- A *guideline value* represents a concentration of a constituent that does not result in any significant risk to the health of the consumer over a lifetime of consumption, usually assessed to be at least 70 years.

- Water that meets the criteria defined by the *Guidelines for Drinking Water Quality* is considered to be suitable for human consumption and for all usual domestic purposes, including personal hygiene. However, water of a higher quality may be required for some special purposes, such as renal dialysis. The Guidelines are not necessarily protective for these special applications.

- When a guideline value is exceeded, this should be a signal that something has gone wrong in the protection system. It should trigger certain actions: (*a*) to investigate the cause with a view to taking remedial action, (*b*) to consult with and seek advice from the authority responsible for public health, and (*c*) to take steps to ensure that the break in the system will not happen again.

- Although the guideline values describe a quality of water that is acceptable for lifelong consumption, they should be considered a minimum for acceptability. Guideline values should not be regarded as a target that is sufficient and that does not require improvement. The quality of drinking water should under no circumstances be degraded to the recommended level from a better level. Indeed, a continuous effort should be made to maintain drinking-water quality at the highest possible level.

- Short-term deviations above the guideline values do not necessarily mean that the water is unsuitable for consumption. The amount by which, and the period for which, a particular guideline value can be exceeded without affecting public health depends upon the specific substance involved and the degree of the deviation.

- It is recommended that when a guideline value is exceeded, the surveillance agency (usually the authority responsible for public health) should be consulted for advice on suitable action. The significance of an excess level may depend in part on the total intake of the substance from all sources, taking into account the intake of the substance from sources other than drinking water (for chemical constituents), the toxicity of the substance, the likelihood and nature of any adverse effects, the practicability of remedial measures, and similar factors.

- In developing national drinking-water standards based on these guideline values, it is necessary to take into account a variety of geographical, socioeconomic, dietary, and other conditions affecting potential exposure. This may lead to national standards that differ from the guideline values.

- In the case of radioactive substances, screening values for total alpha and total beta activity are given, based on a reference level of dose.

Microbiological Standards

Most of the disease agents that contaminate water and food are biological and come from animal or human feces. The contaminants come in the form of pathogenic bacteria, viruses, protozoa or parasites. Those that can be transmitted via the fecal-oral route by drinking water are listed in Table 6.2, together with a summary of their health significance and main properties. These pathogens present a serious risk of disease whenever they are present in drinking water. Many of these pathogens are also a hazard in food (these are described further in Chapter 7) and include *Salmonella spp.*, *Shigella spp.*, pathogenic *E. coli*, *Vibrio cholerae*, *Yersinia enterocolitica*, *Campylobacter jejuni*, *C. coli*, the viruses listed in Table 6.2, and the parasites *Giardia*, *Cryptosporidium*, *Entamoeba histolytica*, and *Dracunculus*

TABLE 6.2
WATERBORNE PATHOGENS

Pathogen	Health Significance	Persistence in Water Supplies	Resistance to Chlorine	Relative Infective Dose	Important Animal Reservoir
BACTERIA					
Campylobacter jejuni, C. coli	High	Moderate	Low	Moderate	Yes
Pathogenic *E. coli*	High	Moderate	Low	High	Yes
Salmonella typhi	High	Moderate	Low	High	No
Other salmonellae	High	Long	Low	High	Yes
Shigella spp.	High	Short	Low	Moderate	No
Vibrio cholerae	High	Short	Low	High	No
Yersinia enterocolitica	High	Long	Low	High(?)	Yes
Pseudomonas aeruginosa	Moderate	May multiply	Moderate	High(?)	No
Aeromonas spp.	Moderate	May multiply	Low	High(?)	No
VIRUSES					
Adenoviruses	High	?	Moderate	Low	No
Enteroviruses	High	Long	Moderate	Low	No
Hepatitis A	High	?	Moderate	Low	No
Enterically transmitted non-A, non-B hepatitis viruses, hepatitis E	High	?	?	Low	No
Norwalk virus	High	?	?	Moderate	No(?)
Rotavirus	High	?	?	Moderate	No(?)
Small round viruses	Moderate	?	?	Low(?)	No
PROTOZOA					
Entamoeba histolytica	High	Moderate	High	Low	No
Giardia intestinalis	High	Moderate	High	Low	Yes
Cryptosporidium parvum	High	Long	High	Low	Yes
HELMINTHS					
Dracunculus medinensis	High	Moderate	Moderate	Low	Yes

Source: WHO, 1993d.

medinensis. Most of these pathogens are distributed through water worldwide, however, outbreaks of cholera and infection by the guinea worm *D. medinensis* are regional. Other pathogens are accorded moderate priority in Table 6.2 or not listed because they are of lower pathogenicity. These parasites often cause disease opportunistically in persons with low or impaired immune systems, for example, in elderly people or people with AIDS.

Acceptable Daily Intake and Guideline Values for Chemicals

How are the risks of different chemicals determined? There are two principal sources of information on health effects resulting from exposure to chemicals that can be used to develop guidelines. The first is to be found in studies on human populations, studies that are often limited by a lack of quantitative information on the concentrations to which people are exposed. The second is found in toxicity studies on laboratory animals and is the source that is used most often (see Chapter 3). In the WHO's *Guidelines for Drinking Water Quality* (WHO, 1993d), the following formulas are used to determine tolerable intake of various chemicals, and these should be consulted for an in-depth discussion of the formula derivations. The formulas presented below refer specifically to drinking water, but they use terminology similar to that used for other topics in risk assessment (Chapter 3).

For most kinds of toxic chemicals studied, there is a dose below which no adverse effects have been observed. For such chemicals an *acceptable daily intake* (ADI) can be derived as follows:

$$\text{ADI} = \frac{\text{NOAEL or LOAEL}}{\text{UF}}$$

where: NOAEL = no-observed-adverse-effect level, LOAEL = lowest-observed-adverse-effect level, and UF = uncertainty factor.

The *guideline value* (GV) is then derived from the ADI as follows:

$$\text{GV} = \frac{\text{ADI} \times \text{bw} \times \text{P}}{\text{C}}$$

where bw = body weight (60 kg for adults, 10 kg for children, 5 kg for infants), P = fraction of the ADI allocated to drinking water, and C = daily drinking-water consumption (2 liters for adults, 1 liter for children 0.75 liters for infants).

- The ADI is an estimate of the amount of a substance in food or drinking water, expressed on a body weight basis, that can be ingested daily over a lifetime without appreciable health risk.
- The proposed ADIs are regarded as tolerable throughout life; they are not set with such precision that they cannot be exceeded for short periods of time. Short-term exposure to levels exceeding the ADI is not a cause for concern, provided the individual's intake averaged over longer periods of time does not exceed the ADI.
- It is impossible to make generalizations concerning the length of time during which intakes in excess of the ADI would be toxicologically detrimental. The induction of detrimental effects will depend upon factors that vary from contaminant to contaminant. The biological half-life of the contaminant, the nature of the toxicity, and the amount by which the exposure exceeds the ADI are all crucial.
- The large uncertainty factors generally involved in establishing an ADI also serve to provide assurance that exposure exceeding the ADI for short time periods is unlikely to result in any deleterious effects upon health. However, consideration should be given to the potentially acute toxic effects that are not normally considered in the assessment of an ADI.
- The GV is generally rounded to one significant figure to reflect the uncertainty in animal toxicity data and exposure assumptions made. More than one sig-

nificant figure is used for GVs only when extensive information on toxicity and exposure provides greater certainty.

As noted earlier, carcinogens, which are generally genotoxic chemicals, have no detectable threshold for consumption and consequently may be harmful at any level of exposure. The development of an ADI for these chemicals is therefore inappropriate, as was discussed in Chapter 2. The initiating event in the process of chemical carcinogenesis is the induction of a mutation in the genetic material (DNA) of somatic cells. There are carcinogens, however, that are capable of producing tumors without genotoxic activity, but through an indirect mechanism. It is generally believed that a threshold dose exists for these nongenotoxic carcinogens, but in most cases this threshold has not been determined.

For carcinogens for which there is convincing evidence to suggest a nongenotoxic mechanism, guideline values are calculated using an ADI approach. In the case of genotoxic carcinogens, guideline values were determined by means of a mathematical model, and the guideline values are presented as the concentration in drinking water associated with an estimated excess lifetime cancer risk of 10^{-5} (one additional cancer case per 100,000 of the population ingesting drinking water containing the substance at the guideline value for 70 years).

DRINKING-WATER SUPPLY AND MONITORING

The Source

Proper selection and protection of water sources are critical for the provision of safe water. It is always better to protect water from contamination than to treat it after it has been contaminated. Before determining that a source of water will be used as a drinking-water supply, it is important to ensure that the quality of the water is satisfactory or treatable and that the quantity available is sufficient to meet continuing water demands. Seasonal variations and potential growth of the community must be taken into account to ensure that there are no shortages. Sources of groundwater such as springs and wells should be sited and constructed so they are protected from surface drainage and flooding. Areas of groundwater abstraction should be fenced in and kept clear of garbage.

The protection of surface water is more problematic. Surface water such as streams, rivers, and lakes are more vulnerable to pollution. The water source should be protected from human activities. If possible, the source should be isolated and there should be control over polluting activities in the area, such as dumping of hazardous wastes, mining, and agricultural use of fertilizers and pesticides. Recreational activities should be limited so that they are not likely to introduce contamination. While it may be possible to protect a reservoir from major human activity, this may be more difficult to enforce in the case of a river. Often it is necessary to accept existing uses of a lake or river and design treatment accordingly.

In areas where drinking water is collected from roofs it is important to avoid contamination from paint on the roof or in the storage tanks. In addition, an increase in air pollution may add to poor-quality roof water.

GEMS/Water

The United Nations Environment Program's Earthwatch office and the Global Environment Monitoring System (GEMS), in association with the WHO, UNESCO, and the World Meteorological Organization, have developed a global water quality monitoring network, called GEMS/Water. Initiated in 1977, the network includes 344 monitoring stations—240 river stations, 43 lake stations, and 61 groundwater stations. Rivers such as the Rhine, the Nile, and the Ganges, and lakes, from Lake Tai in China to the North American Great Lakes, are routinely sampled and analyzed. Groundwater, crucial for drinking-water supplies, is sampled in Africa and the Middle East, particularly in areas where no perennial rivers flow. More than 50 water variables are measured, providing information on the suitability of water for human consumption, and for agricultural, commercial, and industrial uses. All data are stored and processed at the GEMS/Water global data bank at the National Water Research Institute in Canada, and summaries of the data are published every 3 years. In 1990, the GEMS/Water Program broadened its scope to include not only monitoring but data interpretation, assessment of critical water quality issues, and management option analysis.

Whereas guideline values have been set for drinking water itself, no firm requirements can be formulated for the source of such water (WHO/UNEP, 1989). Water quality monitoring, however, is in place in several countries through the GEMS project (Box 6.6).

Drinking water can also be produced from seawater through desalination. This is common in countries with little rainfall and large oil supplies, e.g., Bahrain and Curaçao. The process of removal of salt from seawater involves boiling, distillation, or reverse osmosis, all technologies with high energy requirements.

Treatment of Drinking Water

Proper treatment of drinking water protects the consumer from health risks associated with biological or chemical hazards in the water. The quality of the original source of water determines the extent of treatment required. The number of people served by a particular drinking-water supply also influences the treatment process. If the water comes from a source serving only one or a few households, the treatment may take place at the site of consumption rather than at the source or in the distribution system, which is the rule for large population supplies. Water purification filters and disinfecting tablets can be used at the household end. It is even better to protect the household source, such as a well, so that the water can be used directly with minimal treatment or handling.

The most common treatment methods include (*a*) pretreatment in reservoirs; (*b*) coagulation, flocculation, and sedimentation; (*c*) filtration; and (*d*) disinfection (see Box 6.7 and Fig. 6.5). Details of these methods are given in the WHO's

Water Treatment and Chlorination By-Products

A typical water treatment facility, as may be found in large cities in Canada, is shown in Figure 6.5. After water is drawn from a source, large debris is removed via a screen. A disinfectant is then added to reduce bacteria. The process of coagulation, flocculation, sedimentation, and filtration constitutes the treatment process. Through coagulation and flocculation particulate impurities are removed; adding a coagulant causes the particles to clump, whereas flocculation is a slow stirring process during which the particles gather together to form larger particles. Sedimentation is used to remove suspended solids that have been preconditioned by the coagulation–flocculation process, following which a filter completes the process of removing suspended solids. Sometimes a disinfectant is added before the distribution of treated water.

Trihalomethanes (THMs) result from the reaction of chlorine with organic precursors during the water treatment process. Several ecological studies have examined the relationship between THMs and cancer. These studies have generally suggested that there is an association between THMs and cancer of the bladder and colon. Some of the studies have also reported that incidence of cancers of the rectum, stomach, breast, lung, pancreas, and kidney and non-Hodgkin's disease may increase in association with THMs. Some case–control studies have also suggested significant associations for cancers of the bladder, colon and rectum. The sum of the available evidence points to a small increased risk of some cancers associated with consuming water with high levels of THMs.

Characteristics of the treatment process affect the amount of chlorine compounds and organic precursors in treated water. The stage at which disinfection is performed is important in determining the THM level, since other treatment procedures will affect the level of organic precursors available to react with chlorine. For example, when chlorine compounds are added before any treatment, the largest levels of THMs result. This effect is tempered by using activated carbon later in the process, as it has the potential to remove volatile organic compounds. The amount of chlorine by-products in treated water can also be reduced with dechlorination.

It is important to recognize that disinfection is an important component of water treatment. While measures should be followed to reduce cancer risk to a minimum, the health risks associated with failing to chlorodisinfect water far exceed the risks of chlorination, according to current knowledge.

Source: Marrett and King, 1995.

Guidelines document (WHO, 1993d). One of the basic elements of the treatment methods is sedimentation of larger particles in reservoirs, where special screens can further reduce the amount of organic matter in the water. Predisinfection with chlorine compounds can also be used in this process if the water is known to be polluted by sewage. In the coagulation step, aluminium or iron compounds are added, which react with impurities in the water to cause flocculation (creation of slimy particles, called *flocs*, in the water). These flocs will attach to bacteria and other remaining organic material in the water, and the flocs can be sep-

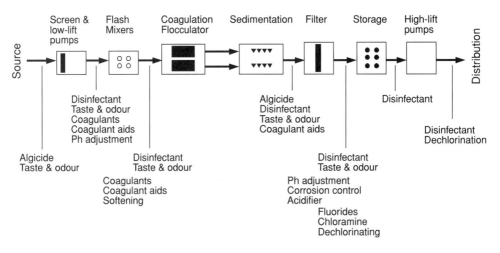

Figure 6.5 Diagram of a water treatment process. From Marrett and King, 1995, with permission.

arated from the water by sedimentation or flotation. To ensure that all flocs and most bacteria are removed from the water, the next step includes filtration in sand. The longer distance of sand the water filters through, the more efficient the filtration. Normally, bacterial counts can be reduced by a factor of about 1000 by a suitable sand filter.

Even after thorough sand filtration, some bacteria and viruses may remain, so a final disinfection is extremely important. The most commonly used methods involve the addition of chlorine or hypochlorite to the water. Disinfection can also be achieved with chloramines, chlorine dioxide, ozone, and ultraviolet (UV) radiation. The latter method has been applied in small-scale solar-powered disinfection units, and this may be the method of choice for remote areas with much sunlight. The chlorination process makes it possible to maintain a certain level of free residual chlorine in the water during its transport through the distribution system. This reduces the buildup of bacterial and algae growth inside the pipes, and it maintains some protection from contamination of the water during transport. In large population supply systems, the water source is often prone to contamination and the storage and distribution systems can be contaminated. Chlorine is preferred because it continues to act downstream. In Box 6.7 chlorination of drinking water is discussed further.

In some countries, fluoridation of drinking water is as an approach to increase the daily intake of fluoride to levels that prevent caries in teeth. This practice has been controversial because excessive intake of fluoride can have detrimental health effects and can discolor teeth (see Chemical and Radioactive Constituents of Water, above). Individual intake is difficult to control. Fluoride in toothpaste provides significant exposure for people who use such toothpaste. The fluoridation of water supplies is nonetheless promoted as an essential intervention for preventive oral health.

Distribution and Storage

Where high-quality piped water is readily available in the home, monitoring of water quality can be done directly at the time of use. According to the WHO's

Guidelines, these conditions are "globally the exception rather than the rule" (WHO, 1993d). Many people worldwide collect water away from the point of use or store water in unsanitary conditions in their homes. In cases where an adequate supply is present, contamination may occur in household storage tanks if they are not property installed and maintained. Contamination can also occur during distribution of water from the source to the household, through the use of dirty containers and/or coverings. Contamination of water in the home may be the most important source of microbiological contamination throughout the world. Educational initiatives on the subject of water handling and the promotion of storage tank maintenance can reduce this risk to human health.

Place of Use

As discussed in Chapter 4, Factors Affecting the Perception and Acceptance of Risk, many organisms present in water have no real health significance but may be important indicators of other problems with either the water supply or the water distribution system. Consumers cannot usually assess the safety of their water systems themselves but their attitude toward their water supply and water suppliers will certainly be affected by what they can perceive themselves. The provision of water that is not only safe but physically acceptable is important to a community (see Other Aspects of Water Quality, above).

Heat kills bacteria and protozoa and destroys viruses. Boiling water is a very effective means of treating water for biological contamination but it is ineffective for controlling chemical contamination. It is also very expensive, especially where fuel is in scarce supply. Water can also be filtered at the place of use. For small volumes, disinfection chemicals can be used to treat highly contaminated water. Small-scale systems based on solar UV radiation as a disinfectant have been developed.

SANITATION

Throughout this chapter numerous references have been made to sewage, excreta, or fecal contamination. The prevalence of waterborne diseases resulting from this type of contamination raises the obvious question of what can be done to improve sanitation. In the 1970s, international agencies began to look at alternative low-cost sanitation technologies for rural and low to medium-density urban settlements. There are now over 20 different excreta disposal systems that offer varying degrees of convenience and protection. One such system, the ventilated improved pit (VIP) latrine, is outlined in Box 6.8 and Figure 6.6. Larger-scale sewage systems for urban areas are described in the section Wastewater Treatment and Reuse, below. Concerted efforts during the 1980s brought improved water and sanitation services to many of the world's poorest people. Although the target of the International Drinking Water Supply and Sanitation Decade (IDWSSD), discussed in the last section of this chapter, was to provide safe drinking water and sanitation to underserved urban and rural communities by 1990, the progress of the decade was not enough.

Most urban centers in Africa and Asia have no sewage system at all, including many cities with a million or more inhabitants (WHO, 1992a). In 1994 at

Ventilated Improved Pit Latrine

A ventilated improved pit latrine (VIP) is an improved version of the traditional pit latrine. The main difference between a VIP and a pit latrine is that a VIP has a vent pipe with a fly screen at the top. The vent pipe and fly screen together have two effects: increased ventilation and fly control. The vent pipe creates a flow of fresh air through the cubicle and pit. As wind blows over the top of the vent pipe, it sucks air up the pipe and out of the pit. Fresh air is then drawn from outside, through the cubicle, and down into the pit. The toilet itself is therefore odorless (see Fig. 6.6a). Flies approaching the latrine are attracted to the odors coming from the pipe, but cannot pass the screen to enter the pit. Flies escaping from the pit are attracted to the light coming down the pipe, but are trapped by the screen and cannot leave. Thus far fewer flies are attracted to and able to breed in the toilet (see Fig. 6.6b).

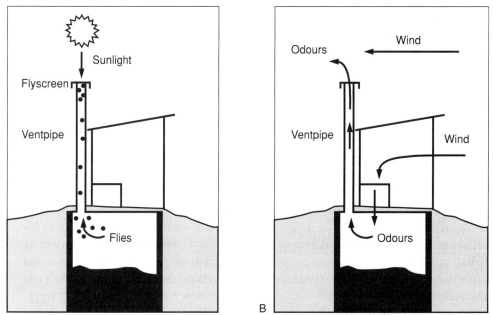

FIGURE 6.6 Ventilated improved pit (VIP) latrine. In addition to the vent pipe and fly-screen, the following are other important features of a VIP toilet: (*1*) Apart from the holes for the vent pipe and the toilet seat, the pit should be completely sealed by the slab to prevent odors (**B**) and flies (**A**) from escaping. (*2*) In soft ground the pit should be lined, to prevent the toilet from collapsing. If the ground is solid, it may only be necessary to line the top part of the pit. (*3*) The superstructure interior must be shaded (i.e., light must not be allowed to enter it directly), as this attracts flies from the pit. (*4*) The toilet must be well maintained and kept clean for it to work properly. Contributed by D. Carter, The MVULA Trust.

TABLE 6.3

URBAN WATER AND SANITATION COVERAGE BY REGION, 1994

Service	Africa (%)	Asia and Pacific (%)	Middle East (%)	Latin America (%)
WATER				
Population covered	68.9	80.9	71.8	91.4
Served by house connection	65	48.4	89.7	92
Served by public standpost	26	24	9.3	3.3
Served by other	9	27.6	0	4.7
SANITATION				
Population covered	53.2	69.8	60.5	79.8
Served by house connection to				
sewer/septic system	53.0	42.7	100.0	91.2
Pour-flush latrine	3.0	43.1	0	2.1
Ventilated improved pit latrine	13.6	2.7	0	0.9
Simple pit latrine	22.4	8.5	0	5.4
Other	2.6	3.0	0	0.4

Reproduced from WRI/UNEP/UNDP/World Bank, 1996, with permission.

least 220 million people still lacked an easily accessible source of potable water (see Table 6.3) (WRI, 1996). Figures for water supply and sanitation often understate the problem because they do not take into account the quantity of water needed by a household for proper hygienic practices. Moreover, figures given for clean water sources or adequate sanitation facilities in a community may also conceal some problems. If people have to wait in long lines for their water, they often reduce their water consumption below what is needed for good health (WHO, 1992a). People who have to walk long distances to use a latrine may end up defecating where it is most convenient to save effort. Improving sanitation will only work if other factors such as personal hygiene and adequate water supply are addressed simultaneously. Improving access to water and sanitation facilities alone can reduce the incidence of diarrheal disease by at least 20% (WRI, 1996).

As noted in *Our Planet Our Health* (WHO, 1992a), capital costs alone are not a sufficient basis for determining the cost of a system because some systems are more expensive than others to operate and maintain. The total discounted capital, operation, and maintenance costs for each household must be calculated to determine the charge that must be levied for the service and establish whether households can afford to pay for the service. If the monthly cost of providing sanitation exceeds 5% of the family income, it may be considered unaffordable. Most low-cost sanitation alternatives come within this range, even for the poorest of communities. Table 6.4 outlines typical sanitation facilities and their costs. Costs are a crucial factor in the choice of sanitation systems, but a number of other determinants such as settlement and population density, ground conditions, and social and cultural practices will also play a role.

TABLE 6.4

CAPITAL COSTS OF SANITATION SYSTEMS (1990 PRICES)

Type of System	Cost (U.S. $) per Household (1990)
Twin-pit pour-flush latrine	75–150
Ventilated improved pit latrine	68–175
Shallow sewerage	100–325
Small-bore sewerage	150–500
Conventional septic tank	200–600
Conventional sewerage	600–1200

Reproduced from WHO, 1992a, with permission.

CONTROL OF WATER POLLUTION

Domestic sewage, stormwater runoff, and industrial wastes have all been mentioned in this chapter as significant contributors to water quality degradation. A few decades ago, it was considered economically acceptable to turn over some water courses entirely to waste disposal, with other water bodies being reserved for drinking water. However, this is no longer acceptable practice. The increase of population density in urban areas, the concern for environmental protection, the greater understanding of the links between the environment and health, and a better assessment of the economic damage of water pollution have all served to motivate an improvement in pollution control practices (Hespanol and Helmer, 1993).

As highlighted in Box 6.5, many of the rivers that flow through the developing world's major cities are little more than open sewers. Untreated industrial and municipal wastes add pollution loads far beyond the rivers' self-purifying capacities. While these rivers and other surface water bodies are highly visible signs of pollution, less visible but equally dangerous is the contamination taking place in groundwater. The attraction of groundwater as a supply source has led to over-exploitation. This in turn has led to a number of quality problems. As the natural water table falls, saline water is drawn in to replace the fresh water. Seepage through the soil can contaminate groundwater with pathogens from sewage, as well as a wide variety of potentially toxic compounds dumped by industry. Improvements in sanitation, wastewater treatment and reuse, and in the regulation of industrial pollution need to be priority areas for controlling the pollution of both surface and groundwater sources.

Industrial Pollution

Industrial wastes degrade water quality when proper disposal methods are not in place. The water may become so polluted that it is not fit for other uses. Many factories in developing countries have been built without effective waste treatment and disposal systems, since costs would increase production costs and accordingly reduce a product's competitiveness on the international market. Industrial wastes, especially those containing heavy metals and organic chemicals, may leave a particularly severe impact due to their persistence, their harmful effects at low concentrations, and their ability to enter the food chain (Hespanol and Helmer, 1993).

Agenda 21 recognizes that "gross chemical contamination, with grave damage to human health . . . and the environment, has in recent times been continuing within some of the world's most important industrial areas. Restoration will require major investment and development of new techniques" (UN, 1993). In every country there must be an appropriate legislative framework developed to support a public administration that can issue and enforce regulations and responsibilities, and develop control policies.

Wastewater Treatment and Reuse

Treatment Wastewater treatment accounts for the largest part of the costs associated with urban sanitation. The level of wastewater treatment established should be consistent with the characteristics of the receiving waters to which the effluents will be discharged after treatment or according to reuse practices. When choosing a treatment system decision makers have to take into account the availability of forms, equipment, and expertise. The system must also be adapted to local climatic conditions, particularly where there is flooding, to support water treatment locally.

There are three levels of wastewater treatment: primary, secondary, and tertiary. In *primary treatment,* sewage is held in settling tanks and solid materials are allowed to settle out of the water. Bacterial action digests organic materials and the sludge that remains is dried and disposed of. Excess sludge from biological treatment plants can be composted to produce a stable biomass that is free of pathogens and can be applied to agricultural land as a soil conditioner. In *secondary treatment,* further degradation of wastewater organics is accomplished by bacteria in an oxygen-rich environment, created by blowing or shipping air into the wastewater. *Tertiary treatment* involves chemical separation of phosphates and nitrates and in some cases further action by bacteria in ponds or through filtration.

The most common tertiary treatment systems used in both developing and industrialized countries are based on processes such as the following:

- stabilization ponds
- activated sludge
- trickling filters and towers
- aerated lagoons
- upflow anaerobic sludge blanket reactors (UASBR).

The choice of treatment depends on such factors as land availability, power requirements, and availability of skilled operators. The UASBRs have low power and land requirements. Stabilization ponds require large amounts of land but are simple and inexpensive to operate. Activated sludge plants require considerable amounts of power as well as skilled operation.

Wastewater is a valuable resource that plays an important role in the management of water resources (WHO, 1980b). Worldwide, water withdrawal for irrigation accounts for nearly 70% of all use. By using wastewater for irrigation, particularly in arid or semi-arid parts of the world, high-quality water currently being used for agriculture could instead be made available for drinking. Reuse of wastewater for irrigation of crops may help to increase food production while improving health and social conditions. The use of wastewater for irrigation or aquaculture can prevent problems associated with the discharge of untreated or partially treated wastewater into rivers and lakes. Additionally, by reducing the dependence on groundwater for irrigation, the use of wastewater helps to diminish the problems of saltwater intrusion into aquifers. Wastewater can be used particularly effectively in forestry and thus be of aid to arid developing areas or countries suffering from deforestation.

If wastewater used in irrigation is not carefully controlled, health problems may result. The following integrated safeguard measures can be used to protect the health of people who may be at risk from wastewater use systems:

- *Wastewater treatment,* to ensure that the wastewater applied to crops has low levels of pathogenic organisms
- *Wastewater application techniques,* such as drip irrigation, that avoid wastewater coming into contact with the edible parts of crops
- *Crop selection,* to limit the use of wastewater for irrigating crops that are not consumed directly (industrial and fodder crops) or that grow well above the ground (tomatoes and chili), or crops not eaten raw (potatoes)
- *Human exposure control,* by advising farm workers, crop handlers, and consumers of potential hazards through programs of health education, by immunizations, by providing treatment and adequate medical facilities to treat diarrheal diseases

RECREATIONAL WATER QUALITY GUIDELINES

Recreational uses of water include swimming, boating and diving. Although water quality for these uses does not have to be as stringent as for drinking water, there must be some controls to prevent contamination and waterborne diseases from recreational water uses. Recreational water quality is becoming an increasingly important issue because of the economic importance of tourism around the globe. Recreational water quality guidelines have mostly been the concern of developed countries. Although acceptable levels of microorganisms and contaminants will vary from country to country, the method of assessing the water quality is fairly standardized among developed countries. The recommended levels given here are from the *Guidelines for Canadian Recreational Water Quality* (Health Canada, 1992). Several aspects of recreational water are examined: presence of pathogens and physical and chemical characteristics.

Indicator organisms are often used for determining the presence of pathogens. These organisms are not toxic in and of themselves but reflect the levels of pathogenic organisms that are probably present in the water. Several organisms lend themselves to this task, depending on the resources available to the tester and the nature of the body of water. In freshwater, fecal coliforms are often measured, but there is some debate about the strength of the correlation between their levels and the risk of disease. It is recommended that levels not exceed 200 fecal coliform/100 ml over a 5-day period. Fecal coliforms are not useful in salt water. Fecal streptococci may be a better choice for both fresh- and saltwater, but at present the methods available for determining their levels are more expensive. Other pathogenic organisms should be measured when there is epidemiological evidence that pathogens are present in a particular body or area of water.

Recreational water quality is also dependent on physical and chemical characteristics. Although water temperature is an important quality aesthetically, and for comfort, humans can tolerate a wide range of temperatures. The optimum for swimming is in the range 18°–25°C. Prolonged submersion into colder or hotter water may lead to some of the physical effects discussed in Chapter 2. Acidic and alkaline pH levels are also a consideration but are not extreme enough to affect humans adversely. The recommended range is between 6.5 and 8.5. Turbidity is important in determining water quality because the presence of pathogens is significantly higher in sediment than in surface water. The maximum suggested level is 50 *nephelometric turbidity units* (NTU). Color and clarity can also be important qualities, but they vary so dramatically among different areas of water, depending on the contaminant, that guidelines are difficult to establish. Oil and grease should not be visible, either on the surface or shore, and no odor should be detectable. Both organic and inorganic contaminants vary dramatically and therefore should be measured and the health risk assessed on an individual basis. Although recreational water does not require the same level of protection as drinking water, proximity to sources of pollutants should also be considered.

ENSURING A SAFE AND SUFFICIENT WATER SUPPLY

The Water Decade, 1981–1990

Drinking-water supply has been a top priority of the United Nations. The United Nations Conference on Human Settlements held in Vancouver in 1976 and the Mar del Plata Action Plan (Mar. del Plata, Argentina March, 1977) set the stage for the launching of the International Drinking Water Supply and Sanitation Decade

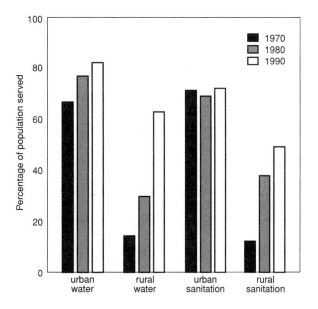

Figure 6.7 Water supply and sanitation access in developing countries. From UNEP, 1992a, with permission.

BOX 6.9

The Mvula Trust: A Community-Centered Approach to Improving Water and Sanitation Services

South Africa had a long history of racial discrimination and inequality. The country had its first democratic elections in 1994. South Africa was left with a huge legacy of inequalities, among them unequal environmental conditions. The challenge of providing the entire country's population with a basic and sustainable level of water supply and sanitation service is enormous. The Mvula Trust is a nongovernmental organization (NGO) dedicated to improving water supply and sanitation services to disadvantaged, poor, and marginalized rural communities. It provides funds mainly to villages that are remote and have low incomes. Local government structures in South Africa are very new, with little capacity to maintain service infrastructure. Overcoming these difficulties to achieve sustainability requires innovative approaches to all aspects of project design and implementation. The technologies installed must be easy for the community to maintain, and they must be affordable. However, the most important element in sustainability is that the community must have a sense of ownership and responsibility for the scheme. For this reason a community-centred approach to project design and implementation is essential. The Mvula Trust has developed an approach based on the following principles.

DEMAND DRIVEN

The Trust only responds to requests for assistance from communities. It does not search for projects, nor does it respond to proposals from consultants unless they are in support of a community application. Without effective, genuine demand for the service and for the level at which it is to be installed, there is unlikely to be a commitment to the smooth implementation of the project and, more importantly, to the maintenance of the scheme.

CONCEPT OF OWNERSHIP

The Trust approach stresses community ownership of the process and the product of the project. The Trust only enters into a contract with the association representing the community, which is then expected to open a bank account, procure materials, employ labor, pay consultants, and set up a tariff collection system.

COMMUNITY IS THE CLIENT

In order for the community to take an active interest in the ongoing maintenance of the scheme, it is essential that the facilities effectively serve their needs. Key decisions regarding the design of the system and the implementation of the project must therefore be made by the community, within a set of clear guidelines, such as the policies of the funding agency. Without this, there is a risk that an inappropriate system will be installed.

COST SHARING

The principle of paying for services is basic to the South African government's reconstruction and development program, which the Trust supports. The Trust expects the community to start contributing cash to a special fund as soon as the pro-

(continued)

(continued)

ject starts. The process through which the association must go to raise the contributions to this fund sets a precedent for the collection of operation and maintenance fees.

CAPACITY BUILDING

A key element in promoting sustainability is to develop the skills needed to take responsibility for the scheme. All Trust-funded projects have a large training component, and the community is given the opportunity to put their training into practice during the course of the project. This develops a strong sense of self-reliance needed to run the project after completion.

The government Department of Water Affairs and the Trust have entered into an innovative agreement. The Trust receives most of its funding from the Department but it is allowed to be separately accountable for public funds. This enables it to retain a flexible NGO structure that can implement rapid, demand-driven processes to support community empowerment.

Contributed by I. Wilson, Mvula Trust.

(IDWSSD, 1981–1990) by the General Assembly of the United Nations in 1980. The main objective of the Decade was to substantially improve the standards and levels of services in drinking-water supply and sanitation by the year 1990.

According to *Saving Our Planet* (UNEP, 1992a), the percentage of the population in urban areas of developing countries with access to safe drinking water increased from 67% in 1970 to 82% in 1990, but access to sanitation services hardly improved at all. In rural areas improvements were more dramatic, with the percentage of people having clean water rising from 14% to 63% and those with access to sanitation services rising from 11% to 49% (see Fig. 6.7). Even so, at the end of the Decade there were still one billion people without a safe water supply and almost 1.8 billion without adequate sanitation. The rate of progress achieved during the Decade would be insufficient to reach the ultimate objective of sanitation for all by the end of the century. The slow progress of achieving the goals of the IDWSSD has been attributed to several factors, including population growth, rural–urban migration, the unfavorable world economic situation, and the debt burden of developing countries. The debt burden has been a major obstacle to investment in infrastructure (UNEP, 1992a).

As discussed in *Our Planet, Our Health* (WHO, 1992a), there are a number of lessons to be learned from the Decade, some of which are outlined below:

- The ability of communities to run and maintain their own sanitation and water systems needs to be strengthened.
- There needs to be greater emphasis on the connections between improvements in water and sanitation and improvements in hygiene and primary health care.
- It is important to involve local populations in decisions regarding design, costs, and management of projects.
- Disease risk and socioeconomic conditions must be considered in the design and delivery of water and sanitation services.

Many development programs have tried to incorporate these lessons into their various projects. The Rural Water Supply and Sanitation Project in Ghana's Volta Region is one example of this approach; many examples are provided in the various international agency publications cited in this chapter. The efforts of the Mvula Trust in South Africa are described in Box 6.9.

Water Resources Management

Consumers, suppliers, industry, and governments all have a role to play in ensuring a safe and sustainable water supply. Leakage is one of the main reasons for the shortfall in capacity of many cities' water supplies. This is particularly true of urban centers in developing countries where typically 30% of the water is treated and pumped into the water supply but as much as 60% is lost on its way. The leakage rate in the United States and Europe is typically around 12%. Proper maintenance of the distribution system is an important way to cut back on water waste. *Pressure* provides the force that moves water through a pipe. When pressure cannot be kept at an adequate level, water cannot be delivered where it is needed and contaminated water outside the pipe can seep into the clean water inside the pipe through leaks. Maintaining adequate pressure requires careful maintenance of pumps and energy to run them. As indicated earlier, governments have an important role to play in the management of water resources, particularly where it relates to pollution control, through appropriate legislative frameworks.

The use of economic devices is also a powerful means of promoting efficient environmental protection and the rational use of water resources by all users, including households, municipalities, industry, and farmers. Public awareness of pricing structures that reflect the real cost of water supply encourages more efficient use of water. Of all natural resources, water is most likely to be consumed at a lower price than the cost to deliver it, as the costs of water utilities are rarely fully recouped from consumers. The most widely known basic principle in this category, the *polluter-pays principle,* is Principle 16 in *Agenda 21* and reads as follows:

> National authorities should endeavour to promote the internalization of environmental costs and the use of economic instruments, taking into account the approach that the polluter should, in principle, bear the cost of pollution, with due regard to the public interest and without distorting international trade and investment.
>
> Source: UN, 1993.

Economic instruments used to put this principle into practice include effluent charges, subsidies to pollution control works, financial enforcement incentives, tax rebates, and budgetary and fiscal mechanisms. Financial incentives that assist polluters to protect the environment, although not universally accepted, are in widespread use. Grants, low-interest loans, and tax credits are incentives given to encourage remedial measures. Financial assistance can be a powerful instrument in environmental protection programs, particularly in developing countries (Hespanol and Helmer, 1993).

Significant progress cannot be made in ensuring water supply and protection without a strong commitment at the governmental level, as large expenditures for infrastructure are required. Some actions can be taken at an *individual* level, however. Water wastage is common in many homes in developed countries. Only 5% of household water consumption in North America is for drinking and cooking; the rest is consumed through toilet flushing (40%), showering/bathing (30%), laundry/dishwashing (20%), and other uses (5%). Most of this water has been treated to a level that is safe to drink, which requires an enormous amount of additional resources. When a lot of treated water is used for purposes that do not require treatment, such as flushing toilets, water and treatment costs are raised. Since it is not generally practical or safe (there is a potential hazard if treated and untreated water lines get crossed) to have a second distribution system for untreated water, the only solution is to minimize the waste.

Study Questions

1. What factors need to be considered to develop an effective strategy to improve sanitation in a rural community of a developing country? Of an urban community?

2. A number of initiatives and suggestions for better management of water resources have been discussed in this chapter. Try to develop other initiatives that could be used to promote water conservation. These could be economic, social, legal, or physical in nature. Think about how these may be implemented.

3. Make a list of ten tips to reduce water consumption in a community affected by water shortage.

7

FOOD AND AGRICULTURE

LEARNING OBJECTIVES

After studying this chapter you will be able to do the following:
- indicate in what ways food may influence human health
- describe the health impacts of nutritional deficiencies
- indicate crucial environmental conditions for food production
- explain the relationship between the environment and food security
- define and illustrate the difference between food poisoning and foodborne infections
- summarize different types of food contaminants, the sources of these contaminants, and their potential health impacts
- indicate various possible routes of transmission of biological food contaminants
- identify the hazards and risks at the various stages between food production and consumption
- describe the impact of the Hazard Analysis and Critical Control Point (HACCP) system on food safety
- illustrate the importance of recognizing differences between perceived risks and objective risk estimations with regard to food safety
- summarize occupational health hazards related to agriculture and indicate risk reduction strategies

CHAPTER CONTENTS

HEALTH AND NUTRITION

Physiological Requirements

Food is a fundamental human need, a basic right, and a prerequisite to good health. The human body depends on the energy, protein, vitamins, and minerals that are found in a variety of foods to survive and remain strong. Studies in Europe in the 1920s showed that in general the poor were short, thin, and suffered from ill health. Their health improved and children grew taller if they were given a diet rich in protein, energy, and vitamins. This diet became the standard for good health and the "balanced diet" became common terminology. A balanced diet could be guaranteed if people ate a plentiful and varied supply of different foods—for example, protein foods derived from animal products or soybeans, energy foods rich in carbohydrate or fat, and protective foods, such as vegetables and fruits, that are rich in vitamins and some minerals.

A variety of nutrients are required by humans to maintain healthy metabolic function. The primary component of our diet is *energy,* expressed as calories or joules. *Energy requirement* is the amount of energy needed to maintain health, growth, and an appropriate level of physical activity. Although the number of calories required varies greatly among individuals, depending on their size, age (all of which influence basal metabolic rate), and level of physical activity maintained, it is commonly based on balancing intake with output. If energy intake and expenditure are not in balance, this imbalance will result in changes in body mass. The conditions of being underweight or overweight both have adverse effects on human health. The health effects of malnutrition and specific deficiency disorders are described below. *Obesity,* defined as a state characterized by excess body fat, is a common cause of severe morbidity and diminished longevity. An association has been found between obesity and hypertension, diabetes, the formation of gall stones, breast cancer, and endometrium cancer. Table 7.1 outlines the basic nutrient requirements and their most common food sources.

Food and Culture

For many years industrialized countries have maintained guidelines for healthy eating. In North America these guidelines are based on the principle of choosing a variety of foods from the basic food groups, including grain products, fruits and vegetables, milk products, and meats (or their alternatives) to ensure intake of

TABLE 7.1

NUTRIENT REQUIREMENTS, RECOMMENDED AMOUNTS, AND SOURCES

Nutrient	Recommended Amount	Common Food Sources
Carbohydrates (sugars and complex carbohydrates)	50%–60% of daily energy intake: (recommended total energy intake: 7–14 MJ or 1700–3300 kcal, depending on age, sex and weight)	SUGARS Fruits, vegetables, honey, milk COMPLEX CARBOHYDRATES Grains, legumes, root vegetables, liver, fruits, vegetables
Lipids	30% of energy (saturated fats and/or trans fatty acids should be <10% of total energy; polyunsaturated fats should be emphasized)	SATURATED FATS/TRANS FATTY ACIDS Animal fat, butter, vegetable shortening POLYUNSATURATED FAT Vegetable oil, milk, fish
Proteins	0.86 g/kg body weight daily (approximation)	Meat, dairy products, eggs, legumes, grains
Electrolytes (sodium, and potassium) and water	—	SODIUM Salt, baking powder and soda, meat, poultry, fish, and eggs POTASSIUM Fruits, vegetables
VITAMINS		
Biotin	No specific recommended amount	Ubiquitous
Folate	No specific recommended amount	Dark green leafy vegetables, meat, fish, poultry, eggs, whole grain cereals
Pantothenic acid	No specific recommended amount	Ubiquitous
Niacin	2 mg/1000 kcal	Meat, poultry, fish, dark green leafy vegetables, whole grain cereal
Riboflavin/Vitamin B_2	0.5 mg/1000 kcal	Meat, poultry, fish, dairy products, eggs, whole grain cereal, dark green leafy vegetables
Thiamine Vitamin B_1	0.4 mg/1000 kcal	Meat, poultry, legumes, whole grain bread, milk, eggs
Vitamin A	No specific recommended amount	Liver, milk, dark green leafy vegetables, deep yellow fruits and vegetables
Vitamin B_6	15 μg/g protein	Meat, whole grain cereal, legumes
Vitamin B_{12}	No specific recommended amount	Meat, fish, eggs, dairy products
Vitamin C	60 mg/day	Citrus fruits, tomatoes, raw green vegetables, some meat, poultry, legumes, whole grain bread, milk, eggs
Vitamin D	No specific recommended amount	Fortified milk, fish, sunlight
Vitamin E	No specific recommended amount	Vegetable oil, whole-grain cereal, legumes, dark leafy vegetables

(continued)

Nutrient	Recommended Amount	Common Food Sources
Vitamin K	1.5 μg phylloquinone/kg/day	Green leafy vegetables, small amounts found in meat, dairy products, cereals, and fruits
MINERALS		
Calcium	—	Dairy products, dark green vegetables, seafood
Chromium	—	Cheese, legumes, nuts
Copper	—	Ubiquitous
Fluoride	—	Fluoridated water, seafood
Iodine	—	Shellfish, saltwater fish, iodized salt
Iron	—	Meat, fish, poultry, eggs, whole-grain cereals, green vegetables, dried fruits
Manganese	—	Ubiquitous
Magnesium	—	Ubiquitous
Phosphorus	—	Dairy products, meat, poultry, fish, legumes, whole grain cereals
Selenium	—	Whole-grain cereals, meat, dairy products, poultry
Trace elements (molybdenum, silicon, boron, nickel, vanadium, arsenic)	—	Variety of vegetables, or seafood
Zinc	—	Plant and animal protein

Source: HWC, 1990.

all essential nutrients. These food groups are considered arbitrary by some investigators, and there is controversy about alleged cultural biases in the recommendations. Many people do not consume products from each of these groups and yet are still in good health. As Table 7.1 indicates, there is a great deal of flexibility when choosing foods that give all the nutrients required. Box 7.1 outlines an example of food consumption that differs radically from the North American model while still providing everything a person requires. Apart from the cultural influences on the dietary composition, factors such as availability, taste, smell, appearance, cost, and convenience are important determinants of food choice.

Effects of Nutritional Deficiencies on Health

Following World War II, protein-energy malnutrition was recognized as a serious health problem throughout the developing world. Simultaneously, it was recognized that communicable diseases were a major cause of death and illness and that nutritional deficiencies weakened the body's resistance to these diseases. The WHO's Panel on Food and Agriculture outlined a number of specific nutritional deficiencies that remain widespread today, usually because of local environment conditions. These are listed below.

BOX 7.1

Inuit Diet

The Inuit are an indigenous people living in northern North America. Their traditional diet consists mainly of sea mammals (seal, walrus, whale, polar bear), caribou, and marine fish, with occasional berries and shellfish. This diet is high in protein and also has high amounts of polyunsaturated lipids (from the phytoplankton consumed by the fish). It has very low levels of carbohydrates and relatively high levels of overall fats, exceeding the recommended amount. Despite these problems and the limited variety in their diet, the Inuit have traditionally experienced good health. Studies of the composition of their marine diet indicate that the animals are extremely rich food sources providing all of the required vitamins and minerals that normally would be achieved only by combining a wide variety of fruits and vegetables. It is gradually becoming clear that native foods can provide all nutritional needs without supplementation.

Iodine Deficiency Disorders Iodine deficiency disorder is a serious affliction in many parts of the world. The Andes, Alps, Great Lakes basin of North America, and the Himalayas are particularly deficient in iodine, although some coastal areas and plains may also be deficient. The most clinically obvious effects of iodine deficiency are goiter and cretinism. Mild iodine deficiency can lead to less obvious conditions such as delayed mental development, reduced intelligence, and diminished work capacity. Some foods, called *goitrogens* (e.g., cassava in central Africa), interfere with the normal uptake and metabolism of iodine from other foods.

Iodizing salt supplies is very effective in controlling endemic goiter, but there are few other practical means of increasing iodine intake. There is some evidence that goiter is increasing in Europe where people are trying to reduce their salt intake. In those areas where intake of iodine from sources other than salt is low, a coordination of policies is needed to control goiter through the iodination of salt without disrupting the control of hypertension by limiting salt intake.

Vitamin A Deficiency Vitamin A deficiency leads to a serious eye disease called *xerophthalmia* and sometimes to blindness. It also decreases resistance to disease and infection and increases child mortality. The availability of vitamin A is limited in some geographic areas and is exacerbated by a diet low in vegetables. In Asia this is a particular problem because the population exceeds the overall availability of vitamin A. Low-fat diets for the prevention of cardiovascular disease are becoming more widespread but if fat intake is too low, it will interfere with intake of vitamin A. By contrast, high dietary supplementation with vitamin A, particularly during pregnancy, may also cause adverse health effects (see Box 7.2 and Fig. 7.1).

Vitamins and Health

Traditionally, health risks related to vitamins are associated with deficiencies. However, the relation between health and the intake of vitamins shows an optimum. Excessive vitamin intake, either through diet or through high supplementation, may result in toxic effects. The margin between physiological need and toxic dose is different for two distinct groups of vitamins: lipophilic (fat-soluble) vitamins (A, D, E, and K) and hydrophilic (water-soluble) vitamins (vitamins B and C, biotin, niacin, pantothenic acid, and folate). For the lipohilic vitamins this margin may be relatively narrow compared to that of the water-soluble vitamins. Whereas vitamin A deficiency may cause xerophthalia or (night) blindness, high doses of vitamin A may result in several other adverse health effects including headache, vomiting, liver damage, and bone abnormalities (see Fig. 7.1 for the health effects of vitamin A deficiency and high dosage). Furthermore, a high incidence of spontaneous abortions and birth defects has been observed among fetuses of women receiving therapeutic doses of 500 to 1500 μg of 13-*cis* retinoic acid per kg body weight. Although the natural content of the diet is not likely to induce toxic effects, it is increasingly important to regulate the standards set for vitamin intake because of the trend toward vitamin supplementation and the use of vitamins as naturally occurring antioxidants in food processing. This is most relevant for the lipophilic vitamins A and D since they may accumulate in the body during long-term consumption of high doses.

Iron Deficiency Anemia is a widespread and persistent problem. Iron is necessary to make blood hemoglobin and is present in the oxygen-carrying red blood cells. Most iron-deficiency anemia in developed countries is the result of iron loss from the body because of internal bleeding. Women are at much greater risk because they lose iron from blood loss during normal menstrual cycles. In some parts of the world, however, the iron intake is also deficient and cannot replace the iron in women or provide sufficient iron stores in children. Certain parasites

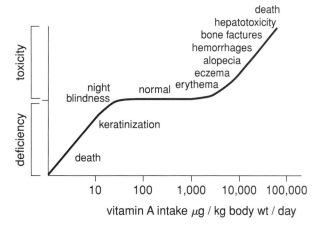

Figure 7.1 Clinical symptoms as a result of vitamin A deficiency and from vitamin A toxicity. From Rutten, 1997 with permission.

also rob the body of iron. Africa and Southern Asia have particularly high levels of iron-deficiency anemia due to a combination of low intake, poor absorption, and parasite diseases. The availability of dietary iron for absorption is affected by both the form of iron and the nature of the foods eaten. The absorption of some iron compounds is strongly influenced by the presence of other factors in the food. Ascorbic acid (vitamin C) and animal foods are known to promote iron absorption. When either of these constituents is missing, a diet based on cereals and legumes may provide only a low level of iron even though the plant foods themselves are rich in iron. Dietary iron intake and low iron stores in the body interact with lead and cadmium intake. Iron deficiency can thus contribute to increased lead and cadmium absorption.

Calcium Deficiency Calcium deficiency causes osteoporosis. *Osteoporosis* literally means "porous bones" and can be defined as a disorder of bone metabolism in which bone mass has been reduced to such an extent that the person is at increased risk of fractures. A shortage of calcium and probably of protein during the growth spurt may contribute to the development of osteoporosis later in life. In addition, the causation of osteoporosis is related to disturbances of the (hormonal) regulatory systems involved in the maintenance of bone mass as well as extracellular calcium concentration. Postmenopausal osteoporosis is the most common form of this disease. At the age of 65 years, 25% of all women have some sign of osteoporosis; at age 85 this amount goes up to 50%. Apart from calcium-deficient diets, the main factors involved in the loss of bone are endocrinological disturbances, the use of corticosteriods, gastrointestinal malfunction, and lack of physical stress to the skeleton. Cadmium and calcium interact so that a high cadmium intake reduces calcium absorption and increases risk of osteoporosis and a low calcium intake increases cadmium absorption and the effects on bones from cadmium exposure.

Other Deficiencies Other nutritional deficiencies are also widespread in some areas of the world. Fluoride deficiencies can lead to dental caries. Rickets and other bone abnormalities are attributable to a combination of insufficient exposure to sunlight and lack of vitamin D in the diet, causing calcium disorders similar to osteoporosis. Ascorbic acid deficiency still occurs in some drought-affected areas, particularly Africa. Vitamin B_{12} deficiency can cause anemia and neurological disorders. People on vegetarian diets that contain no food of animal origin are particularly at risk for B_{12} deficiency.

FOODBORNE DISEASES AND FOOD POISONING

Foodborne illnesses are a common and serious health problem. Statistics underestimate the number of cases of foodborne illness because not everyone affected visits a doctor, and doctors may not report all cases to public health authorities. Some cases of foodborne illness may not be documented because they are not recognized as such. In various developed countries up to 60% of cases may be caused by poor food handling techniques and by contaminated food served in food service establishments. Similar problems exist in the developing world.

Chemical food safety and microbiological food safety are similar but separate issues. Basically, food is a mixture of chemicals (including nutrients), natural toxins, contaminants, and additives. The nutrients account for over 99.9% of the food. Some of these nutrients may also cause adverse health effects in unbalanced diets, as discussed in the previous section, Health and Nutrition. Biological contaminants, additives, chemicals, and radiation will be the focus of this section.

Foodborne biological toxins can originate from two sources: either they are a naturally occurring constituent of the food or they are produced by microorganisms present in or on the food. In the course of evolution, humans have learned through trial and error to select foods that do not cause acute adverse health effects. However, the presence of toxins of microbial origin is not always easy to recognize. Illnesses related to consumption of foods that are contaminated in this way are referred to as *food poisoning*. These illnesses require bacterial growth and toxin production in the food and not in the individual. If the produced toxin is heat resistant, food preparation will not affect the health risks involved.

Natural toxins in food can be acutely toxic. A classic example is ciguetera toxin, a common toxin made by algae in the ocean and contained in the flesh of certain fish that consume the algae. When eaten by humans, the toxin causes severe illness. Natural toxins include venoms and other poisons produced by animals for defense and to capture prey. However, many plants also produce natural toxins in abundance for protection after injury, healing, and defense. Some of these natural products are highly toxic, some of them mimic estrogenic hormones, and some are even carcinogenic. The Nobel prize–winning biochemist Bruce Ames has estimated that the daily human consumption of natural plant toxins may exceed the intake of industrial or synthetic chemicals in almost all societies. Other natural toxins develop when plants are contaminated with fungi that produce toxins, such as peanuts (ground nuts), which always contain small quantities of aflatoxin produced by fungi. But the role of these natural toxins in causing disease, specifically cancer, is very controversial. Ames has argued that the risk of cancer arising from consumption of natural toxins is much greater than the risk associated with exposure to pollutants in the environment, but not all scientists in the field are yet convinced of this (Ames and Gold, 1990).

In contrast to food poisoning, foodborne infections depend on the transfer of viable microorganisms to an individual and the subsequent distribution and multiplication within the human body. The risk of food poisoning as well as foodborne infection is considerably reduced by use of additives aimed at the prevention of microbial spoilage. However, such spoilage can also be avoided by storage of foods at low temperature (refrigeration), proper preparation of the foods, and reduction of the storage time.

Many of the foodborne diseases discussed in this section are an indirect result of pathogens in a community's water supply. Any consideration of foodborne diseases, particularly those of a microbiological nature, should be done concurrently with a consideration of waterborne illnesses.

Substances are also added intentionally to foods to improve their appearance, texture, flavor, and nutritional value. Although the use of food additives is generally strictly regulated and their effects on human health may generally be considered to be beneficial, serious health effects such as allergic reactions have been attributed to these chemicals. Food contamination can also occur through the use of sewage or improperly treated wastewater for irrigation and/or as fertilizer.

Potentially toxic chemicals, for example, those used in agriculture, can find their way into food products, as can insecticides used in the home. These environmental contaminants of both biological and chemical origin will be discussed in more detail below. In addition, physical contaminants (e.g., glass, pieces of metal) must be considered, as these may be inadvertently introduced during food processing.

Biological Contaminants

Biological hazards in food that are of concern to public health include pathogenic strains of bacteria, viruses, parasites, helminths, protozoa, algae, and certain toxic products they may produce (WHO, 1992b). The following four categories summarize the concerns about biological contaminants.

Bacterial Contaminants Biological hazards may act through two general mechanisms in causing human illness. One mode of action is the production of toxins that may cause adverse health effects ranging from mild symptoms of short duration to severe intoxications that can be life threatening or induce long-term health consequences. These toxins are complex enzymes that can destroy protein and tissues. The second mode of action is the production of pathological responses that result from ingestion of viable organisms capable of infecting the host (see Box 7.3). Generally, for foodborne illness to occur, one of the following events must take place: (*1*) bacteria present in the original food source survive food production, including harvesting, storage, and processing stages; (*2*) bacteria enter the food preparation area via the food source or food handler and contaminate other foods that are ready to eat; (*3*) (bacteria in food multiply and are present in sufficient quantities when consumed; and (*4*) bacteria produce a toxin when they multiply and a sufficient level of the toxin is present.

In the case of food poisoning induced by bacterial toxins, threshold levels of concern are much easier to establish than with illnesses resulting from infections. Dose–response data can be obtained and health risks can be assessed by following the quantitative risk assessment paradigm proposed for chemicals (see Chapter 3). To characterize risks from invasive strains of pathogenic bacteria, however, dose–response data only apply to the quantity of bacteria needed to start an infection, and this may vary for the following reasons:

- host susceptibility to pathogenic bacteria is highly variable (e.g., infants, the elderly, or undernourished people are more susceptible to foodborne illness than healthy adults)
- attack rates from a specific pathogen vary widely
- virulence of pathogenic species is highly variable
- pathogenicity is subject to variation resulting from frequent mutation
- antagonism from other bacteria in foods or the digestive system may influence pathogenicity
- food composition will modulate the ability of bacteria to infect and/or otherwise affect the host.

Bacteria Causing Foodborne Infections and Food Poisoning

SALMONELLAE

The bacteria may reach food either directly or indirectly through such channels as animal excreta, human excreta, or water polluted by sewage. The symptoms include diarrhea, abdominal pain, vomiting, and fever. In recent years the contamination of poultry has been a major source of salmonellosis. Other incriminated foods include dairy products, shellfish, and vegetables. This is a classic example of a foodborne infection.

STAPHYLOCOCCI

Foodborne illness due to staphylococci depends on the presence of sufficient toxin in the food. The source of the staphylococci is often food handlers with skin infections (e.g., boils). Symptoms include nausea, vomiting, abdominal pain, prostration, dehydration, and subnormal body temperature. Incriminated foods include ham, poultry, egg salads, produce, and cheese. This is one of the most common examples of bacterial food poisoning.

Therefore, when assessing health risks imposed by pathogenic bacteria, a qualitative risk assessment may be the only feasible method.

Several bacterial diseases are communicable. These include *cholera*, described in Chapter 6, and *typhoid*, which is characterized by fever, headache, cough, enlargement of the spleen, and rose-colored spots on the trunk. There is a greater risk for typhoid in areas where there is poor general sanitation and no water purification. Shigellosis is an acute bacterial disease marked by diarrhea, fever, nausea, and sometimes vomiting and cramps. Humans are the reservoir of infection and the illness is usually passed on by fecal-oral transmission.

Viral and Parasitic Contaminants Viral foodborne diseases are believed to be more prevalent than is documented. Even if a microbiological examination of food and water does not reveal a high number of bacteria, the food may still contain pathogenic viruses. Among the most notable viral foodborne diseases is hepatitis A. Epidemiological evidence shows that the hepatitis A virus is spread primarily through food. However, because the incubation period is quite long (usually 28 to 30 days), outbreaks are difficult to investigate. Symptoms include fever, malaise, nausea, and abdominal discomfort followed by jaundice. Shellfish from polluted areas, water, fruits, and vegetables contaminated by feces, and various types of salad prepared under unhygienic conditions have all been involved in outbreaks.

Parasitic infections of food are difficult to investigate as little is known about the infective dose required or the exact method of transfer to an individual. Contamination may occur from hand to food or directly from polluted water. Prob-

Parasitic Foodborne Infections: Giardiasis and Trichinellosis

Giardiasis is generally characterized by flatulence, belching, nausea, vomiting, fatigue, and cramps, caused by Giardia cysts penetrating the intestinal walls. Giardia is often spread by feces entering water that is later used for washing food, or it may be transferred from hand to mouth (see Fig. 7.2). The disease occurs most often in areas where there is poor sanitation and a lack of clean drinking water. The main preventive measure is the sanitary disposal of feces and the protection of public water supplies.

Trichinellosis is characterized by fever, retinal hemorrhage, diarrhea, muscle soreness and pain, skin lesions, and prostration. It is caused by the migration through the body of the helminth (worm) *Trichinella spiralis*. In the small intestine, larvae develop into mature adults and mate. Female worms produce larvae that penetrate the intestinal wall and enter the bloodstream. The larvae encyst themselves in skeletal muscle. Infection occurs through the consumption of raw or undercooked meat, particularly pork (see Fig. 7.2). Preventive measures are inspection of meat in the slaughterhouse and adequate cooking of pork.

lems arise in many parts of the world where meat and/or fish are eaten raw or undercooked and where people drink untreated water or use it in food preparation. The best protection from parasitic diseases is a safe water supply and adequate cooking and refrigeration temperatures (Jacob, 1989). Two of the most widespread parasitic foodborne diseases are giardiasis and trichinellosis (sometimes called *trichinosis*) (see Box 7.4 and Fig. 7.2).

Mycotoxins Mycotoxins are secondary metabolites of fungi that can exert various types of adverse health effects, including teratogenicity, carcinogenicity, mutagenicity, as well as oestrogenic effects. At this moment several hundred mycotoxins have been documented, and many of them are produced by the genera Aspergillus, Penicillium, and Fusarium. Although toxic syndromes associated with exposure to mycotoxins, also indicated as mycotoxicoses, have been known for many centuries, it was not until the discovery of the aflatoxins in the early 1960s that these dietary risk factors were fully appreciated. Mycotoxin contamination of food items depends on the environmental conditions that may allow mold growth and production of toxins. As with bacterial food intoxication, the absence of live molds in foods does not imply that mycotoxins have not been produced, or vice versa. Toxins may have been formed in earlier stages or during production or storage and, as a result of their chemical stability, may still be present after cooking or other forms of food processing. The aflatoxins, now regarded as the most important mycotoxins, are produced by the molds *Aspergillus flavus* and *A. parasiticus*. Aflatoxins reveal high carcinogenic activity. Before they are biologically active, they have to be metabolized. Aflatoxin B1, the most prevailing

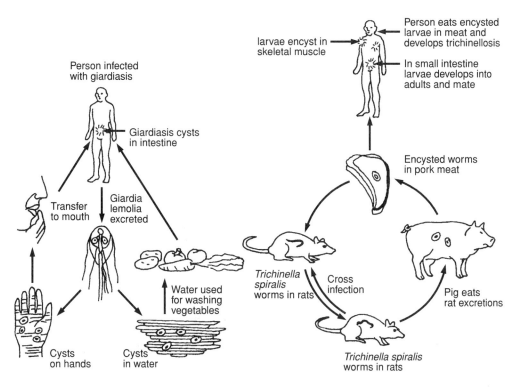

Figure 7.2 Mode of transmission of giardiasis and trichinellosis. From Jacob, 1989, with permission.

form, followed by G1, B2, and G2, has been shown to be a potent hepato-carcingen. Particularly in combination with hepatitis B virus infection, aflatox-ins may lead to primary liver cancer. Aflatoxins are produced both pre- and post-harvest, at relatively high moisture contents and relatively high temperatures. The fungi involved in the production grow best at approximately 25°C and with a relative air humidity of over 80%. Aflatoxins occur on several food products, including oilseed (groundnuts), grains (maize), and figs. Aflatoxin M1 can be found in low concentration in milk samples. Discouraging fungal growth is the most effective way to achieve prevention of aflatoxin contamination. Particularly, adequate post-harvest crop drying is essential to reduce the chance of fungal growth.

Prion Diseases Bovine spongiform encephalopathy (BSE or mad-cow disease) first came to the attention of the scientific community in November 1986 with the appearance in cattle of a newly recognized form of neurological disease in the United Kingdom. Between November 1986 and May 1995, approximately 150,000 cases of this newly recognized cattle disease were confirmed from approximately 33,500 herds of cattle in the U.K. Epidemiological studies in the U.K. at that time suggested that the source of disease was cattle feed prepared from carcasses of dead cattle and that changes introduced in 1981 and 1982 in the process of preparing cattle feed may have been a risk factor (Will et al., 1996). Speculation about the cause of the disease appearing in the food chain of cattle has ranged from spontaneous occurrence in cattle (the carcasses of which then entered the cattle food chain) to entry into the cattle food chain from the carcasses of sheep with a similar disease.

Bovine spongiform encephalopathy is thought to be associated with a transmissible agent called a *prion*, which stands for *proteinaceous infectious particle*, and is yet to be fully characterized. Prions appear to multiply in a very exceptional way, by converting normal protein molecules into dangerous ones by changing their shape. Prions affect the brain and spinal cords of cattle, which develop sponge-like changes visible under an ordinary microscope. It is a highly stable agent, resisting normal cooking temperatures and even higher temperatures such as those used for sterilization, freezing, and drying. The disease is fatal to cattle within weeks to months of its onset.

Bovine spongiform encephalopathy is one of several different forms of transmissible brain disease in animals. Human forms of spongiform encephalopathies also exist. The best-known form, Creutzfeldt-Jakob disease (CJD), is associated with a hereditary predisposition (approximately 10% of cases) and with a more common, sporadic form that accounts for the remaining 90%. Another form, kuru, was identified in Papua, New Guinea, and appears to be transmitted by human ritual handling of bodies and brains of the dead. Symptoms of the human prion diseases are dementia, in combination with or followed by loss of coordination.

One of the conclusions at a 1996 WHO meeting was that the risk of transmission of BSE to humans could be minimized if certain measures were undertaken in the U.K., including the handling and composition of offal in cattle feed given to cattle for consumption, and precautionary measures at farm, slaughter, and meat-processing levels. The meeting also recommended that the WHO encourage research on BSE and its possible implications for public health and continue to provide guidance to countries to minimize the risk of transmission of BSE and of human diseases such as CJD through medical procedures (WHO, 1996).

Chemical Contaminants

There are many sources of chemical contaminants (see Fig. 7.3). Vehicle exhausts and emissions are a common cause of air pollution, and hazardous airborne elements can be deposited onto and absorbed into various crops. Industrial and mining activities that produce poisonous wastes can contaminate plant and soil alike. Because of the complex interrelationships between air, water, land, and plants, the contamination of any one element—from, for example, a chemical leak or a nuclear accident—will have serious implications for the others. Contaminants are often found in animals, particularly as a result of modern farming methods. Drugs used to prevent disease and promote growth in these animals have to be carefully regulated to ensure that levels in meat are safe for human consumption.

Contamination can also occur during food storage. Coatings containing polychlorinated biphenyls (PCBs) have been used inside silos and have resulted in high levels of PCBs in milk. Food processing allows another potential period for chemical contamination. Some processing plants have witnessed instances of heat

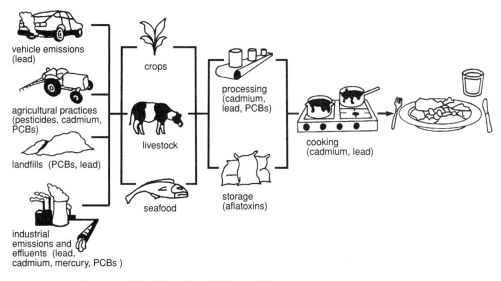

Figure 7.3 Pathways to food for selected chemical contaminants. From UNEP/GEMS, 1992, with permission.

exchangers, transformers, and capacitors containing PCB-based fluids leaking and contaminating food. Both commercial and domestic cooking utensils have been detected as sources of lead and cadmium in foods. Lead-based solder used in food tins is the major source of lead in canned foods (UNEP/GEMS, 1992).

The Global Environmental Monitoring System (GEMS) Food Contamination Monitoring Program was established in 1976 to monitor and report levels and trends of food contaminants worldwide. About 40 countries submit data from national food-monitoring programs; the choice of foods and contaminants that are monitored vary from country to country. From 1971 to 1988, 19 contaminants were monitored through the program. The chemical contaminants that caused the most concern from 1980 to 1988 and the results of the GEMS/UNEP program are described below. (Pesticides were also included in the monitoring program, they will be discussed in Environmental and Occupational Health Hazards, below.)

Polychlorinated Biphenyls *Polychlorinated biphenyls* are fluids that were widely used in electrical transformers, heat exchange fluids, and hydraulic systems. They have other industrial uses and were, for example, added to paints, copying paper, adhesives, and plastics to improve their flexibility. Commercial production of PCBs began in the 1930s but has been drastically restricted in some countries since 1970 when their toxic effects were determined. Contamination of edible oil with PCBs led to large-scale poisoning in Japan in 1968 and Taiwan in 1979. The PCBs are known to suppress the immune system and to induce neurotoxic effects and developmental disorders. Furthermore, studies on exposure to PCBs in the workplace suggest that they may also present a carcinogenic risk to humans. No tolerable intake levels have been established for PCBs internationally, although some countries have drawn up national limits for food products. The PCBs are rarely detected in vegetables, vegetable oils, fruits, eggs, or cereals, al-

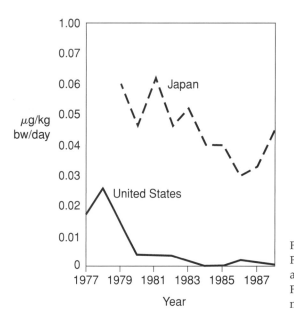

Figure 7.4 Average daily intake of PCBs in adults in the United States and Japan (μg/kg bodyweight/day). From UNEP/GEMS, 1992, with permission.

though there have been reports of high levels in some breakfast cereals, a result of contamination by packing materials. Generally, of all types of foods monitored, fish contain the highest levels of PCBs. As a result, diets consisting of high levels of fish consumption may have a high PCB intake, as seen in Figure 7.4, which shows the difference between average dietary intake of PCBs in the United States and that in Japan, where large amounts of fish are consumed.

Polybrominated Biphenyls Polybrominated biphenyls are compounds similar to PCBs that were extensively used in the past as fire retardants. In 1973, bags of PBB (the hexabromobiphenyl) were added to animal feed at a dairy farm in Michigan. The mistake was caused by a mistake in packaging; the same plant produced both. Dairy cattle ate the contaminated feed and their contaminated milk was widely distributed to people in the region. The PBBs were later identified as possible carcinogens.

Lead Lead produces adverse effects on blood forming tissues, the digestive and nervous systems, and the kidneys (also see Chapter 2). Lead is naturally present in the soil and is introduced into the environment through industry and through exhaust fumes of leaded gas used in vehicles. Lead is found in batteries, solder, dyes, and insecticides and can be transferred to food either directly through personal contact or indirectly through environmental contamination. Lead may be present in drinking water where lead pipes are used for domestic plumbing or where lead-based solder is used on copper pipes. It may also be found in the enamel used for kitchenware, in the glazes used for pottery, and in the solder used for cans containing food or drink.

Fish and shellfish generally have a higher concentration of lead than other foodstuffs; however, in regions where there is extensive industry and mining, vegetables also show significantly high concentrations. Vegetables, grains, and fruit exposed to heavy vehicle exhaust or industrial emissions also contain higher-than-normal lead concentrations.

Because lead accumulates in bone, tolerable levels of consumption are given as a weekly figure to limit intake on a long-term basis. This level is known as the *provisional tolerable weekly intake* (PTWI) and is expressed as micrograms of the chemical per kg of body weight. The PTWI of lead is 50 μg/kg of body weight for adults and 25 μg/kg for children (see Chapter 3 for discussion of acceptable daily intakes [ADIs]).

Cadmium Cadmium is a cumulative poison that affects the kidneys even at relatively low levels of exposure. It also affects placental function, liver function, testes, and formation of bone tissue. In addition, cadmium is a suspected human carcinogen. The main sources of cadmium in foods are industrial emissions and fertilizers. In Japan in the 1950s a number of areas with cadmium-contaminated rice were identified, and similar problems have been found more recently in China. Other potential sources of cadmium in food are kidneys (especially from animals that roam wild), cadmium-lined metal equipment used in commercial food processing, kitchen enamel, pottery glazes, and some plastics.

The established PTWI for cadmium is 7 μg/kg body weight. Data show that average levels were lowest in dairy products, vegetables, fruit, cereals, meat, and fish, whereas a sharp increase in cadmium concentration was found in molluscs and crustaceans and in animal kidneys. Populations in industrial areas showed significantly higher concentrations of cadmium in their bodies.

Mercury Mercury has been used for many centuries and is still commonly used today. It can be found in thermometers, batteries, fluorescent lights, and in many industrial processes including the production of fungicides and paints. Mercury has toxic effects on animals and people. Pregnant women, nursing mothers, and children are particularly susceptible to mercury poisoning. The most toxic form of mercury is methylmercury, which causes damage to the central nervous system.

The PTWI for mercury is 5 μg/kg body weight, of which no more than 3.3 μg/kg should be methylmercury. Methylmercury is often found in fish because of the industrial effluents containing mercury that are discharged into rivers or seas and converted by bacteria into methylmercury (see Box 7.5). The Mediterranean area accounts for half the world's production of mercury and accordingly, mercury levels in fish from this area have been found to be very high. (Aston et al., 1985; Bosnir et al., 1999)

Other areas of naturally high mercury discharge are the mid–north Atlantic ocean and some river systems in North America. Some tributaries of the Amazon have been contaminated by mercury from the use of the metal in gold extraction in primitive gold mining operations. Flooding caused by hydroelectric dams is another source of increased levels of mercury in fish (see Chapter 11, Deforestation and Desertification).

Radioactive Contaminants

On the basis of the non-threshold concept, radionuclides may present carcinogenic, mutagenic, and teratogenic hazards. Several radionuclides have special,

BOX 7.5

Mercury Poisoning in Minamata, Japan

Poisoning from organic mercurial compounds results in a wasting brain disease and loss of control of the motor nerves. This form of poisoning became known as *Minamata disease* because one of the worst outbreaks occurred in Minamata, Japan in the early 1950s. This outbreak alerted the world to the dangers of chemical contamination.

People in the small fishing town suffered progressive weakening of the muscles, loss of vision, and eventual paralysis and coma. Minamata seabirds and household cats that, like the fishermen and their families, subsisted on fish also showed signs of the disease. Several hundred people—40% of those affected—died, and others suffered from permanent damage from the poisoning.

Concentrations of methylmercury were discovered in fish and shellfish taken from the local bay, and in 1968 mercury was officially identified as the cause of the poisoning. The source of the mercury compounds was traced to the effluent discharged from a local chemical company.

Source: Environment Agency, 1975.

strong affinities for specific organs or tissues, resulting in a relative dose that may be several times higher than the ingested or absorbed dose. These affinities may result in accumulation over time. There is no detoxification or elimination mechanism for radionuclides except for excretion or spontaneous decay.

The radionuclides of interest in food safety are the so-called internal emitters that enter the body by ingestion. Naturally occurring internal emitters that contribute to the total radioactive dose in the diet are potassium-40, radium-226, uranium-228, carbon-14, tritium, rubidium-87, lead-210, and polonium-210. In addition to this natural radioactivity, the environment (and therefore also food) can be contaminated with a number of human-made radioactive elements. Small amounts of these elements may be released in the environment by emission from nuclear reactors through their effluents (see below). Furthermore, radioactivity may come from fallout from atmospheric testing of nuclear devices, spills from reactor accidents, and nuclear warfare.

Since the first nuclear reactor was constructed in 1954 in the United States, many other nuclear power plants have been built all over the world. Although relatively small amounts of radionucleides are emitted through the effluents of these reactors into the environment, they are generally considered to be safe. By contrast, the release of radioactive products following a reactor malfunction or explosion is a much bigger concern. Unfortunately, such events have occurred on several occasions, including the accident in the Windscale reactor in the northwest of England (October 1957) and the Three Mile Island reactor in Pennsylvania in the United States on March 28, 1979. Following the Windscale accident, iodine-131 was found in milk produced in the surrounding areas. (Dunser et al., 1959). There was no contamination found in milk or other foodstuffs with other radionuclides. Because of the short half-life (8 days) of iodine-131, its presence in foods is only significant a few weeks after an accidental spill. For instance, 60 days after the event less than 1% of the original amount of iodine-131 was found in milk samples. Also in the case of the Three Mile Island accident, some of the milk samples were found to be contaminated with iodine-131 (Ad Hoc Population Dose Assessment Group, 1979).

In cases such as a nuclear accident of the magnitude of the one in Chernobyl, radioactive contamination can be widespread over many countries (WHO, 1995c). The problems for public health and agriculture at a relatively large distance, referred to as the *far-field*, are completely different from those in the proximity of the nuclear power plant. (Problems in the near-field are discussed in Chapter 9, Nuclear Power). Generally, at a large distance there is relatively little deposition of radioactivity unless the passage of the plume coincides with rainfall. Therefore, contamination of soil and crops can vary substantially from one site to another. Outside these contaminated areas, the exposure in the far-field will occur primarily from the incorporation of the deposited radionuclides in the human food chain.

Control of crops and animal products may have to be exercised for a long period of time since radionuclides deposited on the ground enter the food chain very slowly. Action can be taken to minimize the accumulation of radionuclides in animals or animal products—for instance, by feeding with imported feed or silage from previous seasons, or by preventing consumption of contaminated foodstuff.

FOOD QUALITY CRITERIA

Overview

The quality and safety of the food supply is a topic of continual interest to the media and the general public. The word *quality* has many different meanings and interpretations. The average consumer associates quality with personal preferences and may therefore subjectively interpret the term as indicating whether the food is liked or disliked, good or poor. In addition to these psychological factors, sensory stimulations such as flavor, color, texture, visual appearance, and packaging are important. Also, new developments in food supply prompt discussions about the scientific evidence for safety and the use of suitable control measures. Food quality from a more scientific point of view also includes a number of safety aspects such as the presence of environmental contaminants, pesticide residues, use of food additives, microbial contamination, and nutritional quality. Thus, food quality is determined by four main categories of qualitative properties: (*1*) organoleptic aspects (how it affects the senses; its taste and smell), (*2*) nutritional value, (*3*) functional properties, and (*4*) hygienic properties. A given characteristic of a food is often relevant to more than one of these categories. For instance, a longer shelf life is an important quality relevant to food retailers, as it makes stock management easier. It is also of interest to consumers, as it keeps prices lower and prolongs home storage periods. These advantages refer primarily to functional properties, but they also affect the hygienic properties, for a product with a longer shelf life may present a lower risk of foodborne illnesses.

Nutritional Value

Two types of recommendations for food intake can be employed: dietary standards and dietary guidelines. *Dietary standards* help to determine the amount of a particular nutrient that is adequate for the majority of the population (see Table 7.1). In 1943, the United States Food and Nutrition Board of the National Research Council published a list of recommended dietary allowances (RDAs). These RDAs represented the quantities of nutrients believed to be adequate to meet the physiological needs of the majority of healthy persons in the United States. Thus, RDAs are safe and adequate levels of nutrient intake but are neither minimal requirements nor optimal levels of intake. The RDAs have now been established by scientific committees in many countries but none of these RDAs can be applied globally because of differences in diet and culture in the various countries. Setting RDAs is not an easy task, simply because of a lack of knowledge about human requirements of nutrients. Therefore, different committees may reach different conclusions, resulting in variations in RDAs. Dietary standards such as RDAs are used for: designing nutrition education programs; planning food supplies to subgroups in the population; establishing guidelines for the nutritional labeling of foods; developing new products in the food industry; and evaluating the adequacy of food supplies to meet national nutritional needs.

Dietary guidelines are recommendations for an optimally balanced diet aimed at the reduction of chronic diseases through changing dietary patterns. These dietary guidelines are based on epidemiological studies that have attempted to identify dietary patterns associated with a high or low incidence of diseases. The hypotheses generated by such studies can subsequently be tested in animal studies. However, dietary guidelines have not been very successful in modifying either consumers' choice of food or the composition of the food supplied by the industry.

Food Safety

In practical terms, *safe food* can be defined as food that, after being consumed, causes no adverse health effects. It is clear, however, that absolute safety is an unattainable goal, and safety must therefore be defined in relative terms such that any health risk associated with food consumption is limited to an acceptable level. The risks must also be weighed against the need for the consumption or a range of foods that supply nutrients sufficient for survival and good health. When discussing the toxicological safety of foods it is necessary to discriminate between the various kinds of toxicological risks. Natural toxins, inadvertent contaminants, intentionally added components (additives), and new food ingredients can pose very different kinds of risks.

Safety Standards for Natural Toxins and Food Contaminants Natural toxins and contam-inants are undesirable and unintentionally present in food. These food constituents form a large and very diverse group of chemicals, some of which have already been discussed in previous sections. Again, acceptable intake is based on the toxicological profile of the component in question, defined in a way similar to that described for food additives. In the case of food contaminants, the terms *tolerable daily intake* (TDI) or *provisional tolerable weekly intake* (PTWI) are generally used to reflect the levels permissible in food to maintain a safe supply (see examples in section Nutritional Value, above). In the case of carcinogens, human exposure should be reduced to the lowest practically achievable level.

Safety Assessment of Additives and New Food Components Detailed information about the nutrient content of stored food should be produced on the packaging so that consumers can choose the nutritional balance of their diets. If a traditional food is produced by a new process or a new variety is produced by selective breeding, analysis of the nutrient profile should indicate to what extent the novel food is equivalent to the traditional product. The current concern about genetically engineered food highlights the uncertainties about the safety and acceptability of new food ingredients. New foods may contain natural toxins as well as contaminants. In the event that new contaminants or toxins are detected, the risk involved will have to be assessed. Even if known contaminants or toxins are found, the levels may not exceed the acceptable levels for food.

Before a new food additive can be used, the manufacturer should carry out a hazard identification. The results of the investigations must then be supplied to a regulatory authority that will carry out the risk assessment in cooperation with the company; most countries require this by law. Furthermore, the need for the new additive should be established to ensure that consumers are not exposed unnecessarily to the additional risk of a new chemical if it is of no particular benefit. If the risk is considered acceptable, the company is generally granted permission to use the new additive, which is usually restricted to particular levels in certain food products or food categories. The additive is also subject to a form of post-marketing surveillance in which the occurrence of unexpected effects may be monitored. If new information about the safety of the additive is obtained, its use must be reviewed.

It is beyond the scope of this chapter to give a review of the requirements for the safety assessment of new food components. In principle, a number of actions, including literature research and additional research, must be taken in this assessment, which should result in the determination of a dose–response relationship for any possible toxic effect of the new food additive. Subsequently, the risk assessment is carried out by determining the no-observed adverse-effect level (NOAEL), which is the highest dose in the most sensitive animal species that causes no toxic effects. The NOAEL is then divided by a safety factor to set an acceptable daily intake (ADI) level (see Chapter 3).

Regulatory Authorities and Standard Setting

National regulatory authorities are responsible for food safety standards, thus in principle, every country can have its own standards. To achieve the acceptance of food standards across national boundaries, many countries adopt values proposed by international bodies such as the WHO and the Food and Agricultural Organization of the United Nations (FAO). Through the International Program on Chemical Safety (IPCS), the WHO, UNEP, and FAO play a guiding role in the international procedure of evaluating risks from chemicals and setting levels of tolerance for residues of chemicals in food. Two joint committees of the WHO and FAO function as scientific advisory bodies of what is known as the Codex Alimentarius Commission: the Joint Expert Committee on Food Additives (JECFA), which evaluates food additives, food contaminants, and residues of veterinary drugs; and the Joint Meeting on Pesticide Residues (JMPR), which evaluates pesticide residues on the basis of toxicological and biochemical data and proposes maximum residue limits (MRLs). The Codex Alimentarius Commission has the following goals:

- protection of the health of the consumer and the safeguarding of fair practice in food trade
- coordination of all food regulatory activities carried out by international governmental and nongovernmental organizations
- establishment of priorities for the preparation of provisional standards
- finalizing of provisional standards that will be published in a Codex Alimentarius
- amendment of already published standards, if necessary.

The Codex standards (FAO/WHO, 1989) have been shown to be of great value in bringing food standards into accord, even though the Codex standards have no legal status (see Box 7.6). The Commission's system is unique in that it provides industry leaders the possibility to participate in pre-Codex meetings and to join the debate, although industry representatives have no voting rights in these meetings. Furthermore, industry representatives are offered the opportunity to comment on decisions made about safety evaluation during specially organized JECFA, JMPR, or European Community (EC) hearings.

The harmonization of food standards is also one of the objectives of the EC. Within the EC the safety evaluation of food additives or other substances in food is formally carried out by several working groups of the Commission of the European Communities. Once a proposal is enforced by the Council of Ministers, it is mandatory for the regulatory authorities in the member countries.

FOOD QUALITY ASSURANCE

To ensure high quality of the food supply, a number of parties must play specific roles. The main actors include the government, consumers, and the food industry. The government is responsible for the establishment of standards or codes of practice as well as the enforcement of laws and regulations. Furthermore, it should encourage the food industry to undertake voluntary measures to improve food safety, such as providing advice and guidance. Consumers in turn should be well aware of the quality of the food they buy, prepare, and consume and should adopt appropriate practices of food handling at home. At the industry level, all segments, including agriculture, should establish some system for safety assurance of their products and employ appropriate procedures and technologies.

The flow of raw food materials to actual consumption is schematically presented in Figure 7.5, including the accompanying hazards and risks. In principle, the same flow scheme applies to both the food industry and to locally produced

Thailand: A Success Story for Food Standards and Export

Like many developing countries in tropical regions, Thailand has had a great potential for improving its food export business. This Southeast Asian country grows pineapple and other tropical fruits, cashew nuts, many types of mushrooms and baby corn. It also harvests shrimp and other marine products, and its rice is considered by many to be the best in the world. Since the establishment of its National Codex Alimentarius Committee in 1969, Thailand has seen its food export grow nearly 12-fold to more than U.S. $4000 million. However, the growth has been haphazard: exports increased by about 30% between 1980 and 1981 but then dropped back to less than the 1980 level for the next 4 years as food products were continually rejected by foreign countries. Noting that products were being refused because of contamination and improper labeling, the country called upon the Food and Agricultural Organization (FAO) and the United Nations Development Program for help. Experts from the FAO were sent to the country, as they often are upon request. Using Codex Alimentarius standards and guidelines, they set up a pilot export control program, trained inspectors, designed voluntary inspection systems, and brought in laboratory people to train Thai workers. Video programs were developed for training projects, and a Memorandum of Understanding ensuring inspection and certification procedures for monitoring and sampling was signed with one of the world's major importing countries. At the same time, WHO experts assisted Thailand in building up its domestic food safety capabilities. Thailand's food exports grew from U.S. $2000 million to U.S. $4800 million between 1985 and 1989, contributing greatly to the country's 10% economic growth rate during the period

Source: (FAO/WHO, 1994).

foods for private consumption, although in the latter case the food processing, storage, and transport stages will be relatively short. In such a situation, adequate monitoring of food quality is usually more difficult to achieve. All steps in this process and possible preventive measures for ensuring food quality at various stages are briefly presented here.

Production of Raw Materials

To ensure safe food production, it is important to look at the agricultural level and improve the hygienic quality of raw foods. By improving the conditions under which animals are raised, the hygienic quality of raw food products can be significantly improved. Furthermore, use of both pesticides and fertilizers should be reduced, and residue levels of toxic chemicals used to improve crop production should be systematically monitored. Food safety at this stage can also be improved through measures aimed at reduction of industrial and vehicle emissions and disposal of hazardous waste materials that can enter the food chain.

Biotechnological methods can be used to develop crops that are more resistant to pests and thereby decrease the need for pesticide use. However, such ge-

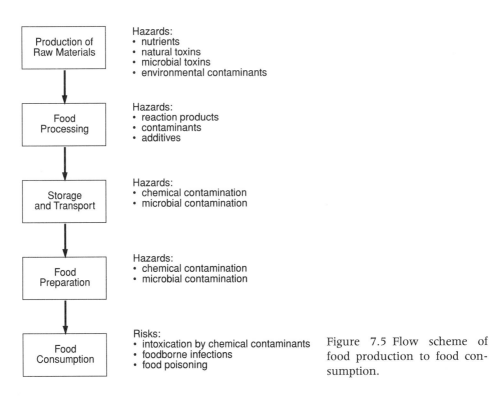

Figure 7.5 Flow scheme of food production to food consumption.

netically engineered foods may include new toxins and the plants may grow in uncontrolled ways creating new weeds. More research on the safety of these genetically engineered crops is needed. These biotechnological methods for food production have been challenged on ethical grounds, as genetic engineering can be seen as the development of unnatural plant species with unpredictable ecological consequences.

Food Processing

Greater demands are being made on the food-processing industry as a result of increasing urbanization. As consumers continue to move further away from the sources of production, they will require an effective and safe food distribution system. This separation of the consumer from the production sector also means a loss of the traditional methods used by the consumer to ensure the safety of food.

Substantial losses of food by contamination and spoilage can be prevented through the use of carefully controlled technology and well designed food processing infrastructure. In addition, modern technologies can be used to prevent or reduce the formation or use of chemicals in food. For example, crops can be dried to prevent mold growth and production of mycotoxins during storage. Irradiation can replace the use of potentially harmful chemicals used for disinfection and inhibition of sprouting. Traditional approaches to food safety, hygiene, protection, and sanitation have their limitations and do not always guarantee reduction to the desired level of reported foodborne diseases, even in developed countries. The potential formation of reaction products from irradiation has not been fully investigated, however, and new health risks cannot be entirely excluded.

TABLE 7.2

HAZARD ANALYSIS AND CRITICAL CONTROL POINT (HACCP) SYSTEM

Determine hazards and assess their severity and risks
Identify critical control points
Institute control measures and establish criteria to ensure control
Monitor critical control points
Take action whenever monitoring results indicate criteria are not met
Verify that the system is functioning as planned

Source: Bryan, 1989.

The mainstay of microbiological food safety programs has been inspection. Inspection programs have serious limitations, however, as they sometimes overlook critical factors that are not part of the inspection protocol. Inspection services are usually inadequate or nonexistent in developing countries, where inspectors, scientists, and regulatory authorities are sorely lacking. Industrialized countries need to standardize regulations to ensure the free flow of food among all the countries of the world (WHO, 1992b).

A different approach to safety in modern industrial food production is the Hazard Analysis and Critical Control Point (HACCP) system, which is attempting to make a significant impact on the prevention of foodborne diseases. The HACCP system consists of a series of interrelated actions that should be taken to ensure the safety of all processed and prepared foods at critical points during the stages of production, storage, transport, processing, preparation, and service. The elements of the HACCP system are summarized in Table 7.2. The applications of this system are discussed in *Microorganisms in Food* (1988 International Commission on Microbiological Specifications for Food, the *Hazard Analysis Critical Control Point Manual* published in 1989 by the Food Marketing Institute of the U.S. [Bryan, 1989], as well as in a WHO report, Bryan, 1992).

Food Preservation and Storage

The aim of food preservation is to eradicate or prevent the growth of harmful pathogens during manufacturing so that food will remain safe to eat for longer periods of time. Bacterial growth is enabled by a number of conditions, the most important being the presence of a good substrate (in this case a food item); an infection with viable bacteria; a temperature that allows bacterial growth; proper pH; and sufficient water for bacterial growth. To guard against bacterial growth, at least one of these conditions should be prevented.

Food irradiation is one method of improving the keeping properties of certain high-value perishable foods, thereby facilitating international trade. It consists of exposing food to gamma rays, X-rays, or electrons over a limited period of time, which kill the present pathogens. Irradiation is the most recent addition to the various types of food preservation that also include pasteurization, blanching, canning, freezing, and dehydration. It is recognized as a safe method of preserving food and one that can contribute to the promotion of safe food supplies as long as the occupational radiation hazard is properly controlled (WHO, 1988). The advantages of irradiation over conventional food processing methods are that (*a*) foods can be treated after packaging; (*b*) fresh foods such as meat, fish, fruit, and vegetables that would otherwise be frozen or canned can be kept in the fresh state; (*c*) perishable foods can last longer without loss of quality; and (*d*) the cost and energy requirements of the process are lower than those of many conventional methods (WHO, 1988).

Handling food may result in changes in its original composition. It is well known that a relationship exists between certain processing techniques and the quality and safety of the products. For instance, the heating of lipids and exposure to oxygen are known to result in the formation of highly reactive oxidation products. Polyunsaturated fatty acids (such as linoleic acid) are especially susceptible to thermal and oxidative decomposition (rancidity). Another example of the formation of toxic compounds during food processing is the *Maillard reaction,* a well-known but complex browning reaction of sugars and amino acids. Animal studies have indicated that these reaction products may induce liver damage and disturb growth as well as reproduction. Furthermore, specific Maillard reaction products may result in allergic reactions. The formation of Maillard reaction products can be inhibited during food processing through regulation of the pH, temperature, and water content. Polycyclic aromatic hydrocarbons (PAH) are pyrolysis products that occur in food heated at temperatures over 300°C. Benzo[a]pyrene, the most potent PAH carcinogen, has been found in the charred crusts of biscuits and bread, barbecued meat, broiled mackerel, and other broiled, baked, or roasted foods. Heterocyclic amines represent yet another group of carcinogens formed during preparation of meat and fish at high temperatures (>150°C). Exposure to these compounds is found to be particularly associated with colon cancer risk.

Food Preparation in the Home

The household is perhaps the most relevant place for developing strategies to combat foodborne illness, as it is the location where the consumers can exert the most control over what they eat. Clearly, one of the most significant components of keeping food pathogen-free in the household is maintaining a clean and hygienic environment in the kitchen or other food preparation areas. Proper sanitation facilities, cleanliness of household members who prepare the food, and control of pests are all essential for the preservation of acceptable food. Many bacterial pathogens are able to multiply in food because of the temperature at which the food is stored. Figure 7.6 shows the temperatures at which bacteria can be killed or controlled.

Refrigeration is one of the most effective means of stopping bacteria from multiplying on or in food. Although bacteria are not killed, their growth is stopped; they will start to multiply when the food is taken out of the refrigerator into a warmer environment. Refrigeration does not change the nature of the food itself, and food kept in the refrigerator will only remain in good condition for a limited time. Most foodborne pathogens stop multiplying at temperatures below 5°C. Therefore, for normal short-term storage of food, temperatures should be kept below this temperature. Freezing food does not kill most microorganisms. When frozen food is thawed, bacteria that were already there will begin to multiply again unless the food is immediately cooked or held below 5°C.

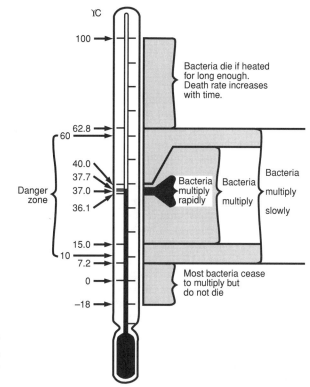

Figure 7.6 The control of pathogenic bacteria by temperature. From Jacob, 1989, with permission.

Fresh food, cooked and eaten while still hot, will not cause foodborne infection. Even though many raw foods are contaminated with pathogenic bacteria when they are purchased, thorough cooking should kill the bacteria. If the cooking is not thorough enough, bacteria can incubate within the food and produce foodborne infections. Some bacteria give rise to spores that can survive cooking and will develop into bacterial growth if the food is cooled too slowly or if it is stored at kitchen temperature for too long.

The chemical risks in food preparation at home are the same as those present during food processing. The general public should be made aware of these risks, such as frying at high temperatures (grill or barbecue), which results in toxic reaction products. Consumers should be advised not to use utensils that may contain toxic materials, e.g., lead-glazed containers.

Food Preparation in the Food Services Industry

The consequences of improper food preparation in food services such as canteens and restaurants can be much greater than that in the household, simply because a larger number of individuals may be simultaneously exposed to unsafe food items. It is essential to have a quality control program that will ensure the maintenance of food product standards during all stages of handling, processing, and preparation; it must also be applied to all areas and equipment that come into contact with food and beverages. Management of small or medium-sized establishments is not always in favor of the implementation of such programs, finding them to be too time consuming and expensive or too complicated. As a re-

Street foods can be defined as ready-to-eat foods and beverages prepared and/or sold by vendors outside and in other public places (WHO, 1992c). Such street foods are an affordable source of nourishment for people on low incomes and in many countries these people would be worse off if these foods were not available. The street food industry has undergone remarkable expansion particularly in Asian, African, and South American countries. Although this industry employs 6%–25% of the workforce, authorities remain hesitant to recognize it as a formal sector of the food industry. As a consequence, this route of food supply may be ignored in food control programs and specific regulatory structures remain to be developed. Health hazards related to street foods comprise all types of hazards discussed earlier in this chapter. Cholera, hepatitis A, typhoid, and other diseases of microbiological origin can be transmitted through such foods. In principle, foods that are thoroughly cooked and consumed on the spot are safe, whereas precooked foods stored at ambient temperatures of 5°–40°C for more than 4 hr present a considerable microbiological risk.

Hazardous chemicals and additives, notably unauthorized colorants and preservatives, have been found in street-vended foods. Regulation of street-vended foods should aim at ensuring safe, wholesome, reasonably priced food at convenient places, without diminishing the economic, employment, and other benefits of this trade. An extensive list of essential safety requirements for street foods has been established (WHO, 1992b), including recommendations regarding raw material and ingredients, place of preparation and sale, water, waste disposal, and preparation and processing. Perhaps the most crucial point is the training of handlers, which has the potential to be a more successful means of safeguarding food quality than punishment of vendors, and should therefore receive more attention.

sult, the emphasis of quality control is often placed on the quality of the incoming product, leaving a wide gap between the initial phase of quality control and service to the consumer. Street foods are particularly prone to lapses in safe food preparation, as discussed in Box 7.7.

GLOBAL FOOD PRODUCTION CAPACITY AND FOOD SECURITY

World Food Situation

Without adequate food and nutrition, there can be no sound social and/or economic development in a community. Healthy nutritional status is best understood as the complex interaction between our health, the food we eat, and our surrounding environment. At the beginning of the 1990s, a worldwide average of 2670 calories of food products per capita was consumed on a daily basis—a level considered nutritionally adequate. However, this global average has little meaning when inadequate food consumption levels are the norm in a significant number of developing countries; there is a gap of 965 calories per capita, be-

BOX 7.8

Malnutrition

While the world's most profound nutritional emergency is visibly exhibited in only 1 or 2% of the world's children, an estimated 190 million children under age five are chronically malnourished. The causes of malnutrition are complex—many households run short of food between harvests, or amid drought and war. Many malnourished children, however, live in homes with adequate food supplies and need only a very small proportion of a family's intake to remain adequately fed. Often low birth weight and specific practices such as bottle feeding contribute to malnutrition in these cases. However, the main cause is the pattern of disease, especially diarrhoea, that thrives in poor communities lacking proper water and sanitation (see Chapter 6).

When nourishment runs low, the body makes concessions to keep itself going. These compromises may be invisible—the only outward sign is lethargy, as the body attempts to conserve energy. To compensate for fewer nutrients, the body's metabolic rate drops, as does blood pressure. If body fat is low, it borrows from its reserves, thereby depleting muscle instead of fat and damaging bone growth. Malnutrition amplifies all other illnesses and the risk of dying from some other disease is doubled for mildly malnourished children and tripled for moderately malnourished children. Good nutrition, by contrast, is excellent protection against disease.

Source: UNICEF, 1994.

tween the developed and the developing countries (3399 and 2434 calories per capita, respectively). There are also wide gaps between and within developing countries (UNEP, 1992a). Some people have too much food and suffer from an unbalanced diet, whereas other people do not have enough to eat and suffer from malnutrition. For a large part of the world's population, malnutrition remains the major cause of mortality and morbidity (Box 7.8) and significant percentages of the world's populations remain undernourished (Table 7.3).

Crucial Conditions for Food Production

Considering the large number of undernourished and/or malnourished individuals in the world, it is hard to believe that there is enough food being produced to meet the world's needs. Nonetheless, according to a report by the WHO's Panel on Food and Agriculture, that is the case. Globally, food grain production has been rising faster than the rate of population growth, and current and emerging food production and preservation capabilities have the potential to produce an adequate supply of safe, nutritious food for all the people of the world, both now and up to the year 2010 at projected rates of population growth (WHO, 1992b). Much of this production capability exists in developing countries where the greatest percentage of malnutrition occurs. In fact, the potential of many developing countries to increase their own food production through increases in yield, arable land, and cropping intensity is considerable. Together with the increased production of

TABLE 7.3

PREVALENCE OF CHRONIC UNDERNUTRITION IN DEVELOPING REGIONS

Region	1969–71		1979–81		1988–90	
	Millions of Under-nourished	Proportion of Total Population (%)	Millions of Under-nourished	Proportion of Total Population (%)	Millions of Under nourished	Proportion of Total Population (%)
Africa	101	35	128	33	168	33
Asia	751	40	645	28	528	19
Latin America	54	19	47	13	59	13
Middle East	35	22	24	12	31	12
Total Developing regions	941	36	844	26	786	20

Seventy-two countries with a population of less than 1 million, representing 0.6% of the developing world's population, were excluded from the table totals.
Source: WRI, 1994.

food, storage facilities and distribution systems should be improved. Three elements must be in place for the production of food: land, water, and fertilizers.

The total area of potential arable land in the world is about 3.2 billion hectares, about 46% of which is already under cultivation. Although large areas of new land could be brought under cultivation, unused arable land is not always available to those who need it most, and opening up new areas is an expensive means of increasing agricultural production. Soil that was once fertile is being degraded through erosion, salinization, and pollution. In areas where fertile land exists, water is often too scarce to properly irrigate it.

Worldwide, about 2700 cubic kilometers of water were withdrawn for irrigation in 1990, or about 70% of freshwater use. As discussed in Chapter 6, freshwater resources are becoming more scarce, requiring increased wastewater reuse and better maintenance of irrigation systems. In arid and semi-arid zones, the problem of water scarcity for food production is particularly acute.

The increased application of fertilizers to supply plant nutrients (nitrogen, phosphorus, and potassium) is an essential component of modern agriculture. Worldwide consumption of fertilizers has been increasing over the last two decades (UNEP, 1992a).

Despite the appearance of global food sufficiency, the global economic climate has changed for the worse so that for some countries the coming years will bring a deteriorating food situation. In every country, there are both rich and poor, urban and rural, and industrialized and agrarian communities; even where national food supplies are adequate, large sections of the population may still not have enough food for their needs. Over the next two decades, food production will have to keep pace with an increasing world population. The challenge for governments and food producers will be to ensure food and nutrition security without placing undue pressure on the environment and perpetuating different types of health problems (WHO, 1992b). Estimates of possibilities for increased food production are shown in Figure 7.7.

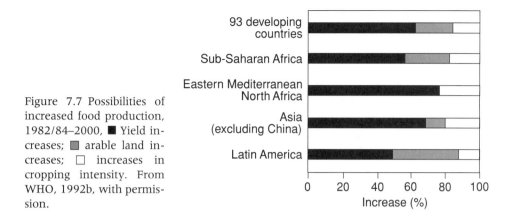

Figure 7.7 Possibilities of increased food production, 1982/84–2000, ■ Yield increases; ▨ arable land increases; ☐ increases in cropping intensity. From WHO, 1992b, with permission.

Environment and Food Security

The continued supply of most staple foods and many other agricultural products is dependent on the sustained productivity of a number of land-based ecosystems. Some land-based ecosystems are of profound, though indirect, importance to the growing of food and agricultural production; they protect water basins from floods and erosion, provide biodiversity or habitats for natural enemies of pests, and regulate the microclimate.

In addition to land-based agriculture, fish farming is a large and important industry. The fishing industry contributes substantially to global food production and provides many people with jobs and financial income. Of course, the quality of fishing waters relates directly to the quality of fish and other seafood. The stability of maritime and other aquatic ecosystems is thus of crucial importance to ensure continued food supply from this source. Overfishing is the most serious threat to aquatic ecosystems. Therefore, actions to protect the water quality as well as regulation of fishing intensity are required.

Unfortunately, increasing numbers of productive ecosystems are being degraded and eventually lost due to human-induced environmental stress (WHO, 1992b; Box 7.9). Land degradation is a major environmental threat to food security. The depletion of the ozone layer and the changes occurring in the global climate also pose a threat to the sustainability of ecosystems. Intensive use of fossil fuels is regarded as the major source of greenhouse gases. Any changes in the climate as a result of the greenhouse effect, including temperature and humidity, can have devastating effects on ecosystems and on the well-being and livelihoods of people, particularly those dependent on natural systems. Similarly, the depletion of stratospheric ozone, which absorbs much of the sun's ultraviolet rays, can be particularly damaging to phytoplancton and may also affect crops (WRI, 1994).

Global Trends

The most important factors that influence consumption and demand for food and agricultural products are population growth, income distribution, and increased urbanization. Most of the changes in consumption of food and agricultural products are due to growth in population and incomes. At constant per-capita incomes, the demand for food and agricultural products was expected to increase at about 1.7% annually during the 1990s. The greater part of this increase was to occur in developing countries, with sub-Saharan Africa showing the largest percentage increase (WHO, 1992b).

Only in recent decades have research findings confirmed the suspicion that dietary preferences may influence the onset of many diseases, particularly those attributed to the so-called affluent diet, a diet consisting of large quantifies of high-fat and high-sugar foods. Examples of these diseases include obesity, heart disease, and certain types of cancer. With about two-thirds of all energy coming from vegetable sources and one-third from foods of animal origin, the developed market economies have reached a level at which no further substitution between the two groups is desired.

While low-income countries have traditionally relied on food from vegetable sources, more animal products are now being consumed. Accordingly, the incidence rates of heart disease, high blood pressure, and cancers are increasing rapidly in some urban communities of developing countries. The relationship between income and meat consumption is reflected in the differences in meat consumption—not only between developed and developing countries but among developing countries at different income levels. Rapid urbanization in developing countries will also result in changes in patterns of consumption. A move from traditional crops such as root crops, maize, and millet to food requiring less preparation time such as wheat, rice, and animal products is already taking place in a number of these countries. As the demand for livestock increases, pressure on agricultural land will become more intense. In addition to having direct environmental effects, intensification of production will increasingly be based on cultivating cereals for animal products that will compete for agricultural resources. The conversion of cereals to animal products will result in large losses of edible energy and increases in resource requirements (WHO, 1992b).

ENVIRONMENTAL AND OCCUPATIONAL HEALTH HAZARDS IN AGRICULTURE

Physical Injuries and Infections

Injuries are the most significant group of hazards for primary food producers. For farmers, most major injuries are caused by machinery or farm vehicles. Unguarded equipment can injure limbs and eyes and can often take lives. Domesticated animals and poisonous insects and snakes can all be a source of injury.

The level of noise produced by agricultural machinery—generators, tractors, and saws—may be loud enough to cause hearing impairments in those workers who are exposed to this noise over a considerable period of time. Vibrating tools and machinery can cause fatigue, impaired balance, and chest pain, as well as chronic health effects such as back pain and degenerative changes in the spinal column and joints. These injuries may be exacerbated by the lifting of heavy objects. Children living in an environment (on or off the farm) with heavy machinery and many chemicals are also at increased risk for injuries.

In addition to the risk of getting injured, the handling of large animals is associated with an increased risk of infection with zoonoses (see Chapter 2). Hundreds of pathogenic organisms have been identified in association with animal contact and a relationship has been established between the occurrence of a number of diseases and the intensity of the contact with animals. Farming in both naturally wet and irrigated areas is also associated with an increased risk of vector-borne infections (see Chapter 6).

Other occupations in the agricultural sector, such as hunting, fishing, and forestry, have their own characteristic risk profiles. Hunters may be attacked by wild animals or get injured by their own knives and firearms. For forestry workers the main risks involve falling trees, saws, and ropes. Seamen are mostly exposed to physical hazards related to machinery and moving objects; they are also at risk of falling overboard.

Pests and diseases have always been a problem in the cultivation certain crops in certain seasons. The factors that have increased output per unit of land—increased use of fertilizer, higher plant population, increased intensity, and new plant varieties—have also increased disease and pest problems. The most common method used to control pests is the application of pesticides. Most pesticides are chemicals used in agriculture to control pests, weeds, or plant disease (Table 7.4). A *pesticide* can be defined as

> any substance or mixture of substances intended for preventing, destroying, or controlling any pest, including vectors of human or animal disease, unwanted species of plants or animals causing harm during, or otherwise interfering with, the production, processing, storage, transport, or marketing of food, agricultural commodities, wood and wood products, or animal feedstuffs, or which may be administered to animals for the control of insects, arachnids, or other pests in their bodies (WHO, 1990a).

The use of inorganic chemicals to control insects has a long history, possibly dating back to classical Greece and Rome. In the middle of the nineteenth century, modern pesticides began to be introduced. They replaced older plant-derived pesticides, such as nicotine, and other chemical pesticides, including the salts of arsenic. Many of the older compounds were highly toxic and their use by the public was restricted in many countries. The introduction of dichloro-diphenyl-trichloroethane (DDT), which was first synthesized in Switzerland during World War II, seemed to be full of promise because of its wide spectrum of activity and relatively low human toxicity. DDT is an organochlorine pesticide that was followed by organophosphorus compounds and the carbamates. The benefits of their use for agriculture seemed remarkable, as both the quantity and quality of crops rose as a result of their use. Eventually, the health and environmental pesticides to the agricultural workers became a major concern (see Boxes 7.10 and 7.11). A wide range of insecticides, fungicides, molluscicides, bac-

TABLE 7.4

GENERAL CATEGORIES OF PESTICIDES

Pesticide	Used Against	Category	Examples
Insecticides	Insects and related species	Organophosphorous compounds	Malathion, parathion, dichlorvos
		Carbamate compounds	Aldicarp, carbaryl, methomyl
		Organochlorine compounds	Aldrin, dieldrin, endrin, DDT
		Pyrethroid compounds	Bioallethrin, cyhalothrin
Rodenticides	Rats, mice, and other rodents	Anticoagulants	Warfarin and derivatives
		Others	Zinc phosphide, thallium
Herbicides	Weeds	Dipyridyl derivatives	Paraquat, diquat
		Phenol derivatives	Pentachlorophenol
Fungicides	Fungi and molds	Dithiocarbamates	Arasan, thiramid
		Phtalamides	Captan
Molluscicides	Snails	Metaldehyde	
Fumigants	Gases used to sterilize products	Ethylene dibromide	
		Methyl bromide	

BOX 7.10

DDT (dichlorodiphenyl-trichloroethane)

DDT, an organochlorine pesticide, was used widely from the 1940s to the 1960s. DDT persists in plants and soil, passes along the food chain, and can thus be present in food for human consumption. In the 1970s, these dangers were recognized and the use of DDT was restricted in many countries. It is still, however, one of the major pesticides in India and is widely used in developing countries to kill mosquitoes and thereby combat malaria. Like other organochlorine pesticides, DDT accumulates in fatty tissue and is therefore found in food with a high fat content, particularly milk and dairy products.

Acute exposure to DDT (or other organochlorine pesticides) causes central nervous system excitation (irritability, excitability, headache, disorientation, twitching). High doses can damage the liver and are suspected to be carcinogenic and may induce xenooestrogenic effects. Apart from its use to increase quality and quantity of crops, DDT has also been widely used to combat malaria. After several years of success in fighting this disease, resulting in significant benefits for human health, the mosquito carrying the malaria developed resistance to the chemical.

Source: UNEP/GEMS, 1992.

tericides, and herbicides, including fumigants, have since become important in agriculture. Without the use of synthetic pesticides the world food situation would have been far more problematic than it is today. Furthermore, pesticide use has contributed significantly to improved human health by reducing vector-borne diseases. After several years of use, however, target pest species began to develop resistance to the most widely used pesticides. Therefore, new compounds with higher acute toxicity to humans had to be introduced, which resulted in unexpected effects on the environment. Since the use of pesticides has become so widespread, and since the general public now has access to such a range of powerful and hazardous chemicals, appropriate control of pesticides is needed. Although many countries have introduced strict regulations and training in the safe and effective use of pesticides, such precautions are not universal.

Populations at Risk for Exposure to Pesticides

The use of pesticides and the incidence of side effects vary considerably among regions and farming systems. The use of pesticides in agriculture in developing countries is very much connected to the type of market for which the farm produces. The very large, monocultural plantation farms are the most likely to use pesticides. Exposure of employees to pesticides will vary according to the management of the plantation. Farms with cash crops are often family run and generally use smaller quantities of pesticides than plantations because of either inaccessibility or prohibitive cost. Subsistence farmers usually do not use pesticides at all because they cannot afford them and thus suffer the consequences of crop losses.

Organophosphate and Carbamate Cholinesterase-Inhibiting Insectides

These substances are the most common cause of acute pesticide intoxication. The organophosphates (e.g., parathion, dichlorvos, malathion) and the carbamates (e.g., aldicarb, carbofuron, carbaryl) share a common mechanism of toxicity—cholinesterase inhibition. The nerve transmitter, acetylcholine, is normally inactivated by an enzyme called *acetylcholinesterase*. The action of this enzyme is blocked through the formation of a pesticide–enzyme complex. The clinical presentation following acute poisoning is easily recognized: neuromuscular paralysis, central nervous system dysfunction, and depression of red cell and plasma cholinesterase activity. The character, degree, and duration of the illness depend on the degree and rate of accumulation of acetylcholine. (Characteristic symptoms include blurred vision, tearing, salivation, nausea, diarrhea, headache) Chronic effects may include dermatitis as well as mood lability, fatigue, and impaired concentration. A delayed neuropathy, rapid-onset distal symmetric sensory motor neuropathy, may also occur.

In developing countries, approximately 63% of the workforce is employed in the agricultural sector. In developed countries, the corresponding figure is 11%. Thus, even if pesticide use in developing areas is low, relatively more people are involved in the handling of pesticides. About 60% to 70% of all cases of unintentional, acute pesticide poisoning are the result of occupational exposure. Pesticide use in agriculture puts farmers and their families at risk for exposure. Workers may be put at risk in other occupations as well, including pesticide manufacturing, and as vendors, transporters, mixers, loaders, operators of application equipment, growers and pickers, and rescue and clean-up workers. Chemical burns of the eye, skin damage, neurological effects, and liver damage are among the acute symptoms of occupational exposure. Chronic effects are more difficult to identify, and there are varying degrees of evidence that different types of pesticides are carcinogenic. For example, there is strong evidence that pesticides containing arsenic are associated with cancer in human subjects, whereas the evidence for the carcinogenicity of organochlorine pesticides is not strong.

Although only a small proportion of the general population is likely to receive a pesticide dose high enough to cause acute severe effects, many more may be at risk of developing chronic effects, depending on the type of pesticide to which they have been exposed. Epidemiological studies of people who have been exposed to low doses of pesticides are quite limited. The chronic effects suffered by these people are often not specifically associated with pesticide exposure, and the exposure levels are often immeasurable. Individuals who receive very high levels of exposure usually belong to well-defined groups, such as people using pesticides with insufficient protective gear, people attempting to commit suicide, or people exposed through the consumption of highly contaminated food or beverages (see Fig. 7.8).

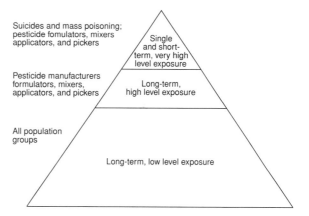

Figure 7.8 Population groups at risk of exposure to pesticides. From WHO, 1990a, with permission.

The width of the triangle indicates the approximate size of the exposed groups

The general population may be exposed to pesticides in several ways, the main routes being ingestion via food and drinking water, inhalation via air and dust, and skin absorption via clothing or direct contact. The most common cases of acute accidental poisoning by pesticides are those in which grain coated in pesticides has been eaten. Other accidents have occurred when insecticides that are effective against one type of pest were used incorrectly against other types, such as bedbugs and lice. The use of old pesticide containers for household food and water storage is another source of poisoning. Pesticides that are improperly stored have been consumed by unknowing children. Studies of any link between pesticides and cancer in the general population are difficult because generally the exposure levels are low.

Toxic Effects of Pesticides

Acute toxic effects are fairly easy to recognize, whereas the effects that result from long-term, low-dose exposure are often more difficult to identify. Most pesticide preparations include carrier substances, active ingredients, and compounds that improve absorption. Many of these inert ingredients have severe side effects that are often worse than those of the active ingredients. For example, carbon tetrachloride and chloroform, both strong agents that are toxic to the liver and central nervous system, may be used as inert ingredients without ever being mentioned on the product label. For most pesticides, a dose–effect relationship has been defined in which the early effects of pesticides may be detected by measuring minor biochemical changes before adverse health effects occur.

The severity of any health effects from exposure to pesticides depends on the dose, the route of exposure, the type of pesticide, the absorption of the pesticide, and the health of the affected individual. Pesticide uptake occurs mainly through the skin and eyes. Individuals in developing countries, are particularly prone to exposure through skin absorption, as protective clothing is often not worn. The vapors of pesticides may be inhaled, and pesticides may be ingested through the consumption of contaminated food. Within the body, the pesticide may be metabolized, stored in the fat, or excreted unchanged. DDT and hexachlorocyclohexane (HCH) are examples of organochlorine compounds that are not readily metabolized and end up stored in fatty tissue.

TABLE 7.5
TYPES OF TOXIC EFFECTS OF PESTICIDES

Biochemical Changes	Reproductive Effects	Skin Effects	Neurological Effects
Enzyme induction	Sterility	Irritant-contact dermatitis	Behavioral changes
	Fetal death	Permanent hair loss	Lesions of the central nervous system
	Fetal toxicity	Allergic-contact dermatitis	Peripheral neuritis
	Teratogenicity (fetal malformations)	Photoallergic reactions Chloracne Deep scarring, skin atrophy	Peripheral neuritis

In addition to the toxic effects listed in Table 7.5, effects on human reproduction have been shown for a number of pesticides, including sterility, fetal death, fetal toxicity, and teratogenicity (fetal malformations). Other recognized effects of certain pesticides include cataract formation, cellular proliferation in the lungs, and damage to the immune system.

Integrated Pest Management

Pest management may consist of many different methods ranging from routine applications of pesticides to measures for ecological management. Pest control based solely on the application of pesticides is now increasingly rejected in most countries. Instead, many approaches that can control pests while reducing pesticide use are employed. In a pest management system, all suitable techniques and methods are used in as compatible a manner as possible, and the pest population is maintained at levels below those causing economic losses (WHO, 1990a). Approaches that minimize pesticide use include plant disease forecasting methods to minimize use; better formulation and placement of chemicals so that smaller amounts are used; alternative farming systems to minimize pest attacks; and repeated field visits to determine whether pest levels necessitate spraying.

A number of other pest control strategies are also increasing in significance, including the use of biological insecticides based on insect pathogens; the release or encouragement of predators of pests; release of sterile male insects to limit the reproduction of pests; planting of crop varieties that are resistant to pests; and planting of trap crops to lure pests away from the principal crop (WRI, 1992). Furthermore, modern biotechnological techniques offer the possibility to transfer genes from one species to another, making crops more resistant to plagues. For instance, it is well known that the bacterium *Bacillus thuringiensis* produces a toxin that kills larvae and insects. Using DNA recombination techniques, the gene coding for the bacterial toxin has been isolated and transferred to tobacco plants, where it is expressed. When insects eat from such a transgenic plant, they die rapidly. However, these techniques are not yet widely accepted by society and there is considerable reluctance to accept genetic engineering because of fears of unanticipated effects and cultural concerns about the ethics of manipulating life.

Fertilizers

Although the per-hectare use of fertilizers is currently much higher in developed countries, the rate of use in developing countries has been rising rapidly. Most fertilizers used are nitrogenous fertilizers, followed by phosphates and potash. About 50% of the fertilizers used benefit the plants; the remainder is lost from the soil system by leaching and runoff, often causing contamination of ground and surface water. As a result, the local or regional ecosystem will be disturbed and specific forms of life may disappear. This type of pollution is also quite common in areas where animal wastes are applied to agricultural land. The problem has been particularly acute on crop-livestock operations where farmers spread large quantities of nitrogen-rich animal manure and continue to apply synthetic fertilizers at the same rate that would be required without manure (WRI, 1992). In many developing countries fertilizer subsidies have led to inefficient application with consequent economic losses and increased environmental damage on and off the farm (UNEP, 1992a).

Extensive use of fertilizers may also result in increased levels of nitrate in ground and drinking water. One of the health consequences of high intake of nitrates is the formation of methaemoglobin, resulting in a decreased oxygen transport capacity of the blood. Infants are at increased risk for this adverse effect, known as the *blue baby syndrome*. High nitrate intake may result in increased formation of nitrosamines in the stomach. Nitrosamines have been shown to exert genotoxic effects.

Some alternative farming methods minimize the need for chemical fertilizers. Legumes in a crop rotation—the successive planting of different crops in the same area—can help to fix nitrogen to the soil and thus reduce the need for additional nitrogenous fertilizers. Alfalfa, chickpeas, and various clovers are among the nitrogen-fixing plants; under proper management, soybeans can also add nitrogen to the soil (WRI, 1992).

Modern Intensive Farming Methods

The mass housing of animals in modern intensified agriculture may lead to an increased exposure to dusts, toxic gases, and zoonoses. For example, intensive poultry rearing brings large numbers of animals into close contact with each other, resulting in an increased likelihood of infection in the herd with pests such as Salmonella mites. In addition, intensive pig rearing in confined spaces leads to the buildup of high concentrations of carbon monoxide (CO), ammonia (NH_3), and dust. Such farming methods require adequate disposal systems for slurry. Intensive pig rearing has also been shown to result in noise levels of up to 102 dB(A), a level at which hearing protection equipment is required in the working environment (see Chapter 2, Physical Hazards).

A number of infections, including brucellosis, leptospirosis, and chlamydiosis, are also encountered in intensive farming. Brucellosis, a chronic bacterial infection, is characterized by joint pains, depression, and mood changes. In some countries this disease is now virtually eliminated by testing and slaughter regulation program. The zoonoses, leptospirosis, and chlamydiosis continue to pose a health threat, thus further study and measures to prevent their spread are required. The spirochaete associated with leptospirosis is transmitted by animal urine, particularly that of rats. Various types of leptospirosis infections, which all differ in the severity and type of symptoms, occur in farmers and farm workers. Sugar cane harvesting is a particularly risky setting for leptospirosis. Some types of leptospirosis may be spread to people in dairy farming through contact with cow urine. Outbreaks of chlamydiosis have been related to poultry as well as to rearing of sheep. Women are at increased risk for this infection because they often help with lambing. The placenta of the ewe may be heavily infected, which then becomes an important source of human infection.

Apart from diseases related to cattle or livestock, farmers are at increased risk for certain respiratory diseases. The inhalable substances to which farmers are exposed include organic antigens such as pollen, fungal spores, animal allergens, grain dust and mites, as well as chemicals such as nitrous oxide, hydrogen sulfide, methane, CO, and ammonia. Some respiratory diseases are associated with silos. Three main types are recognized. Silo filler's disease is due to a toxic effect of nitrogen dioxide and results in acute irritation and may cause pulmonary edema, dyspnea (labored breathing), cough, and fatigue. Silo emptier's disease (pulmonary mycotoxicosis) is a reaction caused by overwhelming concentrations of fungal spores. Symptoms include upper respiratory irritation, dyspnea, malaise, and fever. Farmer's lung disease and allergic alveolitis may occur after exposure to moldy grain silos, barns, and stocks.

Prevention and Control

In addition to integrated pest management, there are a number of techniques that can reduce accidents and chemical exposure, including adherence to good agricultural practices such as crop rotation, avoidance of excessive fertilizer application, the use of proper dosages for pest control, and the correct use of agricultural tools and machinery. Personal protective devices can also help prevent accidents and chemical exposure. These include protective clothing and goggles, respirators in dusty atmospheres, gloves, steel-toed boots, and hearing protection. Medical precautions include vaccinations of both humans and animals against diseases such as tetanus, yellow fever, and rabies. Illnesses should be treated early, before they become established in the individual or are transmitted to others. Finally, the education of workers and others who are particularly vulnerable to agriculture hazards (families of workers, for example) is needed on an ongoing basis (WHO, 1992b)

<u>Study Questions</u>

1. How can the HACCP concept be used to reduce the formation of Maillard reaction products?

2. Many different actions can be taken to improve the safety and quality of our food. Prepare a summary of these actions, indicating (*a*) the level at which this action should be taken and (*b*) the type of contaminant (biological or chemical) involved.

8

HUMAN SETTLEMENT AND URBANIZATION

LEARNING OBJECTIVES

After studying this chapter you will be able to do the following:

- describe human settlements as ecosystems and name the basic requirements for their optimal functioning
- discuss the principles governing healthy housing
- discuss the health problems related to urbanization
- describe the principles of "healthy city" planning, and understand how strategies are developed and implemented.
- indicate the factors leading to urbanization
- summarize health hazards characteristic of the urban environment

CHAPTER CONTENTS

Human Settlements as Ecosystems

Chapter 1 introduced the concept of ecosystems. Before we discuss the health requirements of settlements, it will be useful to think about human settlements as ecosystems. An *urban ecosystem* is an urban nexus of dynamic conditions among inhabitants and activities within urban areas or regions (Guidotti, 1995). In a stable, sustainable urban ecosystem, one group of persons or activities does not destroy or harm the natural or human-made environment that supports and enhances the living conditions of other groups or systems of plants, animals, or humans within that locale. Box 8.1 outlines the complexities of urban ecosystems.

Universal principles for sustainable urban ecosystems include the following:

1. Ensure adequate water supply. In order to be sustainable, each urban ecosystem should use only its fair share of regional freshwater and should not have a negative impact on other ecosystems, either upstream or downstream.

2. Maintain vegetation cover. It is important to maintain and enhance the natural environment, including treed and watered areas. This involves provision of shade and cooling for people, plants, and animals; protection of banks and slopes from erosion; and protection of topsoil from natural forces such as wind, rain, heavy snows, and other storms. For example, heavily treed hillsides and embankments will dramatically reduce the effects of flood-producing storms and rapid runoff.

3. Preserve quality soils. As far as possible, the best soils should be preserved for agriculture uses and lesser soils should be used for urbanization, including buildings and infrastructure. The best soils need to be preserved for both present and future food supplies.

4. Ensure sustainable conditions for wildlife. Protect natural open space systems surrounding urban areas, including treed and watered areas, to support wildlife habitat and environments for all creatures. These are also important sentinels for future environmental well-being of both humans and other species.

5. Maintain regional food production potential. To ensure that urban ecosystems can be self-sustaining with respect to at least certain aspects of their fresh food needs, it is essential to maintain and enhance local food production potential within the region of each urban ecosystem.

6. Create an urban environment on a human scale. Adapt the transportation system, land use patterns, architecture, and governance of cities so that they are convenient and energy efficient, responsive to the needs of residents, attractive to live in, and diverse in cultural and socioeconomic terms.

Basic Health Requirements of Settlements

Both rural and urban settlements must meet many requirements to provide adequately for the needs of economic, physical, and psychological health. The family dwelling not only serves as shelter but is usually the focus of people's emotional life. Settlements furnish a larger dimension of shelter, including basic communal services such as water supply, waste disposal, communications, roads

BOX 8.1

A Framework for Ecosystem Health

As humans have become more alienated from their natural environment, the biofeedback mechanisms that throughout time have regulated human–ecosystem interactions have become more obscured. To provide a comprehensive explanation of the intimate relationship between humans and their surrounding life-supporting environment, a holistic transdisciplinary "ecosystem health" approach must take into account the circumstances of these rapidly expanding built environments.

Urban settlements, ecosystems created by and inhabited by humans, consist of both the built and human-modified physical environment. Thus they include the processes of social aggregation, migration, modernization and industrialization, and the circumstances of urban living. These human-created urban ecosystems exist within a larger frame of reference—the bio-regional and planetary "natural" ecosystems that ultimately provide fundamental life support. The social and economic development that has played a central role in improved population health historically is built upon those natural ecosystems, their resources and the "free" eco-services they provide. Human health, thus, cannot be maintained if ecosystem health is not sustained.

DIMENSIONS TO CONSIDER

The relationship between the built environment, the natural environment, and human health is closely intertwined. Analysts such as Trevor Hancock (Hancock, 2000) have drawn attention to six distinct dimensions of urban ecosystem health:

1. Health status of the urban human population in terms of its physical and mental well-being, including health equity, the distribution of health, and well-being across the different segments of the community;
2. Social well-being within the urban community, including social, economic, and cultural conditions, the effectiveness of the processes of governance (including education, participation, and access to decision-making power), and social equity, the distribution of these and other determinants of health;
3. Quality of the built environment, including aspects of housing quality, transportation, sewage and water supply, roads and public transport systems, parks and recreation facilities, and other civic amenities;
4. Ambient environmental quality within the urban environment in terms of air, water, soil and noise pollution;
5. Health of the biotic community, including aspects of habitat quality and genetic and species diversity;
6. Impact of the urban ecosystem on the wider natural ecosystems of which it is a part, as measured by environmental sustainability concepts such as the urban "ecological footprint."

Adequacy of urban ecosystems can be assessed in relation to their capacity to support a liveable, viable, and sustainable quality of human life. By liveable, built environment components such as the quality of housing stock and basic physical infrastructure, such as water and sewerage, roads and public transportation, etc., and maintenance of public safety should be considered. By viable, basic life support parameters should be taken into account. By sustainable, the impact of the urban ecosystem on its surroundings is called into question.

(continued)

Ecosystem Dimensions	Social Well-being	Built Environment	Environmental Quality	Biotic Community	Ecological Footprint
Driving Force		Urbanization (Migration etc.)			
Pressure	Development/Equity Culture Education/ Governance	Infrastructure Created/Maintained /Absent	(Polluting Sources)	(Habitat Enhanced or Threatened)	e.g. Resource Demands, Greenhouse Gas Emissions
State	Capacity to Prevent, Cope or Mitigate; Social Capital	e.g. Sanitation/ Microbiological Contaminants	Deteriorating AQ, WQ, IAQ, Soil Q	e.g. Contamination of Land/Habitat	e.g. Deforestation
Exposure	Socio-Economic Determinants of Health	e.g. Access to Potable Water	e.g. Particulate, Microbiological Contamination	e.g. Contamination of Produce/Animals	e.g. Increased Likelihood of Adverse Events (e.g. Floods)
Effect	e.g. Psychosocial	e.g. Diarrhea	e.g. Respiratory	e.g Poisoning	Impacts on Ecosystems (e.g. Climate Change)

Health Status of Urban Population

From Spiegal et al., 2001, with permission.

(continued)

In the developed world, the long-term sustainability of current patterns of resource consumption has been repeatedly called into question and questions of eco-toxicity (e.g., endocrine disruptors, persistent and cumulative exposures) have been frequently raised. Nevertheless, improvements in environmental protection achieved over the last quarter of the twentieth century have contributed to create generally liveable conditions, albeit with threats to viability and sustainability. However, in the developing world, there are many indicators of distress—and the ability to provide liveable and viable conditions is under considerable strain. Frameworks developed to assist decision-makers understand the relationship of human-ecosystem interactions are especially valuable in understanding dynamic relationships between driving forces, pressures, states, exposures, and effects (DPSEEA) within this environment. The figure in this box builds upon Hancock's urban ecosystem dimensions (Hancock, 2000), utilizing the DPSEEA framework discussed elsewhere in this text. It shows how each dimension ultimately impacts human health, albeit mediated by different pathways and determinants.

One example of how this framework is being applied within an urban ecosystem community is in Centro Habana, Cuba, in which an extensive series of health interventions were implemented in an inner-city community to try to improve the quality of life and ecosystem health. The interventions addressed areas that the community perceived as being of highest risk, including housing conditions, environmental sanitation, lifestyle concerns, social environment issues and immediate threats to health. The results to date indicate the strong capacity-building nature of applying such approaches (Yassi et al., 1999; Fernandez et al., 2000). In fact, the development of analytical indicators collaboratively with the community is itself a principle that has received recognition as an element consistent with an ecosystem analysis (Spiegel et al. 2001).

Contributed by Dr. Jerry Spiegel.

and public transportation, and the production and distribution of consumer goods like food and clothing. They also enable the provision of services such as education, health, and law enforcement, as well as provide infrastructure and support for cultural, religious, and recreational activities. Settlements also give assistance to vulnerable groups, such as elderly people.

In effect, a symbiotic relationship exists between family dwellings and community settlements, in which the values of both enhance each other. The family dwelling is not just a place in which to eat and sleep but is also where people store their possessions, relax, study, procreate, nurture and educate their children, and often die. It is usually the most important focus of a person's life. Settlements provide an umbilical cord of support for families and individuals.

Shelter requirements are to a large degree dependent on climate. For example, in extreme northern and southern latitudes, shelter from cold is of central importance, while in hotter regions protection from heat is essential. In low-lying coastal or tropical regions, hurricanes, monsoons, and tidal waves are serious problems for communities, while in some inland regions, sandstorms, tornadoes, and blizzards present different problems. In regions where seismic activities are possible, volcanoes and earthquakes pose a potential threat to communities. Each of these conditions has inspired different designs for both dwellings and settlements with regard to ideal infrastructure and housing needs.

Although some variation in infrastructure does exist among settlements, there are several universal requirements. All people require access to a safe and permanent supply of water and food as well as to appropriate household energy for cooking, heating, lighting, etc. All humans produce fecal waste and generate at least some food and other waste that require management. Additionally, most communities have several features in common that require management. For example, most have some connection to industry and must provide protection from pollutants, and most have motorized traffic, which creates pollution and injury risks. When communities are unable to meet these requirements, the result is often health problems for community residents.

If housing design and development are to be effective, they must be based on appropriate community standards and have the means to enforce them. Enforcement of standards is particularly difficult for poorer communities, those in developing countries, and in informal communities sometimes known as *shantytowns*. These hastily improvised communities spring up along the margins of many big cities, usually in areas not designated as residential neighborhoods, and they suffer greatly from substandard housing construction and maintenance. They are usually exposed to industry and are isolated from both basic services, such as water supply, and more complex ones, such as cultural venues. Often these communities often cannot turn to government for intervention and assistance either because they are technically illegal or the residents are disenfranchised politically in settlements that are barely tolerated. They must therefore rely on community initiative to address issues of concern.

The quality of housing from a health perspective can be assessed using a number of indicators (Box 8.2) categorized according to the driving force-pressure-exposure-effect-action (DPSEEA) framework (see Chapter 3).

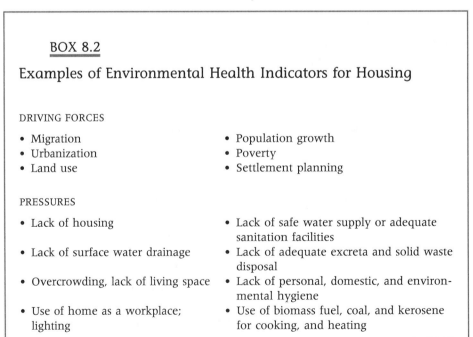

BOX 8.2

Examples of Environmental Health Indicators for Housing

DRIVING FORCES

- Migration
- Urbanization
- Land use
- Population growth
- Poverty
- Settlement planning

PRESSURES

- Lack of housing

- Lack of surface water drainage

- Overcrowding, lack of living space

- Use of home as a workplace; lighting

- Lack of safe water supply or adequate sanitation facilities

- Lack of adequate excreta and solid waste disposal

- Lack of personal, domestic, and environmental hygiene

- Use of biomass fuel, coal, and kerosene for cooking, and heating

(continued)

(continued)

- Use of unsafe food preparation facilities
- Lack of structural safeguards
- Safety, chemical and fire hazards
- Lack of lighting, ventilation, and insulation
- Lack of open spaces and greenery
- Inadequate siting, inadequate protection from floods, landslides, industry, and traffic

LOCAL HAZARDS

- Microbiological and chemical contamination of water supplies (recreational and drinking water)
- Contamination of food supplies
- Refuse and wastes
- Dampness, odors
- Indoor air pollution
- Standing water (vector breeding sites)
- Pests, rodents, vermin, pathogenic organisms
- Fires, explosions

EXPOSURES

- Proportion of households to people with inadequate water supplies, sanitation facilities, and refuse removal services
- Proportion of households to people using coal, kerosene, or biomass fuels for heating, cooking, and lighting
- Proportion of households to people exposed to varying levels of indoor air pollution from indoor fires and environmental tobacco smoke
- Proportion of households with high levels of radon, leaded paint, lead water pipes, asbestos
- Proportion of households to people exposed to dampness, odors, or high levels of noise
- Proportion of households to people exposed to pests, rodents, and vermin
- Proportion of households to people exposed to shelter that is structurally unsafe or sited on unsafe land, in close proximity to pollution-producing industry
- Proportion of people living in overcrowded conditions, with poor domestic and environmental hygiene
- Proportion of households to people exposed to inadequate ventilation, lighting, and insulation

EFFECTS

- Skin conditions (eczema, dermatitis, lice)
- Violence, crime, abuse, drugs, alcoholism
- Prevalence/incidence of accidents, injuries, and burns in the home, or traffic accidents
- Gastrointestinal diseases, parasitic diseases, tuberculosis, measles, and other communicable diseases
- Lead poisoning, neurobehavioral disorders, and other chronic, ill health–related conditions
- Psychological/mental health conditions (stress-related, anxiety, depression)
- Environment-related respiratory conditions

ACTIONS

- Land-use planning and zoning measures
- Conservation measures
- Improved stove programs

(continued)

(*continued*)

- Land and housing tenure measures
- Housing legislation, standards, and enforcement measures aimed at incremental improvements in living conditions
- Impact assessment procedures for housing schemes
- Low-cost housing provision, housing upgrading
- Social and economic improvement programs
- Intersectoral programs for housing and health
- Community participation and action program support
- Education measures and advocacy programs for housing and health
- Adult literacy and empowerment programs for women
- Surveillance and monitoring programs, health risk assessment programs
- Service provision measures (e.g., water and sanitation, electricity, preventive and curative health services, community services, emergency services).

HOUSING AND HEALTH

Housing, Communicable Diseases, and Infections

Housing conditions play a crucial role in the control of many diseases, especially in the transmission of communicable diseases; a number of these factors have been discussed in detail in previous chapters (Table 8.1). The home can both protect from disease or facilitate disease. Of all the factors listed in Table 8.1, water supply and sanitation facilities often appear to be the most important in determining a community's health. Efficient drainage of surface water helps to control communicable and vector-borne diseases and reduces safety hazards and property damage. Lack of, or a breakdown in, drainage systems can result in vector-breeding sites. Flooding can result in similar problems. Appropriate solid waste disposal and storage can discourage insect and rodent vectors of disease and reduce population exposure to urban conditions likely to cause problems. Solid waste management is even more crucial when excreta are among the waste products. Waste disposal problems tend to exist predominantly in urban settings, where there are space constrictions, crowding, and greater consumption. The urban poor are especially at risk because of their dependency on scavenging for their livelihood, placing them in direct contact with all types of waste materials.

Personal and domestic hygiene is crucial to the reduction of numerous infections, including skin complaints such as sepsis, dermatitis, and eczema, or eye

TABLE 8.1

HOUSING FACTORS INFLUENCING HEALTH

Safe and adequate water supply
Sanitary disposal of human and animal excreta
Efficient drainage of surface water
Appropriate solid waste disposal and storage
Personal and domestic hygiene
Safe food preparation
Housing structure and maintenance

TABLE 8.2

FEATURES OF HOUSING DESIGN THAT HELP PREVENT DISEASES

Design Feature	Diseases Combated or Prevented
	STRONG ASSOCIATION
Adequate supply of water	Trachoma, skin infections, gastroenteric diseases
Sanitary disposal of excreta	Gastroenteritis and intestinal parasites
Safe water supply	Typhoid, cholera
Bathing and washing facilities	Schistosomiasis, trachoma, gastroenteritis, skin diseases
Means of food production	Malnutrition
Control of air pollution	Acute and chronic respiratory diseases
	FAIRLY STRONG ASSOCIATION
Ventilation of houses (especially if indoor fires)	Acute and chronic respiratory diseases
Control of house dust	Asthma
Siting housing away from vector-breeding areas	Malaria, schistosomiasis, filariasis, trypanosomiasis
Control of open fires, away from kerosene or bottled gas	Burns
Finished floors	Hookworm
Screening	Malaria
	SOME ASSOCIATION
Control of use of thatch material	Chagas' disease
Rehabilitation of housing	Psychological disorders
Control of heat inside shelter	Heat stress
Adequate food storage	Malnutrition
Refuse collection	Chagas' disease, leishmaniasis

Source: Stephens et al., 1985.

disease such as trachoma and conjunctivitis, or contagious diseases such as tuberculosis (TB) and meningitis. Good hygiene is impossible to maintain without adequate water supply. Features of housing design and the diseases they may help to overcome are listed in Table 8.2.

Communicable Diseases If there are not sufficient rooms in a house to allow for separation of sick people from healthy inhabitants, contagious diseases are more readily transmitted. Overcrowding is therefore an important factor in the spread of a number of communicable diseases. Additionally, housing with no adequate sunlight and ventilation facilitates the spread of disease by increasing available breeding sites of vectors. This is especially true for (TB, one of the more common killers globally. Tuberculosis is a contagious disease that flourishes in crowded, unhygienic environments. It is caused by bacteria that produce lung lesions, which eventually impair lung function sufficiently to cause death. Once in place in the human body, the bacteria are very resilient to treatment with antibiotics, making the cure of patients with TB difficult and expensive. Elimination of the spread of the disease, however, may be as simple as placing the sick person in a space with adequate ultraviolet (UV) light and ventilation. As TB makes its way into poor urban environments, it has the potential to have disastrous effects on many inhabitants in both the developed and developing world because of overcrowding.

Meningitis is a communicable disease that kills many people worldwide. Like TB, it is spread by airborne transmission and is linked to overcrowding and poor-quality housing. Meningitis can be caused by many different viruses and bacteria when they are able to penetrate the blood-brain barrier, which is normally impenetrable. There is no external cure for the viral form of the disease, meaning that patients' chances of surviving depend on the state of their immune systems. The bacterial forms can be treated by antibiotics, but the disease is fatal and may develop rapidly, and it requires rapid and extensive treatment that is not always successful. Other diseases, such as influenza, may also be transmitted more readily if housing is inadequate.

Poorly maintained, unhygienic buildings also provide excellent breeding grounds for many insect vectors, particularly in tropical regions. For example, Chagas' disease is caused by a parasite transmitted by the Vinchuca bug, which lives in the dark cracks and crevices of poorly built and maintained homes in certain parts of South America. Its bite leads to a specific type of heart disease that is usually fatal within 10 years for adults and in much less time in children.

The poor are especially vulnerable to inadequate housing conditions. Just as they cannot afford adequate housing, they also are generally not able to afford proper nutrition, education, and health services. They are also more likely to be exposed to dust, pollution, noise, and the hazards of climatic extremes because of the nature of their economy and often flimsy housing.

Home Accidents and Toxic Exposures

Housing should also protect its inhabitants against physical hazards and toxic exposures; this depends on both the structure of the facility and the behavior of the people using it. In the planning of housing, many factors must be taken into consideration to protect residents against these hazards, including structural features and furnishings. Poorly designed or inadequately built homes increase the risk of accidents and injuries, particularly for children.

A variety of injuries can be due to poorly designed or maintained housing. Makeshift buildings that collapse on top of their inhabitants in earthquakes, heavy rains, storms, or mudslides are common in the poorest areas of many countries. Even under "normal" conditions, makeshift buildings made of poor materials result in a high number of injuries in or around the home. In more affluent countries, elderly people and young children tend to suffer more severe injuries from falls down stairs, particularly if proper safety precautions are not incorporated in housing. Elderly people often stumble on thresholds, carpets, or other flooring hazards, causing hip fractures, one of the more common and costly injuries among elderly people. Other injuries related to unsafe housing include burns from contact with unprotected fireplaces or stoves or from house fires when occupants cannot escape in time. Fires in factories, hotels, and other buildings where large groups of people congregate can have disastrous consequences if buildings are not suitably designed, lack fire protection or fire-fighting equipment such as extinguishers or sprinklers, or have insufficient emergency exits and evacuation planning.

In many communities, indoor air pollution presently poses a much greater health risk than outdoor air pollution. Residents dependent on open fireplaces or unventilated stoves in their homes are most vulnerable, and the resulting respiratory diseases in children are responsible for as many fatalities globally as diarrheal diseases (WHO, 1997). Biomass fuels are used extensively for domestic purposes; in some settings the associated health risks are severe (see Chapters 5 and 9). Fossil fuels are also commonly burned domestically and poor combustion technologies expose people to harmful emissions of carbon monoxide (CO), nitric oxides (NO_x), dust (suspended particles), and volatile organic compounds (VOCs). Lack of ventilation, proper stoves, and chimneys greatly compounds the risks associated with both fuel types. Additionally, construction materials and furnishings are often a source of indoor pollutants, releasing a wide variety of airborne contaminants (e.g., formaldehyde, asbestos). Cigarette smoking also contribute to air pollution, and the effects of environmental tobacco smoke (ETS) can be severe.

Pollutants from the environment surrounding dwellings can also become a problem. In a number of countries the natural leakage of radon and radioactive gas has caused high levels of exposure inside dwellings and thus an increased risk of lung cancer. Air pollution builds up in urban areas from the concentration of population and industry. The heating of houses with wood or coal fires is a major source of outdoor urban air pollution in some countries.

Lead-based paints are a source of lead poisoning, especially in children. Aging water pipes made of lead or which have lead soldering in them are still in use in some parts of the world.

Cottage industries, where the home is used as a workplace, carry an associated risk of contaminant exposure. Home industries often involve the use of hazardous materials and produce noise and/or waste contaminants (either solid or airborne). These risks are compounded in an urban setting, where, in areas of high-population density, accidents such as fires can affect an entire community.

In some industrialized countries, the problem of sick building syndrome (SBS)—or *building-related illness,* as it is sometimes called—is common. The fact that most people spend 80% to 90% of their time indoors underscores the importance of dealing with this problem. When the oil crisis in the early 1970s sent the price of energy skyrocketing, industrialized countries put a priority on making new buildings as airtight as possible. It was soon noted that gases given off by construction materials and other pollutants could become trapped inside these airtight environments, resulting in a range of health problems among those living or working inside. Throughout the next two decades, the incidence of complaints regarding air quality in homes, schools, office buildings, and other workplaces increased dramatically. The term *tight building syndrome* was originally coined to describe this phenomenon.

Often SBS-related complaints are general and nonspecific. Symptoms typical of SBS are shown in Table 8.3. Causes of SBS include inadequate ventilation (estimated in the United States in the mid-1980s to be responsible for 50% of cases); some source of environmental contamination, from either inside or outside the building (30%); and unknown causes (10%). Building materials, humidity, molds, cigarette smoke, noise, and illumination account for the rest (10%). In

TABLE 8.3

TYPICAL HEALTH COMPLAINTS ASSOCIATED WITH SICK BUILDING SYNDROME

Nasal congestion and sinus problems
Headaches
Fatigue/drowsiness
Eye irritation
Respiratory difficulties (e.g., chest tightness, exacerbations of asthma, increased number of upper respiratory tract infections)
Skin problems (e.g., eczema and other rashes)

addition, inadequate humidification can cause dry air (a known cause of irritation to eyes, skin, and throat), static electricity, and temperature fluctuations.

Sources of environmental contamination include off-gassing from new furniture or carpeting, cleaning materials, chemicals from adjacent offices, unclean ducts, fibreglass, and cigarette smoke. Virtually all dusts, vapors and aerosols that can react with proteins can cause an allergic reaction. Generally considerable exposure is required to become sensitized. However, once the individual has become sensitized to any of these, allergic reactions may be elicited after only a brief and low-concentration exposure.

Psychosocial Problems

Reducing psychosocial stress is a vital role of proper housing, as the link between a good psychological environment at home and health is strong. Poor psychological health makes people generally more susceptible to many communicable and chronic diseases and there are numerous other health problems that accompany poor psychological health (e.g., psychosomatic illnesses, substance abuse, mental illness, and violent behaviors). Increasingly, housing in urban settings fails to serve the role of psychosocial haven, as overcrowding and the stresses of urban life produce exactly the opposite effect. Urban housing, with its model of individual family homes (transplanted from the developed world to communities all over the globe), often tends to break down traditional community structures that existed in rural environments, increasing individual alienation. The urban poor have the additional burden of living in insecure tenant situations and being subject to exploitation in their housing environments. All of these problems are experienced most keenly by those making the transition from rural to urban life. The trend toward urbanization makes this problem urgent. Many factors involved in housing can reduce these problems to a minimum, some of which are listed in Table 8.4.

TABLE 8.4

FACTORS AFFECTING CONTROL OF PSYCHOSOCIAL PROBLEMS

Living space should be sufficiently large and reasonably private and comfortable.
The housing environment must be safe and conducive to community interaction.
Recreational space must be available to neighborhood residents.
Neighborhoods should be protected against traffic noise and industrial pollution.
Parks, playgrounds, and other community amenities should be easily available.
Housing should be easy to maintain and keep clean.

Trends in Urbanization

Urbanization, the process by which an increasing proportion of the population comes to live in urban areas, has become a worldwide problem. Urbanization is a reflection of population growth and opportunities in cities. A population can grow, only through increase in births, decrease in deaths (the natural increase); or increased immigration. Decreased emigration may reduce the loss of population if the rate of immigration does not also fall. Urban areas of the world are now experiencing both a natural increase and an increase in net migration to the cities.

In 1999 the world's population reached 6000 million people—more than three times the population of 100 years ago. A 30% rise is predicted by the year 2010. Of this predicted growth, 90% is expected to occur in countries that are presently classified as developing countries. Urbanization is also occurring at a dramatic pace. The urban populations of developing countries will double in the 20 years from 1990, which means that by 2010, well over half the world's population will be in urban centers, or about 4000 million people (UNEP/WHO, 1992c). By 2025 it is expected that more than 5000 million will live in urban areas, as shown in Figure 8.1 (WRI, 1996). Urbanization has been growing in developing countries at a much faster rate than in developed countries. It is estimated that by 2010, 60% of the developing countries' urban population will be living in shanty towns or informal settlements.

Of special concern in this global trend of urbanization is the growth of megacities, or cities with a population of 8 million or more; it is projected that by 2015 there will be 36 megacities (UN, 1997). The largest cities are listed in Table 8.5. Megacities warrant concern because their sheer size creates great challenges to human health and the environment.

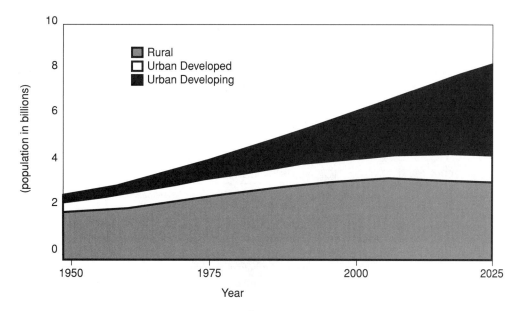

Figure 8.1 Urban population growth, 1950–2025. From UNDP, 1995, with permission.

TABLE 8.5

THE WORLD'S LARGEST CITIES, 1995 AND PROJECTED 2015

	Population (millions) 1995	Population (millions) 2015
Tokyo, Japan	26.9	28.9
Mumbai (formerly Bombay), India	15.1	26.2
Lagos, Nigeria	10.3	24.6
São Paulo, Brazil	16.5	20.3
Karachi, Pakistan	9.8	19.4
Mexico City, Mexico	16.6	19.1
Shanghai, China	13.6	17.9
New York, U.S.A.	16.3	17.6
Calcutta, India	11.9	17.3
Delhi, India	10.0	16.9
Beijing, China	11.3	15.6
Metro Manila, Philippines	9.3	14.7
Cairo, Egypt	9.7	14.4
Los Angeles, U.S.A.	12.4	14.2
Jakarta, Indonesia	8.6	14.0
Buenos Aires, Argentina	11.8	13.9
Tianjin, China	9.4	13.5
Seoul, Republic of Korea	11.6	13.0
Rio de Janeiro, Brazil	10.2	11.9
Osaka, Japan	10.6	10.6
Paris, France	9.5	9.7
Dhaka, Bangladesh	7.8	9.5
Moscow, Russian Federation	9.3	9.3

Source: UN, 1996.

Migration to Urban Centers

People migrate from rural to urban areas for a variety of reasons. As life expectancy increases and the birth rate rises, single farms may not be able to support all family members. In addition, rural customs and discriminatory inheritance laws can encourage or force migration from rural areas. Improved survival of children has created a rapid growth in the number of young people without sufficient land to support them.

TABLE 8.6

FACTORS AFFECTING REGIONAL URBANIZATION

Changes in a region's economic or employment base often lead to increased employment opportunities in urban centers.

Areas with unequal income distribution, where only a few individuals are affected by economic growth, experience significantly different urbanization patterns than areas where many people have access to economic benefits.

Political structures can affect the distribution of poverty and hence urban development areas.

Government macroeconomic policies may favor urban centers, and thus increase urbanization rates.

World markets, which influence national economies, necessarily influence urban systems.

Economic and political factors greatly influence migration patterns (Table 8.6.) Many developing countries, for example, Cote D'Ivoire, Indonesia, India, Mexico, Brazil, and Thailand, are expanding their economies rapidly and along with this expansion are experiencing very high rates of urbanization. An increased economy means more industry. Jobs follow industries, and people often follow jobs. People thus migrate to cities to seek work, better living standards, better education, and other facilities and services. Population movements to the cities have also been accentuated in many countries, e.g., in Somalia in the 1970s and Ethiopia in the 1980s, as a result of famine, drought, and other natural hazards in rural areas. Additionally, wars, natural disasters, and ecological crises can have a large impact on urbanization trends of specific regions. By contrast, many countries with stagnating economies, falling public expenditures, and enormous debt burdens have experienced much slower urban growth than predicted.

In developed countries, a shift away from urbanization to suburbanization is occurring as people and industries seek locations just outside major cities. These cities may be becoming too expensive for people and industries. Advances in transport and communications and changes in economic structures (e.g., away from heavy industry and toward the service sector) enable rural areas and small towns to attract enterprises and inhabitants that were previously located only in cities. As more of this suburbanized population commutes to the city to work, rural populations in developed countries tend to be less agriculturally based. It should be emphasized, though, that the net shift in populations in developed countries is toward urbanization (WHO, 1992c).

RURAL ECONOMIC AND SOCIAL DEVELOPMENT

Differences of Time and Space

Rural communities undergoing development must deal with realities of time and space that are different from those of urban communities. In rural areas, distances between suppliers and consumers are greater, transportation takes longer, and the density of population is much less than in a city, so there is less efficiency in conducting business. Because the density is lower, and usually more evenly distributed than in an urban area, it is often more practical to do business by bringing people together at a particular time, rather than in a particular place. This is the basis of the traditional marketplace, where people come on a particular day to buy and sell goods and to conduct their personal business. Fairs, festivals, and expositions accomplish the same purpose. Many cities began as permanent settlements that grew on the sites for such markets and fairs. (To get an idea of how common this was, one need only look at a map of England. Most country towns and all cities ending in "chester" started this way, as well as many others.) Prices for local commodities and land (except in agriculturally rich areas) tend to be lower in rural areas than in cities, but the cost of construction and transportation can be much higher.

Dependence on Primary Industries

The economy of most rural areas is based on agriculture and resource industries such as mining, forestry, and fishing. Agricultural commodities and fishing may help to sustain a community, but most rural areas survive economically by selling these commodities or trading for the goods they need.

Because commodities produced in the rural area must be sold or traded, rural areas tend to be susceptible to changes in prices. If the demand for their commodity drops, prices may fall abruptly, as has often been the case for crops such as coffee or cacao. This means that rural areas are often highly dependent for their prosperity on goods that have fluctuating prices, and this leads to economic instability. Diversification of the rural economy has therefore been a goal in many countries. Where the density permits, some limited manufacturing can be supported, as with township industries in China where the rural districts are much more densely populated than in most countries. In developed economies, industries based on information services are now increasingly common in rural districts because improved communications make it easier to live farther away from customers.

The economy in rural areas tends to be seasonal. Crops are planted, tended and harvested by the time of year and weather, and fishing may occur only during certain times of the year. Many rural residents make their living by selling crafts or working in industries such as mining during the off-season, and farm or fish when they can. As a result, a farmer in a rural area may be accurately described as someone who does many jobs, among them, farming.

Development and Ownership of Land

In developing countries, rural areas are often less developed than cities. The infrastructure is often relatively poor because the investment is less productive in less dense settlements and the area to be served is much greater. Rural poverty is a common problem that is aggravated if the rural area is remote from industries that could provide employment or if agriculture is weak or commodities unstable.

Land ownership, an important issue in agricultural communities, often lies at one of two extremes: (1) widespread ownership of small plots of land that are too small to be economically productive or (2) concentrated ownership of very large areas of land in the hands of a few people or families. Concentrated ownership is often associated with social unrest, exploitative labor practices, and over-reliance on cash crops that are dependent on commodity prices. In such societies, the tension between land owners and a class of resident farmers who work the land and are required to pay rent is often the basis for social unrest.

Conservative/Traditional Values

Socially, rural areas tend to be conservative and traditional. Families, clans, and neighbors are very important where there are few social institutions that can guarantee security and when communities are small. This conservatism is not absolute, and the influence of modern communications and transportation has clearly reduced the isolation of many rural areas. Likewise, the need to pay attention to commodity prices has made many rural residents experts on the operation of international markets. Overall, however, rural areas tend to be places where traditional values are held for a long time and where change is resisted. Consequently, more and more rural young people leave the area to try their luck in the city.

Mixed Implications of Environmental Protection

Environmental protection has mixed meaning for rural areas. To the extent that environmental protection preserves the advantages of rural life and makes life in villages and isolated communities safer, it is welcomed. However, environmental protection may be perceived as threatening to a community if it changes farming practices, removes resources from economic use, or interferes with the construction or development of infrastructure. Villagers that make their money during a certain season from, for example, wood cutting or catching fish may not accept that it is necessary to preserve the forest, reduce the catch, or save the soil.

URBANIZATION AND HEALTH

The Urban Poor

Globally, urban residents enjoy better health than rural populations. This fact does not take into account, however, the differences within cities between wealthy and poor populations, which can be staggering. In many cities, poverty among urban residents is widespread. In developing countries it can affect the majority of the residents, and in developed countries it is on the rise. Poverty is a major factor in exacerbating the risks discussed earlier. The health situation of the urban poor is often worse than that of people living in rural areas. The urban poor must endure the difficulties of rural life (lack of services, decreased access to health care) along with many urban hazards (crowding, stress, and exposure to industrial hazards). Figure 8.2 illustrates that a large proportion of residents in the major cities of developing countries live in poverty. These figures are from 1988; the situation is worse today.

The process of urbanization has often been haphazard and chaotic. Most of the urban poor live in low-quality, overcrowded, self-made forms of shelter that are only marginally served by the public utilities taken for granted by others. In many cities, a majority of people live in shantytowns, or informal settlements, which in turn account for more than half the built-up areas. Informal settlements can account for up to 90% of low-income settlements, as they do in Addis Ababa and Yaounde.

There are two important points to note about these settlements. The first is that they are not a temporary phenomenon brought about by a dysfunction in the development process, but rather a product of low wages and the inability of governments and agencies to provide adequate settlements. The second point is that these settlements differ widely around the world with respect to culture, legal status, tenure, levels of home improvement, age, physical structure, community involvement, immigrant status, and major health problems facing them. They should not be treated as a homogenous population (UNEP/WHO, 1987a). Nonetheless, there are certain infrastructural requirements and problems that apply to all such settlements.

Infrastructural Requirements of Urbanization

The process of urbanization has significant requirements, including the provision of water safe for household consumption and sanitation purposes, solid and liq-

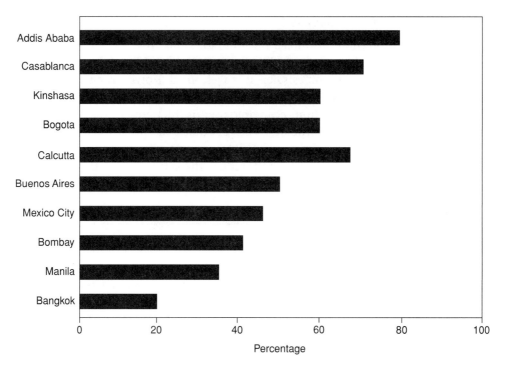

Figure 8.2 Percentage of people living in slums and squatter settlements in some urban centers (1988). From UNEP, 1992a, with permission.

uid waste management, and housing and transportation networks. All of these are energy-expensive but they must be met, at least to some degree, to ensure a minimum standard of health. The rapid pace of urbanization in many areas has virtually outstripped the ability of local governments to provide these services adequately. Additionally, promotion of economic growth has led to industrial expansion that frequently overwhelms the existing urban services. Several of the health-promoting housing design features listed in Tables 8.1 to 8.4 relate directly to urban infrastructure.

Air Pollution

As discussed in Chapter 5, air pollution is one of the many problems modern cities experience, no matter what their level of economic development. In the past, air pollution was often considered a matter of aesthetics and quality of life, but not of survival or health. Increasing scientific evidence has shown that the effects of air pollution on health are considerable, even in developed countries where the levels of air pollution have been largely controlled. This has led to a reexamination of the need for air quality management. The negative effects of air pollution are now taken much more seriously. The annual sulfur dioxide (SO_2) and suspended particulate matter (SPM) levels in cities involved in the Global Environmental Monitoring System (GEMS) are shown in Figures 8.3 and 8.4.

The principal sources of emissions into the air are the direct products of economic activity in cities: transportation, power production, home heating and cooking, and industrial production. The costs imposed by air pollution are most

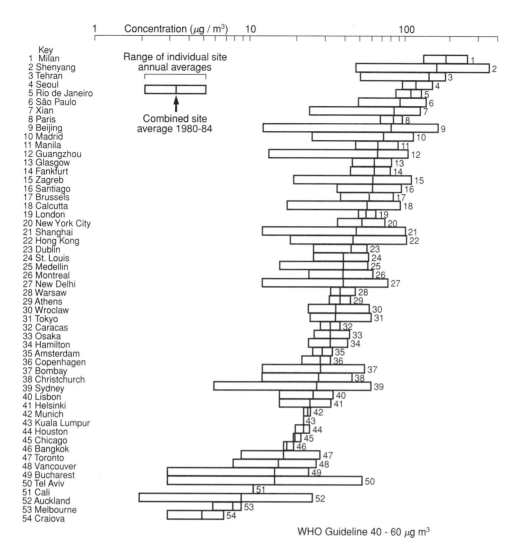

Figure 8.3 Annual SO_2 measures in GEMS/Air cities, 1980–84. From UNEP/WHO, 1987b, with permission.

obvious in cities as well: human health problems, destruction of materials, plant and animal damage, poor visibility, loss of appeal for tourists, and reduced quality of life for residents.

City and regional planning can make a great difference in determining air quality. The provision of energy-efficient mass transportation, for example, can greatly reduce air pollution from motor vehicles. However, if the city is large and spread out, mass transit may not be practical, and if it is too expensive, it may not be used. The location of industry in or near residential communities or in valleys, basins, or other landforms that collect pollution can aggravate the problem. Box 8.3 presents some major accomplishments in promoting the use of nonmotorized vehicles that have occurred across the globe. Housing that is energy-efficient and power supplies that are both energy-efficient and reliable may reduce the amount of air pollution, but these require an investment in infrastructure.

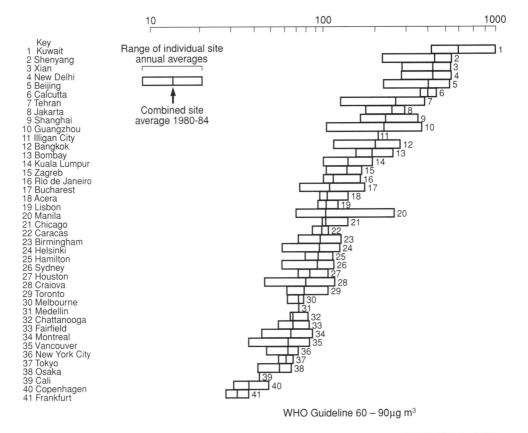

Figure 8.4 Annual SPM measures in GEMS/Air cities, 1980–84. From UNEP/WHO, 1987b, with permission.

In recent years, it has become obvious that poor communities tend to be more affected by air pollution than those with higher average incomes. This observation has been followed by a number of studies that have shown that exposure to pollution tends to accompany poverty, marginalization from society, and lack of access to social services and health care. The likely explanation for this is that people who have access to personal resources are more likely to live together, avoiding unhealthy or unpleasant neighborhoods. However, there is also evidence that factories, power plants, or other facilities that may be sources of pollution are more likely to be built in or near poor communities in the first place. The problem of equity in environmental risk, called *environmental justice,* is an issue of serious concern in discussions and policies regarding air pollution, contaminated water supplies, and hazardous waste disposal.

Noise

The major sources of noise are road and air traffic, construction, industry, and people. These types of noises are generally on the rise as urban centers become more dense, industry expands, and the need for transportation increases. Noise is of most direct concern in the workplace, where hearing loss most commonly occurs. (Industrial noise and its control are also discussed in Chapters 2, 4, and

BOX 8.3

Examples of Success in the Use of Nonmotorized Vehicles

In many countries of the world, governments have actively promoted bicycle commuting. For example:

- In China, where 50%–80% of urban trips are by bicycle, the government offers subsidies to those who bicycle to work. It has also allocated extensive urban street space to bicycle traffic.
- Prompted by Cuba's petroleum crisis, car traffic has been reduced in Havana by 35% and bus traffic by 50%, and bicycle use has been actively encouraged. Now, one of every three trips in Havana is made by bicycle. The city government reduced car speeds to improve safety conditions, and in addition to offering bicyclists subsidies, has constructed bike lanes.
- In developed countries, Denmark and The Netherlands have done a great deal to promote bicycle use. The Dutch National Transportation Plan aims to increase the amount of cycling by 30% by 2010, by providing new bicycle routes, parking at railway stations and bus and tram stops, and additional safety measures, despite the fact that bicycle use is already very high in this country.
- In several cities in Canada and Australia, extensive bicycle paths have been introduced.
- In Seattle, all buses in the Metropolitan Transit System are now equipped with bicycle racks.

These examples illustrate how, if properly promoted and encouraged, bicycles can provide access to shopping, schools, and work. This can help reduce air pollution and the other problems associated with motorized vehicles described in this chapter. In addition, bicycle use is a form of active transport that gives much-needed physical exercise to sedentary populations of developed countries.

Source: WRI, 1996.

10.) However, as rates of urbanization all over the globe exceed the ability of city planners to protect residents from noise, increasingly it has become a generalized urban problem.

As discussed in Chapter 2, noise may cause physical, physiological, and psychological effects in humans. The physical effect of sound waves against the ear drum resulting in hearing loss is sometimes referred to as a *direct effect*. The physiological changes that may register cognitively include sleep disturbance and psychological damage, and are considered *indirect effects*. The dose–response relationship between noise and hearing loss was discussed in Chapter 2.

Environmental noise, (also called community noise) is often complex (Rylander, 1992; Berglund et al., 1999). Acoustical patterns are traditionally expressed as the summation of sound energy over a certain period of time. Various methods of calculating an average have been developed, such as the noise pollution level, the average day and night level, and the equivalent sound level

(Leq) for different parts of the day. (For a complete review of noise-related issues, the reader is referred to the Guidelines for Community Noise produced by the WHO [Berglund et al., 1999].) The concept of average level has two critical features. A few events with a high noise level will have the same Leq as a large number of events at a lower noise level. However, it is unlikely that these two noise scenarios will cause an equal effect in the exposed populations. A second critical feature for the average noise level relates to the number of events. If, for example, the noise increases because of an increase in the number of cars, the Leq will gradually rise, even though the noise level from each car is still 65 dB(A).

There is no strong documented evidence that environmental noise generally or road traffic noise in particular can cause long-term hearing damage; levels in the general environment do not reach those that will induce hearing damage, even in areas close to traffic along heavily congested streets. This is important to bear in mind when assessing exposure and estimating risk. The interaction of noise from road traffic with other sounds in the environment is nonetheless important. Noise levels causing speech interference are often present in areas close to heavy road-traffic and air-traffic. Vulnerable groups in the population include school children in noisy classrooms who may experience performance, attention, memorization and reading problems than children in quieter rooms (Berglund et al., 1999).

As noted above, the immediate response to a noise stimulus often comprises a startle and a defense reaction. The startle reflex may be accompanied by an increase in blood pressure and pulse frequency of a very short duration (up to 30 sec), and in extreme situations, an increased secretion of stress hormones. A review of the cardiovascular effects of noise reported that of 55 studies that assessed the relationship between noise and blood pressure, about 80% reported some form of positive association (Dejoy, 1984). The author noted, however, that there is a lack of quantitative data and it is difficult to assess strength of association or to derive a dose–response relationship. In any case, it would be difficult to distinguish the influence of noise from other environmental stress factors, which could also produce a slight increase in blood pressure.

Exposure to noise can induce disturbance of sleep through causing difficulty in falling asleep, alterations of sleep rhythm or depth, and being awakened. Evidence suggests that sleep disturbance is one of the major adverse effects of environmental noise, and this may seriously impede normal functioning and health in exposed populations. Noise can also give rise to headaches, fatigue, and irritability. The exact conditions under which sensitive individuals become vulnerable are not known, but it is conceivable that other environmental strains could act synergistically with noise. A discussion of a dose–response relationship between the intensity of noise and the extent of nonspecific nuisance, disturbance of night rest, disruption of conversations, and shock or startling reactions is presented in Box 8.4 and Table 8.7.

Annoyance with noise is widespread in urban centers and around airports. According to the definition of health cited in Chapter 1, subjective annoyance should be considered an important health effect, an adequate rationale for taking action against noise. A practical means of confronting the problem is to make the subjective interpretation of noise the primary criterion. Noise standards could

Noise and Nuisance

Noise may affect health by inducing nuisance. Nuisance is a difficult concept to measure objectively and has many of the characteristics of psychosocial hazards discussed in Chapter 2. For instance, the extent to which a person is aggravated is not merely determined by the type and intensity of the noise but also by personal characteristics or circumstances. Nuisance may be rather specific—for instance, when a conversation is interrupted by a passing train, but it can also be nonspecific and give a general feeling of annoyance, discontent, or even fear. Apart from the intensity of the noise, other physical characteristics such as frequency and rhythm (impulse versus nonimpulse sounds) are of relevance. Noise with low frequency components, for example, require lower guideline values. For impact noise, both the maximum sound pressure and number of noise events must be considered.

During the day, few people are annoyed at noise levels below 50 dB(A). However, sound levels during the evening and night should be 5–10 dB lower. A WHO expert panel (Berglund et al., 1999) developed the guidelines in Table 8.7 for community noise in specific environments.

therefore relate to the extent of the impact on the population, i.e., the proportion the population suffering from serious sleep disturbance, the most serious adverse effect of noise. According to the principles of risk assessment, health effect data constitute the necessary background information for the formulation of standards. The WHO suggests that from a medical point of view, the proportion of very annoyed people in the population of urban centers should not exceed 5% (Rylander, 1992). Politicians and administrators who are responsible for setting noise standards should bear this suggestion in mind, as well as the guidelines in Table 8.7.

Many things can be done to alleviate noise-related problems. Residents can be protected from industrial noise by zoning laws that prohibit the mixing of industry with residential areas. (This is particularly important for informal settlements, which are often forced to develop in industrial areas because these areas are the only viable option for the very poor.) Zoning laws can also separate residential areas from major transportation routes and airports. Municipal bylaws can prevent people from making unnecessary or excessive noise. Regulations can also place restrictions on motor vehicles, specifying that they must be in good running condition and that they must have appropriate mufflers. The difficulty with all of these solutions is that they require active participation on the part of government. Large-scale changes in laws are notoriously difficult and slow to be implemented.

There is little residents can do independently to reduce the amount of noise in their lives. Hearing protectors can be worn to reduce the likelihood of direct hearing loss, and they may reduce sleeplessness due to background noise. But

TABLE 8.7

GUIDELINE VALUES FOR COMMUNITY NOISE IN SELECTED ENVIRONMENTS

Specific Environment	Critical Health Effect(s)	Leq [dB]	Time Base [hours]
Outdoor living area	Serious annoyance, daytime and evening	55	16
	Moderate annoyance, daytime and evening	50	16
Dwelling, indoors	Speech intelligibility and moderate annoyance, daytime and evening	35	16
Inside bedrooms	Sleep disturbance, night-time	30	8
Outside bedrooms	Sleep disturbance, window open (outdoor values)	45	8
School classrooms and preschools, indoors	Speech intelligibility, disturbance of information extraction, message communication	35	during class
Preschool, bedrooms, indoor	Sleep disturbance	30	sleeping-time
School, playground outdoor	Annoyance (external source)	55	during play
Hospital, ward, rooms, indoors	Sleep disturbance, nighttime	30	8
	Sleep disturbance, daytime and evenings	30	16
Industrial, commercial and traffic areas, indoors and outdoors	Hearing impairment	70	24
Ceremonies, festivals and entertainment events	Hearing impairment (patrons: <5 times/year)	100	4
Public addresses, indoors and outdoors	Hearing impairment	85	1
Music and other sounds through headphones/ earphones	Hearing impairment	85 (under headphones)	1

Adapted from WHO, 1999.

this solution does not address the real cause of the problem and brings new problems of its own (discomfort, inability to hear important low-intensity noise).

Motor Vehicle Accidents

Motor vehicle usage has increased dramatically around the globe. In 1950, there were approximately 53 million cars on the world's roads; this has increased more than eightfold over the last four decades, with the global automobile fleet now over 430 million. This represents an average growth of approximately 9.5 million automobiles per year (WHO, 1992c). While the growth rate has slowed in the highly developed countries, population growth and increased urbanization and industrialization have accelerated the use of motor vehicles elsewhere. The growth of motorization exceeds the growth of population—5.2% per year be-

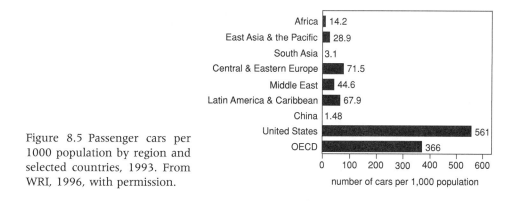

Figure 8.5 Passenger cars per 1000 population by region and selected countries, 1993. From WRI, 1996, with permission.

tween 1960 and 1989, compared to 2.1% per year, respectively. By early next century, if current trends continue, the rapidly developing areas of the world (especially Asia, Eastern Europe, and Latin America) and the Organization of Economic Cooperation and Development (OECD) Pacific region will have as many vehicles as North America and Western Europe, although per-capita rates will remain substantially lower. Figures 8.5 and 8.6 show the 1993 per-capita number of passenger cars in selected regions and projected trends in worldwide motor vehicle ownership, respectively.

In 1993 an estimated 885,000 people died in traffic accidents (WHO, 1995a). Globally, this makes traffic accidents the second-leading cause of death for people aged 5 to 44. With the majority (70%) of these deaths occurring in developing countries, in some places it is the number-one killer for this age-group. For example, in Nigeria, motor vehicle accidents account for one-half of the total deaths for this age-group.

In developed countries, the mortality rate for motor vehicle accidents has been dropping over the last 70 years, even as the rate of vehicle ownership has dramatically increased. This has been attributed to the gradual improvement of road conditions, the establishment of higher vehicle safety standards, and increased driver training. In developing countries, however, the opposite has occurred. The rate of fatal injuries per registered vehicle climbed to 300% since 1968 in Africa. One reason for this is that each incident frequently affects many people—for example, when a motor vehicle accident involves a crowded bus. Moreover, mo-

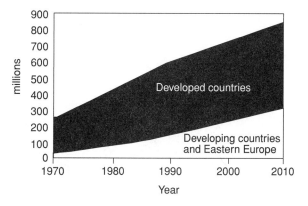

Figure 8.6 Worldwide motor vehicle ownership, 1970–2010. From WRI, 1996, with permission.

torized vehicles have been introduced over a relatively short time span, and governments have been unable to implement the necessary safety measures quickly enough, resulting in an increase in the associated mortality rates.

Globally, two-thirds of motor vehicle–related fatalities involved pedestrians, predominantly children and the elderly. Several factors contribute to this phenomenon. One is that pedestrians sustain greater injuries and are more likely to be injured or killed in an accident than passengers of enclosed vehicles, even if the accident is not particularly severe. Second, in poorly planned urban areas (especially in developed countries), roads are used by all forms of traffic with little or no separation of vehicles and pedestrians. This naturally increases the risk of pedestrian involvement in motor vehicle accidents. Additionally, children or elderly pedestrians may be more vulnerable because of their decreased sensory perception. Children are often unable to identify the source of a sound and they have difficulty making simple distinctions in direction. They are also greatly disadvantaged by their lack of experience with motor vehicle traffic. The elderly frequently suffer from a decreased ability to see and hear and walk slower. They also may experience mental confusion and are often unable to cope with the rapid changes in their environment, making it more difficult to navigate their way through traffic.

Mortality and morbidity rates for particular countries are also associated with motorcycle/bicycle ownership rates. Drivers and passengers of these types of vehicles experience the same kind of vulnerability to serious injury or death as pedestrians. For bicycles, those most at risk are again children and the elderly, for many of the same reasons that they are at risk as pedestrians. For motorcycles, those most at risk are 15–25 years old.

THE "HEALTHY CITIES" APPROACH TO PREVENTION

Promoting Urban Health

Rapid urbanization has made it increasingly important to deal with issues that affect the health of urban populations. It is estimated that by the end of this decade, roughly half of the world's population will live in urban centers. The basic idea behind the Healthy Cities Program is to improve urban health by starting intersectoral action for health at the local level WHO, 1995b; Hancock, 1996. Therefore, the major objective of this program is to place health promotion high on the political agenda of municipal governments. In addition to this local political commitment, the cooperation with various community groups, neighborhood associations, and health care providers is essential.

The healthy city concept refers to a process, not just an outcome. A healthy city is not necessarily one that has achieved a particular health status. It is conscious of health as an urban issue and tries to improve its environments and expand its resources so that people can support each other in achieving their highest potential. This general principle is expressed more specifically in a description of the 11 qualities that a healthy city should strive to achieve, as indicated in Box 8.5. Thus, any city can be a healthy city if it is committed to health and has a structure and process to work for its improvement.

The Qualities of a Healthy City

A city should strive to provide the following:

- A clean, safe physical environment of high quality (including housing quality)
- An ecosystem that is stable now and sustainable in the long term
- A strong, mutually supportive and nonexploitative community
- A high degree of participation and control by the public over decisions affecting their health and well-being
- The meeting of basic needs (for food, water, shelter, income, safety, and work) for all the city's residents
- Access to a wide variety of experiences and resources, with opportunity for ample interactions
- A diverse, vital, and innovative city economy
- The encouragement of connection with the past, with the cultural and biological heritage of city dwellers, and with other groups and individuals
- An optimum level of appropriate public health and sick care services accessible to all
- High health status (high levels of positive health and low levels of disease)

Source: WHO, 1995b.

Characteristics of a Healthy Cities Program

Political commitment is the first step in working toward a healthy city. Cities that have entered the WHO network have been requested to make such commitments. They have been asked to formulate intersectoral health promotion plans with a strong environmental component and to secure the resources for implementing them. These should include an intersectoral political committee, mechanisms for public participation, and a program office with full-time staff. Central to the initial commitment to the WHO is an agreement to report back regularly on progress and share information and experience. Since each urban center has its own specific health problems and will therefore emphasize their most relevant actions to improve health, all Healthy Cities programs will be different with regard to their content. However, the framework of each program is identical and all healthy cities share a number of important characteristics:

- All programs are based on a commitment to health. The holistic nature of health is affirmed and the interaction among its physical, mental, social, and spiritual dimensions is recognized. It is assumed that health can be improved through the cooperative efforts of individuals and groups in the city, if promotion of health and prevention of disease are recognized as priorities.
- Each healthy city requires political decision making for public health. City government programs such as those addressing housing, the environment, edu-

cation, and social service have a major effect on the state of health in urban centers. The aim of Healthy Cities programs is to strengthen the contribution of such programs to the promotion of health by influencing the political decisions of the city council.

- The programs stimulate intersectoral action. The intention of Healthy Cities programs is to mediate between all parties that influence the determinants of health, including industry, various city departments, and other bodies, and to bring them together to negotiate their contribution to improve the urban environment. In this way, organizations or individuals working outside the health sector change their activities so that they contribute more to a healthy environment. An example of such intersectoral action is urban planning that supports physical fitness by encouraging the linkage of "active" transport with public transport and by providing ample green space within a city for recreation.
- The programs promote a more active role for the general public. The program provides the means for having a direct influence on the activities of city departments and other organizations. In addition, health can also be promoted on the individual level by changing individual views on health issues, lifestyle choices, and use of health services.
- All programs strive to promote health by stimulating the constant search for new and innovative ideas and methods. The success of Healthy Cities programs depends upon the ability to create opportunities for innovation. This can be achieved by spreading knowledge of innovative methods, creating incentives for innovation, and recognizing the achievements of those who experiment with new policies and programs.

All of the above indicated actions (political decisions, intersectoral action, community participation, and innovation) contribute to the outcome of a program: a healthy public policy. The success of a Healthy Cities program is reflected in the degree to which policies that create settings for health are in effect throughout the city. Program participants have achieved their goals when homes, schools, workplaces, and other parts of the urban environment become healthier settings in which to live.

From Program to Movement

The dissemination of Healthy Cities strategies has been greatly accelerated by the growth of national and subnational networks. Although the Healthy Cities program was introduced in Europe, the influence of the program extends beyond the boundaries of this region. Regional networks have been developed in Australia, Canada, the Maghreb region (Northern Africa), Iran, Malaysia, the United States, and Middle and South America. Participation in Healthy Cities programs in developing countries is also encouraging (WHO, 1995b). Through the success of the developed networks, the number of communities cooperating with the official programs is becoming a sort of movement that is growing far more rapidly than expected.

In 1996 World Health Day was dedicated to the Healthy Cities program and about 1000 cities committed themselves to urban health promotion. In addition, a Safe Communities Network has grown up as well, and the United Nations Environment Program (UNEP) is monitoring a Sustainable Cities network based on similar principles.

Healthy City Actions

There is no ideal model for a healthy public policy, and the type of actions taken or emphasized is quite different among projects. A number of actions are briefly illustrated here.

1. Actions for equity: Inequities are caused by economic factors as well as by the use of skills that people have to take advantage of life opportunities. Inequities in access to a healthy physical environment are as important as socioeconomic inequities. They are reinforced by standard town planning regulations or through the absence of policies focusing on equal access to city amenities. A number of cities have taken action to improve such equity, including Liverpool and Milan. Liverpool is one of the European cities that has been hardest hit by economic recession, resulting in the socioeconomic inequities of unemployment and racial tension. In this city a wide range of integrated activities has been undertaken that affect the environmental, social, and health services components of the prerequisites for health of the district population. In Milan it was found that women and foreigners had substantially less access to a broad range of health and social services. Milan tried to tackle the problem by conducting information campaigns that targeted specific groups and by functionally improving the accessibility of services.

2. Actions for supportive environments and sustainability. The environments in which people live determine their quality of life, health, and well-being. Some Healthy Cities programs try to inform people about their environments and some explicitly try to transform and improve environments. In Denmark, a good example of supportive environments is the Horsens initiative to build a new block of houses to promote integrated living. In the new living area, houses and flats for people with disabilities are located next to housing for those without disabilities, and old people will live together with younger generations. Furthermore, houses are built in a way that conserves energy, and sufficient green spaces are provided. In Sofia, the old diesel-powered public transport was replaced by trolley buses and electric trams to diminish air pollution.

3. Actions for community involvement. If people actively participate in determining actions for health, they will ensure that services and activities undertaken are appropriate, and they will be more satisfied with the result. The Healthy Cities Program in Liège has encouraged community groups and organized meetings in neighborhood centers. A media campaign was started, and people were supplied with brooms, garbage cans, and other cleaning materials to help the municipal services clean up the city. More recently, children have been involved in a number of similar programs. In Seattle children were asked to draw, paint, or write about their neighborhood and how they would like it to be. This type of program has since been carried out in Pécs, Eindhoven, Munich, Copenhagen, Barcelona, and Horsens.

4. Actions for reorienting health services. Because health services are a major concern of residents in cities, many cities are making a major effort to reorient health services to meet the needs of the population. However, in some countries, health services are a regional or national responsibility and city administrations cannot interfere with the quality and quantity of health services. Nevertheless, some cities have initiated innovative programs to improve health services in urban areas. For instance, in Sofia, actions have been undertaken to renovate primary health care facilities for children with chronic diseases. Bremen has developed an action plan for elderly people through an intersectoral and integrated policy to improve the accessibility of services, provide support systems, and facilitate self-help groups.

Study Questions

1. Is urbanization occurring in your area? If so, why? If not, why not, and do you think it will occur in the near future?

2. Is noise a problem in your area? If so, what are the main sources?

3. Outline what you would do to decrease the incidence of road injuries in your jurisdiction.

4. How would you apply the principles of "Healthy Cities" in your jurisdiction?

9

HEALTH AND ENERGY USE

HUMAN ENERGY NEEDS

Energy Needs for Health and Sustainability

Energy can have direct and indirect, beneficial and detrimental, effects on health. It is essential for socioeconomic development. Without it, communities would not be able to cook their food, and would be more susceptible to infections and food poisoning. Nor could they maintain systems for heating, transportation, communication, and the production of materials. Energy requirements are summarized in Table 9.1.

TABLE 9.1

SUMMARY OF ENERGY NEEDS

Basic human needs (heating, lighting, cooking)
Agriculture (irrigation, mechanization)
Urbanization (basic services)
Transportation
Industrial production

The patterns of energy use and production are key characteristics of all societies. The challenge is to produce the amount of energy needed while imposing the least possible health risk and environmental detoriation. The availability of energy often determines the nature of a region's socioeconomic development. For development to be sustainable, energy sources must also be dependable, safe, and environmentally sound.

It is widely accepted that an assessment of the total risk of an energy source must include an evaluation of all the risks across the *energy cycle*: (*a*) material acquisition and construction, (*b*) emissions from material acquisition and energy production, (*c*) operation and maintenance, (*d*) energy back-up systems, (*e*) energy storage systems, (*f*) transportation, and (*g*) waste management.

Energy Consumption and Requirement Trends

Various forms of development require many forms of development, resulting in a number of trends in global energy consumption. Overall energy consumption increased by about 2.2% per year before 1950; between about 1950 and 1970, energy consumption increased by 5.2% per year; but since the energy crisis in the 1970s, the demand for energy has slowed back to an increase of 2.3% per year. The total energy consumption over the period of 20 years (1973–1993) was 49% greater than in the previous 20 years (WRI, 1996, see Fig. 9.1).

Although the developing world's population far exceeds the population in industrialized countries, the latter consumes far more energy. In 1991, the industrialized countries of the Organization for Economic Cooperation and Development (OECD) accounted for 52.4% of the world's total energy consumption, while they were responsible for only 37.4% of global production (WRI, 1994) and have only about 22% of the world's population. These ratios have remained reasonably con-

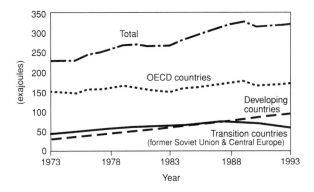

Figure 9.1 Trends in energy consumption, 1973–1993. From WRI, 1996, with permission.

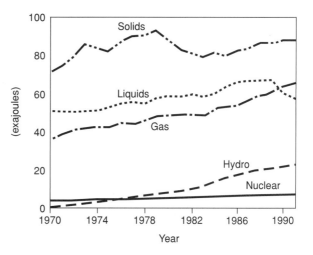

Figure 9.2 Commercial energy consumption by source, industrialized countries, 1971–91. From WRI, 1994, with permission.

stant since 1965, although some current projections suggest that the energy consumption growth rate will be highest in the developing countries over the next several decades (4.5% per year versus 1.5% per year in developed countries) (UNEP, 1992a). In fact, according to the U.S. Office of Technology Assessment, commercial energy use in developing countries could triple over the next 30 years. In some countries demand is growing more than 10% annually (OTA, 1992).

With industrialization, there is a trend away from reliance on biomass and other renewable energy sources and toward dependence on fossil fuels, which are nonrenewable. About 100 years ago, noncommercial sources of fuel (fuel wood, agriculture [e.g., dung]) accounted for about 50% of the total energy used in the world. Today, this type of fuel only comprises about 12% of the total energy use in the world, although about two billion people depend on noncommercial products for their fuel. This percentage has remained constant since about 1970 (UNEP, 1992a).

Figures 9.2 and 9.3 show how the use of various energy sources has changed between 1971 and 1991 in the industrialized countries, and developing countries

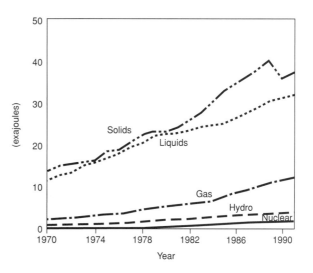

Figure 9.3 Commercial energy consumption by source, developing countries, 1971–91. From WRI, 1994, with permission.

respectively; it should be noted that there are wide variations by region within these groups. Solid energy sources include wood, other biomass, and coal. The various uses of energy, and typical sources for these uses, are summarized below.

Basic Human Needs (Heating, Lighting, Cooking) Approximately 50% of the global population, predominantly in developing countries, is dependent on biomass fuels (i.e., wood, crop residues, animal dung) for domestic tasks. Other domestic energy sources include fossil fuels. Some of these are burned raw, like coal or lignite ("brown coal"), and others are processed, like kerosene and oil. Some households use electricity produced from fossil fuels, especially in the developed world. A small proportion of households have their energy needs met with electricity produced from renewable sources, such as hydropower.

Agriculture (Irrigation, Mechanization) Only 4.5% of total global energy consumption is due to agricultural use. On a per-capita average, consumption in the developing world is about one-tenth that of the developed world. Most of the energy consumed in agriculture in poorer countries is spent on fertilizers, whereas in richer countries it is consumed by farm machinery.

Urbanization (Basic Services) Urbanization is often accompanied by industrialization, as industry requires the pooling of resources and labor. Energy needs in urban areas are therefore greater than in rural areas, because of industrial requirements and the provision of basic services (i.e., water, water disposal) to urban populations is energy-intensive. Statistics on the energy costs of urbanization are difficult to establish, but it is clear that in the developing world, where many basic urban services are not provided and industry is not as prevalent, energy consumption is much lower than in equivalent urban centers in the developed world. On the other hand, energy efficiency may be much lower in rural areas and in developing societies.

Transportation Energy consumption by transportation is tightly linked to urbanization and industrialization, as the need for movement of goods and services into and out of urban/industrial areas is greater than in rural areas, which are traditionally fairly self-reliant. The major user of energy in transportation is the motor car.

Industrial Production Socioeconomic development is linked to industrialization, which is greatly dependent on energy. In the developed world, where industry is entrenched, industrial production uses 40%–60% of the total energy consumed. In the developing world, only 10%–40% of the total energy consumption is accounted for by industry, but this percentage is increasing. The rate of growth, however, is as yet unable to keep up with population growth in these regions. This results in an increase in energy consumption without a corresponding increase in socioeconomic development.

Hydroelectric power is a renewable form of energy that is being increasingly used throughout the world, but it may carry a high cost in ecosystem damage. Nuclear energy, in its traditional form of fission, is nonrenewable but requires only small amounts of fuel. Many countries have come to rely on nuclear energy, including France and the Ukraine. Others, such as Sweden and the United States, have not expanded their nuclear energy capacity in recent years because of concerns over safety and cost. Since the oil crisis in the 1970s, coal use has grown in OECD countries. For their oil-hungry economies, OECD countries depend on imports, primarily from the Gulf states.

As urbanization and industrialization proceed, energy is used increasingly for functions that did not exist or were relatively minor in traditional cultures, e.g., bright lights, illuminated signs, air conditioning, heating of office buildings and shopping malls, entertainment (television, radio), and computers. These cultural changes in energy consumption may have a major impact on global energy requirements. Information technology may increase the efficiency of energy use (e.g., as a result of teleworking, replacing traditional mail and face to face meetings by e-mail and virtual conferences, respectively).

BIOMASS FUELS

Use of Biomass Fuels

Half of the world's population depends on biomass fuel for domestic use. The hazards associated with them have global repercussions. Biomass fuels include wood, logging wastes, sawdust, animal dung, and vegetable matter. These are often the only fuel sources available in the poorest rural areas, and as conditions deteriorate for the urban poor, it becomes their only option as well. Because of incomplete combustion, biomass smoke contains respirable particles, carbon monoxide, nitrogen oxides, formaldehyde, and hundreds of other simple and complex organic compounds, including polycyclic aromatic hydrocarbons. It has been shown in many studies that the concentration of these pollutants often exceeds the WHO guidelines by a factor of 20 or more (see studies cited in Smith, 1991). The pollutant load for each meal cooked is much higher for biomass than for any other energy source (Fig. 9.4). Because of these large concentrations, and the total number of people involved, the total human exposure to biomass pollutants is large. Most studies of the health effects of these air pollutants from energy use have been on ambient (outdoor) air pollution, and extrapolation to indoor air pollution situations is necessary. (Smith, 1991).

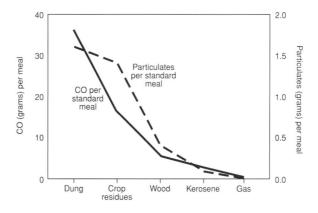

Figure 9.4 Amount of indoor air pollution for each meal cooked. From Smith, 1991, with permission.

Direct Effects of Biomass Fuels

The problems resulting from biomass fuel combustion are worsened in urban areas, as fuel use is often completely contained within the dwelling and is inevitably accompanied by poor ventilation. Populations living in cool regions that use biomass fuels as their indoor heat source are especially adversely affected. Chapter 5 discussed some of the health risks associated with the combustion of airborne contaminants. The greatest health effects are those caused by smoke inhalation. The smoke may come from coal, cooking oil, or wood and may be used for heating or cooking. Indoor air quality is a serious hazard to health in many developing countries, such as Nepal, China, and India. Decreased lung function has been noted in tests on Nepalese women as a result of the time spent near the stove. This was also found in Chinese women using coal stoves compared to those using gas stoves. Respiratory symptoms have been associated with the use of biofuel in India, Malaysia, and in several Chinese studies among different age groups, as summarized by the WHO (1991b). A Nepalese study, for example, also showed that household smoke exposures was associated with an increased rate of acute respiratory infections in children (Pandey et al., 1989), one of the largest causes of mortality in Nepal. A study of pregnant women in India has noted that biofuel smoke was a significant risk factor for stillbirth (Smith, 1991).

Lung cancer and chronic bronchitis are more common among women in some of these societies because of the time they must spend in the home. This has been studied in Nepal, India, Japan, and China (Smith, 1991; WHO, 1992). The resulting respiratory problems tend to compound each other, creating a vicious cycle of pathologies.

Domestic fuel combustion is also accompanied by a risk of accidents due to open fires and poorly designed stoves. Other direct health effects include problems encountered in the collection of fuel and tending of fires. All of these hazards are experienced most directly by women, who are usually responsible for domestic tasks, and children, who spend much of their time in the home and are most physically vulnerable. Tables 9.2 and 9.3 describe the major health risks

TABLE 9.2

ADVERSE EFFECTS OF BIOMASS FUEL PRODUCTION AND COLLECTION ON HUMAN HEALTH

Function	Possible Health Effects
Processing/preparing dung cakes	Fecal/oral/enteric infection
	Skin infection
Charcoal production	CO/smoke poisoning
	Burns/trauma
	Cataracts
Gathering fuel	Trauma
	Reduction in infant/child care
	Bites from venomous snakes, spiders, leeches, insects
	Allergic reactions
	Fungus infections
	Severe fatigue

Source: WHO, 1991b.

TABLE 9.3

ADVERSE EFFECTS OF BIOMASS COMBUSTION ON HUMAN HEALTH

Effects of smoke (acute and subacute)	Conjunctivitis, blepharoconjunctivitis
	Upper respiratory irritation, inflammation
	Acute respiratory infection
Effects of toxic gases (e.g., CO)	Acute poisoning (from CO)
	Cardiovascular diseases
Effects of smoke (chronic)	Chronic obstructive pulmonary disease
	Chronic bronchitis
	Adverse reproductive outcomes
	Cancer (lung)
Acute effects of heat	Burns
Chronic effects of heat	Cataracts
Ergonomic effects of crouching over stove/fire	Arthritis

Source: WHO, 1991b.

associated with the dependency on biomass fuel, addressing adverse effects of fuel processing and fuel burning, respectively.

Indirect Effects of Biomass Fuels

The most significant indirect health effects of biomass fuel consumption arise from the deforestation and greenhouse effect that are caused by this kind of consumption unless the vegetation materials used are replanted at the same rate. These effects will be discussed in Chapter 11.

Less Polluting Household Energy Sources

It is possible to minimize the problems associated with biomass fuel combustion. Almost all biomass fuel combustion is for domestic purposes. The commonly used open fire pits provide the least efficient method of combustion, but unfortunately are often the only option available. Biomass stove technology is well developed (Smith, 1991), and households can reduce the amount of fuel they require by using more efficient stoves. Cutting the amount of fuel required for domestic tasks means less work for the family, and lessens the rate of deforestation. Of most importance for household residents is that better stoves can also reduce emissions, which pose the greatest threat to their health. Indoor emissions can be further reduced with the installation of chimneys and hoods on stoves. There are no studies, though, that definitively measure the improvement by the addition of a chimney, and the costs of adding one can make this option difficult (Smith, 1991). The most cost-effective method of reducing emissions is often simple household rearrangement, by placing the stove or fire in a position where more of the emissions can flow outside. This access to outside air circulation results in less immediate harm to human health.

Although it has been suggested (WHO, 1991b) that alternative fuel sources to biomass fuel, such as kerosene, liquid petroleum gas (LPG), and electricity are good alternatives, each of these has its disadvantages. Air pollution from kerosene stoves (carbon monoxide and particulate matter) may be a considerable problem, and more research is required before substitution programs can be reasonably suggested. Liquid petroleum gas and electricity are both very expensive, making their widespread implementation largely impossible. It is probable that those households now dependent on biomass fuels will continue to use them for the foreseeable future. Biomass fuel upgrading, by the production of briquettes (by compression of charcoal), or biogas (methane from fermentation of various biomass sources) may be an intermediate solution, as they burn more efficiently. Of the two, biogas is the best alternative, as charcoal combustion produces many harmful emissions.

FOSSIL FUELS

Use of Fossil Fuels

Fossil fuels include oil, coal, and natural gas. All of these energy sources are nonrenewable. They are derived from solar energy trapped, due to photosynthesis, in the form of fossilized plants, and were created over millions of years. In 12 months the world consumes an amount of fossil fuels that took one million years to create. Despite awareness of this, and recent conservation efforts, these fuels continue to provide almost 90% of the world's commercial energy. Most of these fuels are converted into electricity before consumption, but some of them are burned raw. Even though there are efforts to convert to alternative fuels, oil is still the principal source of energy, supplying 38% of the world's energy needs. Coal, used extensively during the industrial revolution, accounts for 30%, while natural gas accounts for 20% (WHO, 1992d). Thus, nonrenewable sources of energy account for the vast majority of global energy needs.

In the past three decades, transportation, which is primarily supported by fossil fuels, has expanded rapidly (see Chapter 8). The known reserves of oil and natural gas may be consumed within the next 30 to 40 years. Coal reserves may last another 200 years, but the remaining coal is of very low quality, and its combustion will produce considerably less energy than the coal now being consumed. Along with problems of renewability come multiple health hazards. These hazards exist at every point along the route of fossil fuel consumption, from extraction and processing (Table 9.4) to combustion (Table 9.5), and have both immediate and long-term effects.

TABLE 9.4

HAZARDS ASSOCIATED WITH FOSSIL FUEL EXTRACTION AND PROCESSING

Fuel	Location	Hazards and Effects
Coal	Underground mines	Coal workers' pneumoconiosis (CWP) or "black lung," silicosis, fires/explosions, injuries
	Open-pit mines	Industrial bronchitis, chronic cough, accidents (mining, transport)
Oil	Off-shore developments	Accidents caused by weather, explosions
	Land oil fields	Dermatitis (from long-term exposure to crude oil), accidents/explosions
	Refineries	Exposure to hydrocarbons (known carcinogens)
Natural gas	Deposits	Hydrogen sulfide exposure, accidents/explosions
	Refineries	Exposure to hydrocarbons (known carcinogens), accidents/explosions

TABLE 9.5

HEALTH HAZARDS ASSOCIATED WITH FOSSIL FUEL COMBUSTION

Fuel	Method of Combustion	Associated Hazards and Effects[a]
Coal	Domestic fires (i.e., using raw coal)	Acute respiratory infections, chronic lung diseases, lung cancer
	Industrial consumption	Accident/fire, air pollution effects
Oil	Industrial consumption	Accident/fire, air pollution effects
	Vehicles	Motor vehicle accidents, air pollution effects
	Domestic consumption (e.g., kerosene stoves)	Indoor air pollution effects
Natural gas	Industrial consumption	Air pollutants
	Domestic use (cooking/heating)	Air pollutants, asphyxiation, explosions

[a]The different types of air pollution are discussed in Chapter 5.

Direct Effects on Health

Combustion of fossil fuel is the single greatest cause of atmospheric pollution. As with biomass fuel combustion, the emissions from the incomplete combustion of fossil fuels that are of greatest concern, for both human and environmental health, are sulfur oxides, suspended particulate, nitrogen oxides, carbon monoxide, polycyclic aromatic hydrocarbons, and carbon dioxide. These emissions, and their direct health effects, were discussed in Chapter 5. Indoor emissions of sulphur oxide particulates, nitrogen oxides, and carbon monoxide can be of great concern. This applies to coal especially, but also to natural gas and oil. The more important though less common circumstances affecting human exposure are those in which the combustion products pollute the indoor environment directly, through faulty flues, and from leaks in fixed appliances. The single most dangerous chemical hazard from indoor combustion of fossil fuels or biomass is carbon monoxide. Poor ventilation and inadequate air supply may lead to high levels in closed rooms, enough to cause death. The burning of fossil fuels also exposes the user to the very real risk of accidental fires and explosions. Where stoves and heaters are inadequate, the risk of fires is much greater.

Other direct health effects from fossil fuels include the occupational risks from the mining of coal. These effects range from cave-ins and gas explosions to pneumoconiosis (from the inhalation of coal dust), as described in Chapter 10. Nonetheless, as discussed in Box 9.1, investigations and consequent advancements in coal technology have been made. While the risk of developing these serious diseases has been decreasing recently through the use of modern technologies that protect mine workers, the risks of injury from mining and transportation of coal have tended to change less. Synthetic liquid fuels made from coal, heavy oil, and mineral deposits of hydrocarbon in shale or sandstone (kerogen) differ in the chemical composition of the crude oil that results. They tend to be more toxic and may be more carcinogenic. The synthetic fuels are potentially more hazardous to workers than petroleum, depending on the source, process and exposure.

Risks associated with the petroleum and natural gas industry are less than those of coal production and are most associated with injuries. Generally, it is the exploration for new sources of fuel and the drilling and servicing of wells

The Swedish Coal-Health-Environment Project

In November 1979, the Swedish Government commissioned the Swedish Power Board to investigate and report on how the health and environmental problems arising from an increased use of coal in Sweden could be solved. The project's investigators analyzed the various stages of the use of coal and the disturbances that can arise from such use. The emission of sulfur and nitrogen oxides, toxic metals, and dust is, of course, not peculiar to coal, but can occur to varying degrees in the burning of other fuels.

Large resources of coal, including the much-desired low-sulfur coal, are available in many parts of the world, including the United States, Poland, the former Soviet Union, western Canada, Australia, and Colombia. Coal, like peat and wood, is not homogeneous, but rather contains a varying content of trace elements. Mercury is one of the most important toxicologically.

The occupational hazards associated with coal are well known. Dustiness occurring in the transport and handling of coal can occur particularly in warm and windy weather conditions. The risks of harmful dust can be eliminated or strongly reduced by rational working methods and technical solutions. This also applies to the transport and handling of waste products. Special care must be taken at the point loading takes place at the installation and when loading the products at the dump (see Fig. 9.5). Dry ash should be handled in fully enclosed systems.

The Swedish Project concluded that adverse effects on the respiratory system were not expected to occur with the burning of coal in Sweden, given the use of modern and effective techniques. Investigations into the content of mutagenic and carcinogenic substances in the emissions have shown that the large modern, well-run, coal-fired and oil-fired installations emit only a small quantity of mutagenic materials. However, emissions per energy unit of mutagenic substances can be considerably greater from small installations.

The Power Board considered that the use of coal, which involves replacement of oil, affected the level of methylmercury in fish to a small degree. There is a risk of increased levels in fish in acid-sensitive lakes close to large point sources, such as a coal-fired powered station, if prudent measures are not taken. Siting, local conditions, and the measures taken in such cases determine the extent to which an increased risk occurs. It was noted that tighter regulations in this area can very well prove essential to bring down mercury risks to acceptable levels.

On the assumption that fly ash with too high a radioactivity is not used in building materials for residences, and that drinking-water wells are not situated in the vicinity of waste dumps, the techniques available for transport and disposal of waste products from the combustion of coal were deemed to be sufficient to avoid risks of negative results. The project concluded that coal can be used as replacement for oil in district heating and power stations and within industry, in a way that is acceptable for health concerns, if coal is used in well-maintained installations that are big enough to make it feasible to use environmentally safe technology. The production of electricity in coal-fired powered stations was similarly judged to be acceptable. It was noted that special investigations into local and regional conditions should be conducted at each site before deciding the extent of electricity production that is possible.

Coal, like other fossil fuels, contains compounds of an undesirable nature that are released during combustion. Many of these may affect health. Apart from the annoyance of people, local effects on the respiratory tract, effects on other organ systems, and genotoxic effects (e.g., cancer) can occur. Impurities in effluent from refuse dumps, particularly metals, can lead to systemic effects.

Source: SCHEP, 1983.

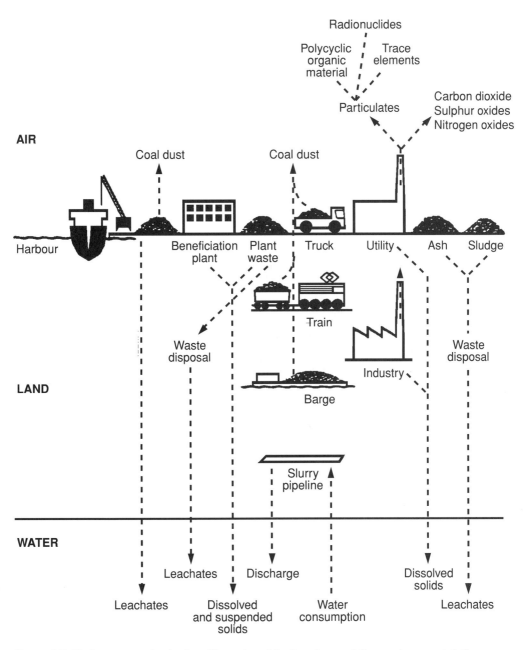

Figure 9.5 Various stages in the handling of coal in Sweden and the environmental disturbances that can occur. From SCHEP, 1983, with permission.

that are the most hazardous. Leaks of crude oil are generally less dangerous than leaks of refined petroleum products, such as gasoline, which can cause explosions, fires and contamination of ground water. *Sour gas*, which is natural gas containing a relatively high content of sulfur is particularly hazardous because it may contain high levels of hydrogen sulfide, a toxic gas.

Large power stations can convert coal, oil, and, to a lesser extent, natural gas into electricity with fewer incomplete combustion products than can individual fires.

The production of wastes at these plants can also be regulated, and they tend to concentrate the ash and waste products, minimizing the impact of such products on the local environment. However, without sufficient pollution control systems, large coal-burning power stations can be some of the most polluting point sources in an area. In Central and Eastern Europe, China and India, for example, the use of coal contributes considerable air pollution, especially SO_2 and particulates; with the use of clean coal technologies, emissions of SO_2 and particulates can be reduced as much as 99% (WRI, 1998). In the Czech Republic, for example, SO_2 emissions were reduced by 36% and dust and particulate emissions by 49% (Havlicek, 1997).

Indirect Effects on Health

Additional problems are created when this pollution becomes transboundary pollution. Large urban centers located along borders are problems not only for the country in which the city is situated but also for their neighbors. The major indirect health effects of the pollution created by energy sources are global warming and acid rain. These are discussed in Chapter 11.

Pollution Prevention Strategies

Mitigation technologies already exist that can greatly reduce the emission of airborne pollutants at the source. Fitting power plants with scrubbers can reduce sulfur dioxide emissions by up to 95%. Similarly, electrostatic precipitators and bag filters can trap large amounts of particulate (dust, ash, soot, and hydrocarbons) in factory or power exhaust gases. What is possibly more important is that new technologies have been developed, such as fluidized-bed combustion, which are capable of burning raw or processed fuels much more efficiently than ever before, greatly reducing polluting emissions. Additionally, more countries are developing cogeneration plants, which produce both heat and electricity for entire cities. In countries such as India and China, natural gas–fired turbines, which are less expensive and more efficient and have fewer emissions than conventional coal-fired power plants, are showing great promise for electricity generation (WRI, 1994). Such improvement in efficiency of energy use not only mitigates air pollution but also conserves resources of nonrenewable fossil fuels (WHO, 1992d).

HYDROPOWER

Use of Hydroelectric Power

For many countries, hydropower is emerging as the favored alternative to fossil fuels. Hydroelectric power accounts for about one-quarter of the world's electricity output. Hydropower has been used extensively in developed countries and developing countries alike. Europe uses about 36% of its potential hydroelectric power, while North America has developed 59% of its potential. The potential for developing countries to harness hydroelectric power is vast. Some investigators estimate that Asia, for example, has harnessed only about 9% of its potential; Latin America, 8%; and Africa, 5% (WHO, 1992d).

Hydroelectricity is a renewable source of energy and is relatively clean, according to its proponents. It must be noted, however, that due to siltation, the life expectancy of a hydroelectric dam is generally measured in decades, rather than centuries. Hydropower is generated by the construction of large dams over fast-moving water, connected to generators. For a country to be able to consider constructing these dams, it must have suitable water resources and it must also have a large amount of money, as these systems are tremendously expensive. There are several serious and significant problems associated with these dams. For the investment in them to be financially viable, the dams must be very large, flooding huge areas of land. This can cause an array of problems in the local environment. For example, when dams fail, although this is rare, they may cause catastrophic flooding and loss of life. Large dams are suspected of causing small earthquakes in some regions prone to earth movement. An ambitious project to build large dams in northern Canada was recently suspended when it was realized that huge tracts of forest (as large as some European countries) would be submerged. Entire ecosystems may be drowned in this way, and residents in the area to be flooded may be displaced at great cost.

Direct Effects on Health

The actual building of the dams can be hazardous to the workers. Over 10,000 skilled and unskilled workers are needed to construct a large dam, and accidents and deaths constitute a significant occupational hazard. Additionally, after the dam is built, the area flooded by dammed water is usually significant, and displacement of the local population can be a problem. For example, two recent dams in India and Thailand displaced 20,000 and 30,000 people, respectively. This displacement can cause psychological stress due to the loss of homes and livelihood, and physical problems from the disruption of usual food supplies and other life supports. Dams have been known to collapse, causing flooding of the area downstream (WHO, 1992d).

On the positive side, hydropower produces large quantities of cheap electrical energy at low cost (after construction of the dam). As with other sources of electricity, this fuel can then be used for refrigeration, health care, and other functions that have a direct positive effect on human health. Also, the dammed water can be used for irrigation purposes, as it has been in India and China, thus having a direct positive effect on agricultural food production. Another positive feature is the ability to breed fish in dams and improve the diet of local people. Of course, the reservoirs behind all dams eventually silt up so a dam has a limited lifetime.

Indirect Effects on Health

The actual process of generating hydroelectric power does not create wastes or other by-products that are detrimental to human health. The accumulation of water necessary to produce this electricity, though, can change the entire biologic local environment. For example, the Aswan dam in Egypt contributed to the spread of the parasitic disease schistosomiasis in the river and irrigation systems in the Nile basin. Shallow waters at the edges of the new lake aided in the rapid growth of freshwater snails, the vector for schistosomiasis. As was described in Chapter 3, the lower Seyhan irrigation project in Turkey is an example of how malaria was introduced into an area where it was not previously endemic by the building of a hydroelectric dam. Again, the vector for malaria, the mosquito, grew rapidly because of the new, almost stagnant, water supply. Other organisms, e.g., algae and midges, may also flourish. Down river, the land is deprived of water, essential for humans and agriculture.

Aquifers downstream are also affected. A hydroelectric dam essentially changes completely the physical environments above and below its structure, and hence changes the lives of the people in those environments. This change often has a negative effect on those living close by. Because large reservoirs are often built in remote areas however, the health impacts of hydroelectric dams have been thought to have only minor effects in many countries (WHO, 1992d).

Another indirect effect can be increased mercury exposure from fish, when the dam creates conditions by which mercury in flooded soils and vegetation accumulates in fish eventually consumed by local people. This has been a particular problem in Canada (JBMC, 1995).

Electricity These possible risks associated with the use of electricity are, of course, independent of the way in which the electricity is generated. Electricity is distributed at high voltage to communities and then stepped down in voltage before delivery to homes. The transformers that convert voltage used PCBs in the past and were a source of heavy exposure for workers. Now, the PCBs have been replaced with mineral oils in most countries. Wiring and appliances must be safety designed and maintained to prevent injury from shock or damage from fires.

An additional concern is that a number of studies have linked electromagnetic fields from the power lines that carry the electricity that is generated, to a number of different types of cancer. These studies have been under recent scrutiny, however, as some researchers question their methodology and conclusions.

Mitigation by Environmental Management

Most of the direct effects on health can be prevented or mitigated by adopting appropriate environmental management practices in the construction and operational stages of the dam. If safety factors are not considered in the construction of large dams, it is usually a result of financial constraints or poor planning (WHO, 1992d). Mitigation factors to reduce the risk of schistosomiasis and mosquito-borne diseases include clearance and leveling; water table and shoreline management practices to discourage the breeding of invertebrate carriers; planning of settlements; the provision of water supply and sanitation to diminish people's contact with infected water to vectors; chemical (i.e., mostly using pesticides) or integrated pest control (i.e., depending less on pesticides and more on environmental management and biological control); and vaccination and other public health practices as required. Health education and the promotion of public participation in the reduction of hazards are of the utmost importance. None of these measures will be effective unless the impacts have been defined at an early stage and monitoring instituted to guide mitigation activities. The WHO/FAO/UNEP/UNCHS Panel of Experts on Environmental Management for Vector Control (PEEM) has developed a number of guidelines and training materials to assist planners and engineers in undertaking these tasks along with representatives from the health sector. Indirect negative health effects associated with the displaced population are more difficult to mitigate and require imaginative project planning (WHO, 1992d).

Environmental impact assessments (as discussed in Chapter 3) should be done on any new project. There has been enough information from previous constructions to be able to predict some of the possible environmental changes that will occur from the dam and its subsequent lake. Small-scale projects have the advantage of offering smaller setup and operational costs, while having less of an impact on the local environment (WHO, 1992d).

NUCLEAR POWER

Use of Nuclear Power

Electrical power generation by nuclear reactors has been growing steadily over the last three decades. By the end of 1989, there were 436 power electricity generating reactors in the world, spread around 26 countries, with a total capacity of 320 gigawatts (approximately 17% of the global electricity production).

The nuclear resources for the production of energy by nuclear fission are uranium and thorium. Uranium production has remained at a fairly constant level of approximately 37 thousand tons per year. Low-cost uranium resources exist in Australia, Canada, South Africa, Nigeria, the United States, and the countries of the former Soviet Union. The geographical distribution of nuclear reactors is not uniform throughout the world; about 95% of the total generating capacity is concentrated in North America, Europe, and Japan.

Currently nuclear power is based on the process of *fission*, the splitting of uranium atoms. Nuclear energy consumes small amounts of fuel and is potentially a very cheap and pliable source of energy. However, several widely publicized incidents in the 1970s (such as Three Mile Island in the United States) and 1980s (such as Chernobyl in what was then the Soviet Union) have caused grave concern over the ultimate safety of this form of energy. Three-Mile Island (TMI) and Chernobyl are the only two recorded incidents in which the effects of an accident in a nuclear power plant were known to have created measurable off-site consequences. While both accidents appeared to have been the result of a combination of design shortcomings and operator error, off-site releases of radionuclides were many orders of magnitude lower in TMI than those from Chernobyl.

At TMI, the core heated and melted, but the pressure vessel and containment structure remained intact. At Chernobyl, the reactor was an obsolete design and was not operated properly. Improper experimentation and operator error provoked a surge in reactor power that could not be controlled, leading to a rapid rise in temperature, explosion of the core, and an intense fire. This accident resulted in the death of 31 emergency workers, the contamination of large areas of the European part of what was then the Soviet Union, and about 1000 thyroid cancers in children so far (WHO, 1995c). In addition, several million people are living in contaminated areas and 100,000 people have been permanently evacuated from a 30-kilometer exclusion zone around the reactor. The Chernobyl reactors have been shut down, although they continue to supply about 10% of the power for Ukrania as late as 2000. Because of safety concerns, many utilities in developed countries have been forced to abandon plans for new reactors. In some countries, including Germany, Sweden, and Canada there has been pressure to close reactors that have already been built and are functioning normally.

It is generally acknowledged that the normal operation of nuclear power plants produces less environmental pollution than many other fuel cycles. Electricity generation in the nuclear fuel cycle does not produce sulfur dioxide, oxides of nitrogen, particulates, carbon dioxide, or other greenhouse gases. However, in a comprehensive picture of the hazards, the entire nuclear fuel cycle should be considered. This includes mining and milling of uranium ore, fuel enrichment and fabrication, reactor operation, spent fuel storage and transport, fuel reprocessing, and finally, the disposal of radioactive waste and decommissioning. The health hazards specific to the nuclear fuel cycle are those due to exposure to ionizing radiation (including radon). An explanation of radioactivity and radiation was provided in Chapter 2. Other hazards, such as exposure to toxic chemicals and dust that occur in other fuel cycles, are also present on a limited scale. These are encountered mainly in stages of the nuclear fuel cycle, fuel fabrication, and fuel reprocessing.

Fusion

An alternative nuclear technology to fission is called *fusion,* in which strong pressures force together hydrogen atoms to release energy. Fusion-based nuclear energy would produce more energy with less risk but the engineering problems are formidable. It is under development in a massive engineering program in the United States along with several smaller projects in the United States, Japan, and Europe. If successful, fusion energy could produce enormous quantities of cheap energy from sea water, but the development costs and engineering obstacles make this a distant possibility, not a likely short-term solution.

Stochastic (Non-Threshold) Effects

Generally, radiation effects can be separated into two sections: health effects that are non-threshold, called by health physicists *stochastic effects,* and health effects that have a threshold, referred to by health physicists as *deterministic effects* (see Chapter 2, Physical Hazards) Cancer and hereditary effects are classified as stochastic effects. The basic question in assessing risks for workers and members of the public, from the routine operation of the nuclear fuel cycle, concerns the nature of the dose–response relationship at low doses and dose rates (see Chapter 3 for information on dose–response curves).

Direct epidemiological evidence of occupational radiation health hazards comes from studies of uranium mining and operation of nuclear installations (WHO, 1992d). Uranium mining has been shown unequivocally to produce an increase in respiratory cancer mortality (Howe et al., 1986; Howe et al., 1987; Kusiak et al., 1993), in addition to the increase in the prevalence of silicosis among the miners that contributes to the risk (Royal Commission, 1976).

As discussed by the WHO (1992d), epidemiological studies provide conflicting evidence of radiation effects in populations residing close to nuclear facilities. An increase in childhood leukemia was reported around two nuclear installations involved in reprocessing nuclear fuel in the United Kingdom. However, other studies, such as those conducted in France around six nuclear installations, did not reveal an increase in leukemia or cancer. A comprehensive study in the

United States examined cancer mortality rates around all 62 nuclear facilities in the country and no increase in cancer mortality was noted. The WHO noted, however (WHO, 1992d) that the U.S. studies included large areas and large populations, so small increases in cancers would be hidden.

Deterministic (Threshold) Effects

Deterministic effects are those that are only seen after an acute exposure to high doses of radiation that exceed some threshold. They include skin burns, damage to bone marrow, and sterility. Such exposures have occurred in survivors of the atomic bomb explosions in Japan and in a few workers in Chernobyl (see WHO, 1995c). Exposures of this magnitude are rare and occur only in occupational settings or after serious nuclear accidents (WHO, 1994b).

Safety Approaches

The United States was one of the first countries to commit to a large-scale program of nuclear power. The costs of building in safeguards and the difficulty in insuring the facilities have essentially stopped the building of new reactors in that country. While these facilities attracted strenuous public opposition, proponents of nuclear energy point out that past problems have been problems of reactor design and that newer models are much safer. However, the extent of public concern in many countries makes it unlikely that fission nuclear power will ever become as widespread as its proponents originally hoped.

As a result of the Chernobyl accident, attention has been focused on the safety of operating older types of reactors. Considerable effort is currently being undertaken to backfit older operating reactors to achieve safety levels compatible with current international standards. Mitigation strategies for nuclear power plants focus on prevention, i.e., building safer reactors. These built-in safety factors include barriers to prevent releases, backup systems for system failures, and quality assurance.

Another major debate concerns radioactive waste. Different stages of the nuclear fuel cycle produce radioactive wastes. At present, there are two approaches to the management of irradiated reactor fuel. These are the temporary or permanent storage of spent fuel and the reprocessing of spent fuel. The latter entails the subsequent recycling of uranium in thermal reactors (WHO, 1992d). Considerations for radioactive waste disposal can be divided as follows.

Low- and Intermediate-Level Waste Disposal Safe methods for the management and disposal of low- and intermediate-level wastes are well established and operational. Essentially safe disposal is ensured by the establishment of effective barriers, preventing significant transfer of radionuclides into the environmental pathways that might lead to excessive human exposures. Typical disposal strategies involve shallow-ground disposal with or without a concrete liner, near-surface engineered structures, or an underground rock cavity repository. Doses to the general public from such waste disposal are likely to be extremely low.

High-Level Waste Disposal High-level radioactive waste is characterized by heat generation and a long half-life. Many of the high-level wastes are produced by reprocessing nuclear fuel and are often in liquid form. Because of the heat generated, these liquid wastes are often stored for a year or more in water tanks to cool down before being processed for ultimate disposal. Once excessive heat generation has subsided, liquid waste is usually solidified prior to disposal. Spent fuel elements disposed of without processing are also classified as high-level wastes. These wastes need to be deposited in deep underground, stable rock formations with multiple engineered barriers to prevent their leakage into the environment. The integrity of these structures must be such that there are no predictable and unacceptable future risks for human health or the environment over a period of thousands of years.

ALTERNATIVE ENERGY SOURCES

A number of energy sources have been developed as alternatives to the previously mentioned sources. The most promising ones include wind, solar, and geo-thermal power. These particular alternatives, are promising because they are generally renewable. They are generally thought to be prohibitively expensive, although as shown in Box 9.2, this need not necessarily be the case. Nonetheless, these sources will not be viable global energy sources for many years to come and still cause health-related problems (see Table 9.6). One of the major problems with *solar-derived energy* is that the generating facilities are individually small and too decentralized for an effective power grid. However, they can be a very useful local power source, meeting local needs relatively cost-effectively, as noted in Box 9.2.

As with any energy source, there are also disadvantages to these technologies. Not all countries have the necessary environmental conditions for their im-

---

BOX 9.2

The Potential for Cost-Effective Electricity from Alternative Energy Sources

Considerable gains in the use of alternative energy sources have been made, despite the lack of commitment on the part of energy planners, technical failures attributable to poor capacity for local maintenance, and the high costs associated with these new technologies. Field experience and technical developments widened the application of wind turbines and solar photovaltaic (PV) arrays in developing countries. These are already cost-effective at many remote sites (Foley, 1992). (Several case examples are provided in *World Resources 1994–1995* [WRI, 1994].) As shown in Figure 9.6, the price of wind energy dropped by two-thirds over the last decade, and some 20,000 electricity-generating wind turbines, as well as large number of wind-powered water pumps, have been installed worldwide (WRI, 1994).

Solar power has also become more cost-effective. The demand for PV assemblies is growing steadily, and prices are expected to fall further. Smaller solar applications, including water heaters, cookers, kilns, and crop dryers, have been successful in India and China.

TABLE 9.6

SUMMARY OF SIGNIFICANT HEALTH EFFECTS OF TECHNOLOGIES FOR GENERATING ELECTRICITY

Technology	Occupational Health Effects	Public Health Effects
Geothermal	Exposure to toxic gases, routine and accidental	Disease from exposure to toxic brines and hydrogen sulfide
	Stress from noise	Cancer from exposure to radon
	Trauma from drilling accidents	Arsenic poisoning from contaminated water
		Mercury poisoning via fish in this water
Hydropower	Trauma from dam failures	Mercury poisoning through mercury contamination of water and fish
	Trauma from construction accidents	
	Disease from exposure to pathogens	Malaria spread to new areas
	Health effects from lifestyle disruption associated with forced relocation	Schistosomiasis
Photovoltaics	Exposure to toxic materials during fabrication, routine and accidental	Exposure to toxic materials during fabrication and disposal, routine and accidental
Wind	Trauma from accidents during construction and operation	Noise disturbance
Solar thermal	Trauma from accidents during fabrication	
	Exposure to toxic chemicals during operation	

plementation. Both wind and solar power are considered to be very environmentally friendly, but the use of *geothermal power* (tapping into the earth's core) requires pollution control measures for the release of hot, mineral-filled underground water to avoid a negative environmental impact, including mercury contamination of fish, arsenic contamination of drinking water, and the effects of heated water on ecosystems.

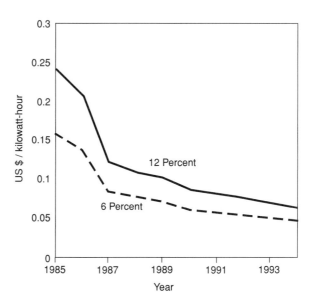

Figure 9.6 Cost of electricity from wind energy at two interest rates, 1985–94. From WRI, 1994, with permission.

The most readily available option in many places is simply to encourage the natural movement of developing countries up the so-called *energy ladder*. The "ladder" is a ranking of fuels from most polluting to least. This process of climbing the ladder has taken many countries from the relatively dirty solid fuels to the higher-quality fuels — gas and electricity. Generally, communities will move up the ladder if fuel is available and affordable. In some areas of the world, the regular supply of alternative fuels is the problem rather than the cost.

COMPARING RISKS

Throughout the 1970s and 1980s, comparisons of risk from different energy sources were investigated. However, these comparisons tended to account short-term local health and environmental effects only and discount the more difficult-to-measure effects, such as the effect of increased CO_2 emissions, which could have global implications. It is also difficult to account for all the health risks that occur across the energy production cycle and to all stakeholders involved.

Unquestionably, reducing fossil fuel consumption will require raising the price of these fuels. Electricity, natural gas and coal are subsidized in most countries; petroleum consumption is subsidized in oil-exporting developing countries (WRI, 1998). The recognition that energy, like water, is a vital resource, underlies these policies. Refrigeration, for example, saves lives from foodborne illness. If prices are changed, the immediate benefits must be weighed against the risks.

The perception of the risk associated with a source of energy is usually more important in the minds of decision makers than the actual risk. A nuclear power station is more likely to be perceived as posing a higher risk than a more common source of energy, e.g., biomass fuels, even though the former has actually caused less mortality than the latter. The factors influencing the perception of risk were discussed in Chapter 4. The subjective perceptions of the risks involved with any given energy source must be taken into account by all those involved.

PRIORITIES FOR ACTION

In 1992, a panel from the *WHO Commission on Health and Environment* (WHO, 1992d) prepared a report on what they considered to be priority concerns regarding energy. The energy-related issues "of the highest immediate and/or future concern for environmental health" were the following:

- exposure to noxious agents in the course of domestic utilization of biomass and coal
- exposure resulting from urban air pollution in numerous large cities of the world
- energy-related climate changes
- serious energy-related accidents with environmental impact.

The first two problems "involve very large groups of people (hundreds of millions) of all ages, mostly, but not exclusively, in developing countries, who are exposed to significant health hazards requiring intensive mitigating action, now."

Health-related problems associated with biomass fuel were discussed above; urban air pollution was discussed in Chapter 5. Climate changes (the greenhouse effect) will be discussed in Chapter 11. Accident-related injuries have been discussed throughout this book.

The indoor use of biomass fuels, with their incomplete combustion, affects large numbers of people in developing countries (actual numbers would be difficult to estimate). Many obstacles exist to changing this major health threat, such as the need to convince local people that it is a threat, the low position women have in many societies (women and children are often the most affected by this indoor air pollution), and economic considerations. Improving smoke stacks, changing fuels, and increasing ventilation are all seemingly simple measures but difficult to apply in practice. Education of the at-risk groups in an appropriate cultural milieu is likely the most important and feasible strategy to overcome this problem.

The major causes of urban air pollution are overwhelmingly related to energy use: production of electric power, transportation (cars, buses, and trucks), home cooking and heating (particularly if coal or biomass is used), and local industry. Global assessments of air pollution have found that well over one-half of the 50 cities throughout the world that they surveyed had higher levels than WHO guideline values (see Chapter 5). This has been estimated to affect approximately one billion people. One of the major difficulties with air pollution control is its high cost. Changing from one fuel source to a cleaner one is expensive, and sometimes the benefits of changing are not immediately seen by industry or governments. Developing countries often cannot afford to import cleaner fuels and therefore rely on domestic coal or biomass.

Climate change is another urgent matter for a different reason (see Chapter 11). Climate change resulting from the use of fossil fuels might be irreversible, and could be devastating.

Severe accidents could occur, with significant adverse health effects in many energy technologies. A comprehensive record of the major accidents in the this field was published in 1990 by the United Kingdom Watt Committee on Energy (WCE, 1990). National strategies must be created to ensure proper maintenance, disaster planning, and data collection.

Study Questions

1. What energy sources are used most heavily in your home town?

2. What do you know about the hazards associated with them?

3. Are there alternatives that should be promoted?

4. What issues/difficulties can you think of in your country concerning the control of the energy-related factors listed above?

5. You are the environmental health officer on duty. You receive a call that there has been a small spill of irradiated water from the nuclear power plant. Using the approach outlined in Chapters 3 and 4, describe the steps you would take to address this problem.

10

INDUSTRIAL POLLUTION AND CHEMICAL SAFETY

LEARNING OBJECTIVES

After studying this chapter you will be able to do the following:

- describe the scope, dimensions, and trends in industrial pollution, including knowledge of the nature of major industrial processes or events that have had significant environmental health consequences
- indicate the scope, dimensions, and trends in occupational diseases
- discuss approaches to managing occupational and environmental health problems
- discuss the issues related to industrial waste management

EXTENT OF INDUSTRIAL POLLUTION

Industrial pollution has grown to be a problem of global proportions, serious enough to pose an immediate health hazard in some areas and a limit to future economic growth. The pollution emissions and resource requirements of industry are substantial, as shown in Box 10.1.

Industrial development is essential to combat poverty and improve the quality of life. Such development may lead to serious environmental pollution and occupational health hazards, however. Measures must be taken to prevent the health problems associated with industrial in development to avoid the kinds of social and environmental destruction that occurred during the Industrial Revolution in Europe in the late eighteenth and nineteenth centuries (see Chapter 1).

Only a few industrial sectors are responsible for most raw material consumption and most pollution. These include food and agricultural processing, metal extraction and processing cement works, the pulp and paper industry, oil refining, and the chemical industry.

The degree to which development can be sustained is highly dependent on the following factors: the technology adopted; the enactment, enforcement of, and compliance with regulations and international treaties; the infrastructure; and the volume of production, which is in turn related to the market being supplied; population; dependence on exports and the stability of markets; the distribution of income, and standards of living. In short, industrial pollution is inextricably linked to economic development, but in ways that are complicated and difficult to separate, as discussed in Chapter 1.

PUBLIC EXPOSURE FROM INDUSTRIAL SOURCES

Industrial Air Pollution

As discussed in Chapter 5, air pollution is an unintended but direct consequence of economic activity. It is generated by transportation, power production, home heating and cooking, and industrial production. Some of the costs of air pollution are shouldered by the industry that may be responsible, in the form of higher costs of production, for pollution control and poor public relations. Much of the cost of pollution control is passed through as higher prices for goods and services to offset costs. However, the cost of the effects of pollution are not accounted for and may be considerably greater. The public bears most of the costs of air pollution: human health problems, destruction of materials, plant and animal damage, poor visibility, loss of appeal for tourists, and reduced quality of life for residents. As many of these costs are not obvious, they are not charged back to the industry that may be responsible. This means that the community subsidizes, or indirectly pays for, the cost of the industry to do business.

The effects of air pollution can be minimized by siting industry away from residential communities or places, such as river valleys, where air pollution can accumulate. The most effective approach to reducing air pollution is usually to control its emission at the source, through a variety of measures that reduce the amount of pollution released to the atmosphere. Industry that is energy-efficient

Industrial Pollution Emissions and Resource Requirements as Proportion of Overall Emissions and Resource Requirements

In the countries of the Organization for Economic Cooperation and Development (OECD), industrial output represents around one-third of the aggregate gross national product (GNP). The pollution emissions or resource requirements of industry in 1987 were the following:

15% of water consumption (excluding water used for cooling)

25% of nitrogen oxide emissions

36% of final energy use

40%–50% of sulfur oxide emissions

50% of contributions to the greenhouse effect

60% of biological oxygen demand and substances in suspension

75% of noninert waste (infectious, toxic, or radioactive waste)

90% of toxic substances discharged into water.

Source: OECD, 1991.

or that uses less polluting technologies may produce less air pollution. This may involve increasing the efficiency of combustion, physically trapping particles before they go into the smokestack, and chemically trapping or scrubbing airborne emissions before they are released into the atmosphere. Much industrial air pollution comes from combustion of coal, oil, or gas. The specific pollution, therefore, often includes particulate matter and sulfur dioxide (SO_2). In addition, many industries emit other specific toxic substances and odors, as discussed in the section Hazards by Industry below.

One of the most effective ways of controlling air pollution at the local level has been to build higher smokestacks at stationary sources (see Chapter 5). Depending on the stack height and the temperature of the emissions, the emissions from the source rise higher in the atmosphere, travel further, become more highly diluted in the atmosphere, and are less likely to affect the local community. The problem with this strategy is that it sends air pollution long distances away from the source. Air movements high in the atmosphere can transport air pollution long distances, allowing the pollutants to fall with rain or snow at locations far away from the source. This is to be one of the more important causes of acid deposition, which has become a problem in recent years (see Chapter 11).

Despite these problems, air quality has improved in many cities of the world (see Chapter 8) and serious air pollution crises, such as occurred in London in the 1950s, are much less common today. However, the control of air pollution is difficult and expensive. It is especially difficult in plants that have not been properly designed in the first place, such as older plants. The cost of air pollution control increases greatly with the degree of control. The cost of reducing emissions by 95% to 99% and then to 99.9%, for example, can be just as expensive as the first 95% reduction. Maintenance of the plant and regular testing of air pollution control devices is critical to ensure that they work properly.

Industrial Water Pollution

As was discussed in Chapter 6, water pollution occurs as the result of the release of a pollutant into a body of water such as a river, lake, or ocean. Much industrial water pollution affects the quality of the water and the biota in the water without having direct effects on human health, as is the case for lignin and wood waste from the pulp and paper industry.

Some pollutants, mostly organic chemicals, will eventually break down as a result of bacterial action and other processes in the soil and water. This process of natural disposal and recycling is called *biodegradation*. Others that are not so easily degraded will persist in soil and sediment. Because bodies of water are home to many microorganisms and invertebrate species, the pollutants are often taken up in the bodies of these species. This is called *bioaccumulation*. Those pollutants that persist in the environment and are not easily degraded biologically tend to accumulate in these species and are concentrated in the bodies of other species that feed on them, such as fish. Likewise, other forms of wildlife, such as bigger fish and mammals, may further accumulate these pollutants. This is called *bioconcentration* or *biomagnification* because at each level the amount of pollutant becomes more highly concentrated in the animal's body. This is illustrated in Figure 10.1, which shows the bioaccumulation and biomagnification of polychloride biphenyls (PCBs) in the Canadian Great Lakes aquatic food chain.

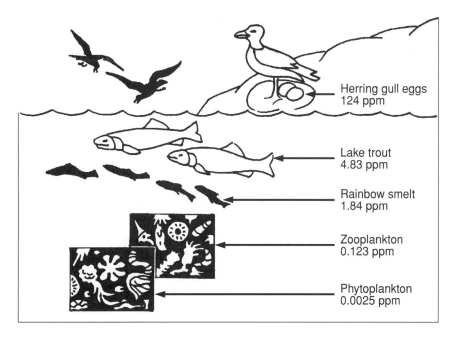

Figure 10.1 Bioaccumulation and biomagnification of PCBs in the Canadian Great Lakes aquatic food chain. From Environment Canada, 1987, with permission.

Hazardous Waste and Chemical Contamination

As noted in Chapter 2, hazardous substances are compounds and mixtures that pose a threat to health and property because of their toxicity, flammability, explosive potential, radiation, or other dangerous properties. Although hazardous substances may be released to the environment during transportation, in the production of goods, during maintenance in service operations and as occupational hazards, their principal impact on the environment comes from the dispersal of waste, after the material has been used or produced as an unwanted by-product.

The storage of large amounts of liquids also creates a risk of continuous smaller leakages of toxic chemicals. These may end up in the ground or local waterways. Many flammable liquids are lighter than water and are quite volatile, meaning that these liquids will seep down to the top layer of the groundwater and from there, the emerging fumes will seep up through the ground, possibly a long distance from where the leakage occurred. To prevent spillage and leakage from reaching the environment, tanks with these types of bulk materials should have walls around them that can contain the spillage (called *berms* or *bunds*) and the ground under the tanks should be provided with drainage that channels the spilled materials into safe storage.

Hazardous waste is not a new threat to health. Exposure to potentially dangerous chemicals has occurred in the smelting of metals and tanning of hides since ancient times; hydraulic mining released heavy metal into groundwater during the nineteenth century; and in the early days of industrialization, urban areas were saturated with pollution, including chemical wastes. Today, however, the problem has assumed much greater urgency as the result of the factors discussed below.

- The number and hazardous nature of toxic substances in common use has changed dramatically. Since World War II, research and development in organic chemistry and chemical engineering have introduced thousands of new compounds into widespread commercial use, including such persistent compounds as the PCBs and more potent pesticides, accelerators, and plasticizers with unusual and poorly understood effects. Compounds for which there has been little time to evaluate are in common use today.
- The production of chemicals has risen dramatically. In 1941 production of all synthetic organic compounds in the United States alone was less than one million tons; since then it has increased 100-fold. Many of these substances are toxic and degrade very slowly, resulting in accumulation in the environment. The environment contains much greater quantities of these toxic chemicals than ever before.
- Toxic chemicals are much more intrusive in daily life. Many chemical plants or disposal sites that were once isolated or on the edge of town have become incorporated into urban areas by suburban growth. Communities now lie in closer proximity to the problem than they have in the past. Some communities are built directly over old disposal sites.

People come into contact with toxic substances in many ways. Exposure may occur at several points in the life cycle of the substance. Some people work in plants that use chemical substances in an industrial process and are not able to change clothes or wash before coming home due to lack of shower facilities. Some people are exposed to chemical substances in household products (e.g., cleaning agents, paints, carpet glues). Sometimes exposure occurs inadvertently, for example, to pesticide spraying or environmental tobacco smoke (previously called *second-hand smoke*). Still others may reside near hazardous waste disposal sites that are illegal or poorly designed, or that provide opportunities for exposure as a result of accidents, careless handling, lack of containment of the substance, or lack of fencing to keep children off the site.

Public attention tends to focus on carcinogens, pesticides, and radiation hazards. However, innumerable compounds that do not fall into these categories can pose a threat to the public's safety and health. Some people appear to react to even very small exposures to chemicals, experiencing what has been called *multiple chemical sensitivity,* (MCS) described further in Box 10.2.

Although we are concentrating here on toxic exposures, we should not forget the substantial problems of safety that appear in many situations. Gasoline, for example, can explode with the destructive force of gunpowder. Fires and explosions also generate their own toxic hazards, depending on the chemicals that were initially present.

Despite the fact that incidents involving hazardous substances take many forms and may be highly individual, the great majority of incidents involving toxic wastes especially seem to involve a relatively narrow range of hazardous substances, which include solvents, paints and coatings, metals, PCBs, pesticides, and acids and alkalis. Solvents, particularly chlorinated compounds, are environmentally persistent, meaning that they tend to remain in the ground or water as contaminants for many years and are concentrated in the bodies of fish, birds, and other wildlife. Many solvents are toxic to human beings in relatively high concentrations and some are known or suspected carcinogens. In addition, these compounds are usually of direct concern for their potential effects on biota and ecosystems. The most toxic solvents have been withdrawn from industry for some years but old waste sites may contain significant amounts of benzene and trichlorethylene. Some of these same compounds, such as benzene and toluene, are also present as combustion products when organic material such as tires are burned. Paints and coatings are of concern primarily because of the solvents and metals they may contain.

Heavy metals are also environmentally persistent and may be highly toxic. Although the chances of significant exposure occurring as a result of exposure in a hazardous waste site are low, this could happen, especially to a young child who is playing in contaminated dirt. Areas contaminated by smelter or lead battery reprocessing operations, where arsenic or lead in the soil may reach high levels, pose a particular problem.

Chlorinated cyclic hydrocarbons, including dioxins, pentachlorophenol, and PCBs, are very damaging environmentally because they persist for long periods and are consumed and accumulated by wildlife. These compounds are capable of causing an unusual and persistent skin rash called *chloracne* that appears on the face and neck of people who are heavily exposed. Some of these compounds cause cancer and adverse reproductive effects in experimental animals. However,

BOX 10.2

Multiple Chemical Sensitivity

Multiple chemical sensitivity (MCS) is the common name for a set of symptoms that occur in the setting of chemical exposure. These symptoms are often vague and nonspecific and do not correspond to the known toxic effects of these chemicals. The symptoms may include fatigue, confusion (called *brain fog* by some advocates), loss of appetite, headache, and nausea. They may occur after the patient has experienced exposure to very low levels of a chemical, well below the levels known to cause toxic reactions. Sometimes they seem to occur at times when exposure is unlikely but sufferers feel that they have been exposed. Some people believe that MCS represents a generalized allergic reaction to all chemicals. The workings of the immune system, however, are highly specific and one normally reacts only to particular chemicals or classes of chemicals. Sufferers of MCS often respond to chemicals of many different types, regardless of chemical composition. The most common chemicals that trigger this reaction seem to be perfumes, pesticides, solvents, tobacco smoke, and food additives. Research on the problem has resulted in many theories, but little firm evidence for a mechanism.

Patients with this disorder may come from all walks of life but most are female, young, relatively affluent, and either work at home or work in office jobs. To determine the cause of their symptoms, they commonly consult practitioners of alternative medicine, some of whom may give them the diagnosis of MCS. The effect of the diagnosis of MCS on them is often quite dramatic. The diagnosis becomes a central feature of their lives. They may withdraw from their usual daily life, quit work, change their diet, change their housing, and require visitors to avoid bringing any chemical into their surroundings, even freshly washed clothes. Many times these changes are very radical and have the effect of isolating them from family, friends, and society. Often they show features of depression or obsessive-compulsive behavior, although it is controversial whether this is a cause or a result of their condition. Alternative treatments are long, involved, and costly, and there is no evidence that they work. Because conventional medicine does not recognize the disorder, there is no obvious medical treatment. Psychotherapy seems to be the most effective form of treatment available. Most patients refuse this, however, and many react angrily to suggestions that their condition may have a psychosomatic dimension.

One of the problems in investigating MCS is that the definition and the terms used change frequently. The leading advocates for the existence of MCS as a distinct clinical disorder once called themselves *clinical ecologists,* and now call themselves *environmental medicine practitioners.* In the past, MCS itself has gone by the names of *chemical sensitivity, twentieth-century disease,* and *environmental hypersensitivity disorder.* Some of these practitioners believe that MCS covers a wide variety of seemingly related illnesses, such as sick building syndrome (which occurs when people working in a building with poor ventilation feel ill; see Chapter 8), chronic fatigue syndrome (another nonspecific diagnosis possibly related to a viral infection), and more conventional allergies and toxicity conditions. Most mainstream medical practitioners strongly disagree that this entity has a distinct pathophysiological basis and believe that a MCS-associated behavior pattern may represent a psychological disturbance on the part of some patients. Some believe that what appears to be MCS is actually a psychosomatic, behavioral response to chemicals in the environment. Others, however, believe that there may be unknown toxicological or immunological responses that underlie the response of some patients to chemicals at low lev-

(continued)

(*continued*)

els but that the responses are not yet understood by current scientific knowledge and, in any case, need not be disabling.

There are many examples in the past of disorders that were once thought to be particular diseases that are now considered psychological responses to stress. These have included hysteria, neurasthenia, and catalepsy—all diagnoses now discarded by the medical profession. (The term *hysteria*, comes from the Latin word for uterus. It is pejorative to women because it implies that women are biologically prone to be emotionally unstable, and thus the term should not be used.) Some physicians feel that MCS, chronic fatigue syndrome, and multiple personality disorder are modern examples of this type of condition. Others feel that some of these patients may well have disorders that medicine cannot yet explain. It is possible that in a few years MCS will cease to be a commonly used medical term and that some cases now called MCS will be found to reflect conventional allergies and toxicities, some will be clearly psychological in origin, and some will remain difficult to explain. Sparks et al. (1994) have provided a useful case definition, and summarized the theories of pathogenesis, diagnostic testing, treatment, and social consideration.

Source: Various summaries produced by the Association of Occupational and Environmental Clinics; See also Sparks, 2000.

humans appear to be more resistant to the effects of these compounds than other species. Even so, these are dangerous compounds to the environment and must be controlled for ecological reasons. We still do not know many of their more subtle effects on humans and it is only prudent that we minimize exposure to humans as well.

Pesticides are particularly dangerous in hazardous waste, especially the relatively toxic class known as the *organophosphates*. Fires involving pesticide storage areas are a particularly dangerous situation, as the pesticides may be converted into even more highly toxic combustion products and substantial amounts of environmentally damaging dioxins and furans may be generated.

Strong acids and strong alkali are commonly found at waste sites and are dangerous if there is a possibility of direct contact or inhalation of fumes. They may cause serious skin and eye burns on contact. Some acids may generate clouds of fumes that may cause lung injury. If mixed together, the acids and alkali may generate intense, possibly explosive heat and substantial dangerous fumes. Two acids that are particularly dangerous are nitric acid and hydrofluoric acid. Nitric acid releases nitrogen dioxide, which may cause pulmonary edema and bronchial irritation. Hydrofluoric acid is used for etching in the electronics industry and is exceedingly dangerous when inhaled or when it touches skin or mucous membranes. On contact with skin or eyes, it causes deeply penetrating burns.

Cyanide is present in some situations, especially gold-plating solutions. Inhaled cyanide fumes from the solution are highly toxic. Cyanide can be released by mixing the plating solution with a strong acid, such as those often found at hazardous waste sites.

A major unresolved issue in municipal solid waste handling is contamination by hazardous waste disposed of by accident or intent. This can be minimized by diverting such disposal into a separate waste stream. Other means have been used to control release of the remaining hazardous substances from a landfill site not constructed to receive such materials, to keep the hazard minimal. Some communities have organized periodic pickup drives for collecting household hazardous wastes to prevent contamination of sanitary landfills. Well-designed hazardous waste disposal facilities, using the best available technologies of recycling, dehalogenation, and containment, are urgently needed.

HAZARDS BY INDUSTRY

This brief summary can only give a snapshot of the types of health hazards that may be related to industry. Information about the specific health hazards and preventive approaches for each industry can be found in publications of the International Labor Office (ILO), particularly the *ILO Encyclopedia of Occupational Health and Safety* (ILO, 1998), as well as documents from the United Nations Environment Program (UNEP) Industry and Environment Office in Paris. A number of major occupational health hazards occur in each of these industries (see section Dimensions and Types of Occupational Health Problems, below).

Materials Extraction

This type of industry is sometimes called *primary industry* and represents the first step in the process of creating manufactured products. It includes mining for metals and minerals, coal and oil extraction, forestry, agriculture, and fishing. Outputs of this type of industry include ore or metal concentrate, coal, oil, sand, wood, fibres (cotton, wool, hemp), grains, and fish. Issues related to the food and agriculture industry are examined in Chapter 7. These primary industries can be found in all countries, but as countries develop they usually tend to represent a decreasing proportion of the overall economy.

The types of pollution and hazards related to the mining industry include dust in air and water pollution from the processes that use water to transport, wash, or concentrate the raw materials. Mines and quarries also create physical scars in the local environment and can cause major emergency pollution risks when *tailings dams* (accumulations of debris that trap water behind them) burst or overflow. Often processing plants for concentration or refining of metals are located together with the mine itself, and these plants can cause major sulfur dioxide or metals pollution, as has happened in a number of places. The sulfur dioxide pollution occurs because the ores of many metals contain large amounts of sulfur. Special problems accompany uranium mining as radioactive compounds can be released to the environment.

Coal extraction is similar to metal mining, except that the coal mines are often colocated with coal power plants, which emit large amounts of particulates (dust), sulfur dioxide, and toxic metals included in the raw coal (see Chapter 9). The amount of pollution will depend on the quality of the coal and pollution control measures. Dramatic air pollution situations related to coal extraction exist, for instance, around coal mines in central Europe, India, and China. Oil extraction involves direct surface oil pollution from spillages, as well as air pollution from the burning (flaring) of excess gas combined with oil or from power stations or petrochemical industries colocated with the oil field.

Although forestry creates mainly physical damage to the natural environment, it can create important health risks if deforestation leads to floods, landslides, or polluted drinking-water sources (see Chapter 11). Other agricultural industries also produce physical changes in the environment, the main threats to health being the use of pesticides and fertilizers. Spraying of pesticides from airplanes can create high exposures to local residents and intensive use of nitrogen fertilizers can pollute groundwater and lead to high nitrate levels in drinking water from wells (see Chapter 7, Modern Intensive Farming Methods). The latter is a major problem in several European countries.

Processing Industries

Industries that process extracted raw materials into concentrated intermediate products are potentially large sources of environmental impact because of the scale and nature of their operations. The metals industries, including iron and steel production, transform metal ores to metal ingots, sheets, and pipes, and can generate considerable air, water, and land pollution. Some metals, such as lead and cadmium, are very toxic, and many incidents of poisoning in populations living around such industries have taken place. Particular problems occur in industries that recycle scrap metal products, as the content of the scrap is not always well known, and a mixture of toxic chemicals may be emitted to the air or water. Lead has been a particular problem in this regard.

Petrochemical industries have already been mentioned. They process oil products into bulk raw materials for the production of plastics and chemicals. These raw materials themselves, e.g., benzene, may be highly toxic. Sulfur dioxide is a common pollutant, as most raw petroleum oil contains sulfur. These industries involve major fire risks, and when a fire occurs, the smoke will contain a mixture of very toxic chemicals. Depending on the wind direction and town planning, population groups may be highly exposed. In some countries, such as the United States and Canada, industry has attempted to address these problems with comprehensive voluntary risk management programs that include public consultation.

The major pollution source in the processing of forestry products is the pulp and paper industry. Large amounts of water are used to prepare the pulp and process it into paper. The lignin (a natural glue that holds together wood fibers) in the wood gets washed out with the water as well as the remains of various chemicals used in the processing. This pollution can seriously affect the water quality as measured by the *biological oxygen demand* (BOD). The BOD is an indicator of the amount of oxygen required to biodegrade all the organic material in water and is the fundamental measurement used to monitor water quality. Mercury fungicides were used in the past to keep the paper pulp from growing moldy. Some of these fungicides ended up in the wastewater and have caused long-lasting pollution of lakes, particularly in Sweden. The sulfate and sulfide processes in the paper pulp industry lead to air pollution of mercaptans and other extremely smelly chemicals. Odor pollution is common, but is often more noticed by people traveling past a plant than those living close to it all the time, because the nose adapts to smells. Another problem in the forest industry is the pesticide treatment of timber or wood products, often carried out under primitive conditions in the forests. Land pollution and occupational hazards result from the use of arsenic compounds and pentachlorophenol to make timber resistant to insect attack.

The processing of plant fibers may lead to problems with dust, mainly in the workplace. *Byssinosis,* for example, is a common occupational lung disease caused by inhalation of cotton fibres in processing plants. The sugar cane industry and other processing industries create major water pollution with the leftover materials and nutrients from the plants, which can damage drinking-water sources. Many of these industries use the leftover plant materials as fuel in water-heating systems, often with resulting severe smoke problems. In addition, these industries use pesticides and process pesticide-contaminated raw materials, which can lead to pesticide pollution of water and land.

Food-processing industries, such as abattoirs and fish-processing plants, cause problems mainly as a result of the organic materials in the large volumes of meat or fish residue that may be discarded. The waterways receiving the pollution can be affected by overnutrition, or eutrophication, as discussed in Chapter 6, and high BOD. The affected waterways are also likely to serve as carriers of any infectious bacteria or parasites that emerge from the slaughtered animals or fish. Odor is also a problem.

Manufacturing

In this type of industry, often called *secondary industry* and common all over the world, raw materials and processed materials are used to create various consumer and industrial products. The largest plants are those that make automobiles, trains, airplanes, ships, and machinery. Occupational hazards are often the main health problems, but air and water pollution can develop in relation to processes that use toxic chemicals. The section Major Chemical Contaminants of Concern in the General Environment and the Workplace gives examples of the major chemical hazards that can be found in the manufacturing industry. Another problem is the storage and disposal of toxic wastes that are produced in manufacturing processes.

In the production of paper, one of the most hazardous processes has been the chlorine-bleaching of paper to achieve a snow-white color. The presence of chlorine and organic compounds has led to the formation of toxic chemicals in effluent from the plant into water, including dioxins and furans. These chemicals have potentially serious environmental effects even though they are only produced in small quantities. They are also suspected to cause reproductive and carcinogenic effects in humans. Fortunately, new technologies in pulp and paper manufacturing do not require chlorine and thus avoid this problem. In the past, mercury has often been used as a catalyst in the production of chlorine. This mercury further contributes to water pollution.

Textile production is a major industry in developing as well as developed countries. Cotton, wool, and synthetic fibers (usually made from petroleum oil) are used to weave fabrics that go into clothes and furniture. Again, the health hazards are mainly occupational, although dying processes and other use of chemicals can lead to severe water pollution.

The production of chemicals carries a great potential for pollution as it requires all of the feedstock chemicals used in raw materials, process chemicals used in the reactions and processes, intermediary chemicals, and the final chemical products. This industry has received considerable attention, particularly in conjunction with serious emergencies, such as the Bhopal accident in India, where more than 200,000 people were poisoned from a cloud of methyl-isocyanate, an intermediary chemical in the production of pesticides (Dhara and Dhara, 1995).

Other manufacturing industries with special problems include the production of electrical batteries (lead or cadmium pollution), electrical transformers (PCB pollution), furniture (paint or solvent fumes), microelectronics (solvents, arsenic, occupational health problems) and glass or ceramics products (lead pollution). Manufacturing of food products involves the production of biological waste. Another sector that is not always classified as manufacturing but nonetheless is associated with environmental hazards is the building materials industry (e.g., cement, asbestos, glues, and paints).

More advanced or refined products of manufacturing, e.g., specialist electronic products such as computers, printed materials, music cassettes, and toys, can involve unusual chemical or physical hazards. Examples of this are found in the rare metals and special solvents used in computer chip production and the lasers used in etching patterns. As mentioned before, occupational hazards often pose the greatest danger in these industries.

A further area of concern related to these special products and some manufactured consumer products is the hazards that may be associated with their use. Malfunctioning or unsafe machines can cause injuries to the user, and improper use of electrical equipment can cause electrocution. Electromagnetic radiation from computer screens or portable phones has been suspected of inducing adverse health impacts, but thus far it appears that the health risks may be low. Paints on toys can cause poisoning in children. A system of consumer protection legislation and monitoring functions has been established in many countries. Countries with a weak system may face difficulties in consumer product safety and in acceptance of their exports by other countries. Some countries have established recognition programs for products that meet criteria for "environmental friendliness" to further encourage the reduction of health and ecological risks (so-called green labeling or eco-labeling).

Service Industries

An increasing proportion of overall economic activity is based on the provision of services, in contrast to the production of goods. This is often referred to as *tertiary industry* and includes restaurant and hotel services, health services, personal services (such as hairdressing), entertainment, travel, tourism, public administrative services, telecommunications, and the new high-tech industries (such as software production). Generally they do not produce much environmental pollution, although all establishments at which large numbers of people are assembled create increased pressures on sanitation and waste management, e.g., tourist resorts create greater needs for sewage treatment. Hospitals and medical laboratories have particular problems with medical waste, which can contain infectious agents and radioactive materials.

Another issue related to concentrations of people is disturbing noise. The travel and transportation industry causes a fair amount of noise around airports, motorways, train tracks, and busy streets in urban areas. The increasing demand for high speed has led to increasing noise pollution levels. In countries with high population densities, such as The Netherlands or Japan, there is often not enough room to provide for wide separation between traffic and residences or schools.

A major concern in service industries is the widespread continuous work at computer keyboards or grocery store check-out counters, which in some countries has lead to "epidemics" of a number of painful hand and arm conditions called *occupational overuse syndrome* (OOS), *cumulative trauma disorders* (CTD) or *repetitive strain injury* (RSI). Stress from high demand for fast service work plays a role in the onset of these conditions. Ergonomically well-designed work stations and limitations of continuous work through regular breaks can prevent the condition (Yassi, 1997, Yassi, 2000).

Another occupational hazard in these types of industries is psychological stress from the demands of person-to-person contact and the economic demands for more rapid decision making and action. Verbal and even physically abusive incidents are of increasing concern in the service sector, especially the health and social service sector (Yassi and McLean, 2001). This industry is also generally very labor-intensive. The varying demands for services can create great uncertainty in the employment prospects of every worker, again leading to stress. Indeed there is growing concern that job insecurity and psychosocial work organization issues, often characterized by high demands and low control, have become the major work-related health hazard in developed countries (Sullivan and Frank, 2000).

MAJOR CHEMICAL CONTAMINANTS OF CONCERN IN THE GENERAL ENVIRONMENT AND THE WORKPLACE

Toxic Metals

The principal toxic metals of concern in industrial pollution are lead, mercury, cadmium, and arsenic, although chromium, zinc, copper, and other metals may be of concern in some areas. It should be pointed out that human exposure to these metals is common both in the workplace and the general environment. In addition, families of workers can be exposed through dust brought home on dirty work clothes. Exposure to toxic metals from food is addressed further in Chapter 7.

Lead Lead is one of the oldest environmental hazards known to society. There are many sources of exposure to lead, with residents in urban areas tending to have lead levels that are higher than those in rural areas. Lead enters the body primarily through the inhalation of tiny particles that contain it or through ingestion of food or beverages that contain it. Absorption of tetraethyl lead gasoline additive through the skin does occur, but such exposures have rarely caused lead poisoning. Petrol sniffing among youth in certain communities has caused significant poisoning problems. Lead remains a serious environmental hazard as well as a serious occupational health and safety problem.

Lead was used long before the Industrial Revolution for making pipes, pigments, and bullets because it is a soft metal, is easily worked, and melts at a relatively low temperature. Industrial pollution by lead has been a particular problem in smelters. Primary lead smelters handle ore that contains high concentrations of lead. Other types of primary smelters may be associated with a risk of lead exposure, because lead is often present in the ores of other metals. The most common type of point source for industrial pollution by lead, however, has been secondary smelters, where old lead batteries are torn apart, melted down, and resmelted. These secondary smelters are often located in populated areas and lead contamination of soil around them can be extensive.

Industrial pollution from lead, however, is a more general problem because of leaded gasoline and lead-containing paints for indoor application. Tetraethyl lead additive was for many years a major contributor to environmental lead exposure in communities. Leaded gasoline has been withdrawn from the market in most countries and where it has, the lead levels in the blood of children have decreased. Another major source of community exposure to lead has been house paint containing lead. Children who eat flaking paint chips or who play on the floor where there is lead-containing dust from disintegrating paint are at risk for lead poisoning. Currently, lead-containing paints are usually restricted to heavy-duty outdoor painting of steel bridges and other nonresidential structures. However, paint stays on buildings for a very long time and any painted building older than 30 years may still have lead paint.

Another important source of lead exposure was (and, in many countries such as Mexico, still is) lead-based glazes on pottery. Lead can enter the food or beverage contained in the vessel, especially if the beverage is acidic. Commercial production of pottery with lead glazes has stopped in most of the world, but the problem is still seen occasionally when a leaded glaze is used by an amateur or when a decorative piece not made for drinking is used as such. Small amounts of lead may also enter the body from food cans or copper drinking-water pipes because solder was used to seal them.

Heavy exposure to lead can result in lead poisoning, which is characterized by anemia, kidney damage, nerve damage and partial paralysis of certain muscle groups, and brain damage. The symptoms of acute lead poisoning are colicky pain in the abdomen, nausea, and weight loss. The effects of lead exposure that cause the greatest concern are those on children. Low levels of lead exposure may cause irreversible brain damage that takes the form of learning disabilities and reduced intellectual capacity. (Chapter 3 illustrated the various dose–response effects of lead in children.)

Mercury Mercury is also an ancient hazard, however, it is much less common as an industrial pollutant than lead. It is unique among metals, being liquid at room temperature and readily volatilizing into a gas. There are many organic compounds of mercury and these are usually more toxic than the metal element itself. Exposure usually occurs through inhalation of mercury vapor or ingestion of mercury-containing food, but mercury can also be absorbed across a wound or damaged skin.

Historically, mercury was primarily an occupational hazard, associated with goldsmithing, mirror-making, explosive detonators, and the many uses of mercurial compounds as antiseptic and antifungal agents. The use of mercurial compounds as an antifungal treatment of seed intended for planting has caused several outbreaks of mercury poisoning, the most famous being in Iraq in 1972 in which hundreds of fatalities occurred among people who used treated seed to make bread. Industrial pollution with mercury was mostly on a small scale until the 1940s, except for some mercury contamination of bodies of water from gold mining. However, industrial pollution on a large scale resulted when the chloralkali process was introduced in paper plants and production expanded during the post-World War II era; this has resulted in substantial mercury contamination in many bodies of water, particularly in the sediment where the mercury accumulates. However, the largest outbreak of mercury intoxication in history was the result of pollution from a vinyl chloride factory that used a mercury catalyst in its production process. This occurred in 1953 at Minamata Bay on the island of Kyushu, Japan, resulting in many deaths and a much greater number of individuals with permanent neurological impairment. Effluent from the factory caused methylmercury contamination of fish, which were eaten by villagers.

Today, in most developed countries, mercury is primarily an occupational hazard in dental clinics (from the use of a mercury-containing amalgam for filling cavities), instrument manufacturing and repair, and smelting. Some cases of mercury intoxication have occurred in homes, for example, where a space heater has been used with a broken mercury-containing switch that was designed to shut the heater off if it tipped over.

In some areas of the world, such as the Amazon, mercury pollution is on the rise. When gold was first discovered approximately three decades ago in Brazil, thousands of impoverished Brazilians began to extract gold from river sediment by mixing in mercury, as the liquid metal binds with the gold. The resulting amalgam is heated, causing the mercury to evaporate, leaving the gold behind. Through this process large amounts of mercury were released into the air as well as into the water.

The effect of mercury on the body can take many forms, depending on the chemical form of the mercury and the circumstances of exposure. Metallic mercury can cause mouth sores, extreme pain and tenderness in the fingertips, tremor, and an unusual, pathological shyness that results from damage to the brain. In the environment, metallic mercury is slowly converted to organic compounds of mercury. Methylmercury compounds may cause severe nervous system damage, both to the brain and the peripheral nerves. This is associated with movement disorders, deteriorating handwriting, slurred speech, and visual abnormalities. The tragic experience of Minamata demonstrated that methylmercury also causes severe fetal poisoning. In the Amazon region, villagers who ate large quantities of fish contaminated by mercury at levels much below international standards were reported to have neurological and cytogenetic damage (see Lebel et al., 1996; Box 11.5).

Cadmium Another metal that has been used in a number of industrial applications is cadmium. It is used as an anti-corrosive coating on steel, and in rechargeable electric batteries. Cadmium compounds have also been used as pigments in plastics, but in some countries restrictions on its use have been regulated to reduce the possibility of environmental contamination by cadmium.

The most famous cadmium poisoning outbreak due to industrial pollution is the "Itai-itai" disease epidemic in Japan, which started in the 1950s (Kjellstrom, 1986a). Water pollution from a mine and lead/zinc refinery caused serious cadmium contamination to downstream irrigated farm fields. The farmers and their families became exposed to high levels of cadmium in rice grown in contaminated water, and hundreds of cases of kidney damage occurred. The most severe cases also developed severe osteoporosis and osteomalacia. A similar combination of kidney and bone disease has occurred in workers exposed to cadmium (WHO, 1992f).

Cadmium accumulates in the body, particularly the liver and kidneys, and the health effects usually develop after many years of exposure. This metal also accumulates in the enviroment and its use in industry and associated pollution has caused indirect exposures many years later. For instance, the mining pollution in Japan took years to build up to a health-damaging level. Similarly, cadmium contamination from industries to sewage water built up in sewage sludge, which eventually was spread on farm fields. The increased cadmium concentrations in soil produced increased concentrations in grains and an increased level of human exposure. Fertilizers with high natural cadmium content add to the problem. Thus some countries are regulating the use of cadmium to reduce human exposure.

Arsenic Arsenic is a more common element in uncontaminated soil than lead, mercury, or cadmium. It is also bioconcentrated naturally in shellfish. As a result, many people have small amounts of arsenic in their bodies. In a number of areas of the world, natural contamination of groundwater with arsenic is a serious problem, e.g., in Bangladesh, India, Chile, and Argentina. In the past, arsenic compounds have been extensively used as antibiotics (particularly against syphilis), as preservatives in tanning and taxidermy, as green dyes for paper, and as antiparasite treatment in sheep dip. In each of these applications arsenic was a serious occupational and consumer hazard. More recently, arsenic compounds have been used in the doping of semiconductors and in other microelectronic applications and present potentially serious occupational hazards to workers. There have been deaths due to the accidental inhalation of arsine (AsH_3) a very toxic gas, in this industry.

Arsenic is a carcinogen to human beings, causing skin cancer and lung cancer. Efforts to duplicate the carcinogenicity of arsenic in animals have not been successful; it is the only known example of a uniquely human carcinogen. In addition, arsenic causes several types of skin rash. Because arsenic has a well-deserved reputation as a potent poison, it is more widely recognized as a hazard than other metals.

Solvents

Solvents are liquids at room temperature that can dissolve other substances without necessarily reacting with them chemically. While water is by far the most common solvent, there are numerous other compounds that are used in industry as cleaners, degreasing agents, extraction solvents, viscosity modifiers, constituents of glues and paints, and paint or coating removers. These mostly organic chemicals are also widely used for many nonsolvent applications as fuels, pesticides, or chemical production feedstocks. The most familiar organic solvents are also important constituents of water and air pollution, frequently as the result of trace contamination from other sources or secondary chemical reactions. Nonsubstituted hydrocarbons, ketones, and aldehydes occur in air pollution. Hydrocarbons, halogenated and nonsubstituted, are important in groundwater contamination and water pollution.

Solvents can be categorized according to physical properties or chemical structure. The basic physical properties of solvents can be described according to their capacity to dissolve substances that carry a polar charge (typically, these compounds are easily dissolved by water) or to dissolve nonpolar substances (such as oils) (see Chapter 2). These characteristics of solvents are important determinants of their human toxicity in the workplace, but they are not as important in environmental exposures where the concentrations are much lower.

The various classes of solvents share a number of common characteristics when it comes to human toxicity. Most solvents evaporate easily and are therefore easily inhaled in the workplace. Nonpolar solvents, those that dissolve oils and fat, penetrate the skin very easily because much of the skin itself is fat; this often leads to problems with skin rashes. Many solvents have essentially identical toxic effects on the central nervous system. They act as anesthetics and intoxicants at high concentrations (ethyl ether and chloroform were the first anesthetics used in surgery) that may cause a complete loss of consciousness if the fumes accumulate in confined spaces, but often lead to a clinical condition sometimes called *painter's syndrome* because it often affects painters. In this syndrome, the worker feels lightheaded then euphoric, loses coordination and acts intoxicated, and finally becomes sleepy or very fatigued (*acute central neurotoxicity*).

In addition to the hazard of toxicity, workers may be more prone to injuries and errors of judgment when under the influence of solvents. After exposure stops, the worker will begin to feel depressed and often gets a severe headache or feels ill. After many repeated exposures, the worker will become moody and show a change in personality, becoming more irritable, and experiencing a loss of short-term memory and eventually permanent brain damage. These symptoms are similar to those from intoxication with alcohol, except that the brain damage typically occurs sooner than with alcohol. Certain compounds exert their toxic effect on peripheral nerves, causing a loss of sensation or a burning sensation in the feet and hands. This condition is called *peripheral neuropathy* and it can also occur as a result of alcohol abuse. Likewise, many solvents are highly toxic to the liver and can bring about all the features of liver damage that can be caused by ethyl alcohol, including cirrhosis. Cancer is a known risk for a few of these solvents and is a theoretical risk for others. There is a large and conflicting literature on the possible cancer risks of particular solvents; for solvents it is not clear whether they represent a significant hazard or not. A number of solvents, particularly the glycols, are also highly toxic to the kidneys. (see *Environmental Health Criteria* documents published by the WHO through its International Programme on Chemical Safety—see the website www.who.int/pcs/for online publications.) These injuries may occur among workers who use these solvents on the job without adequate protection; these effects are particularly seen in workers on spray-painting operations. All of these effects can be prevented by limiting exposure in the workplace to existing occupational exposure standards. Nonetheless, cases of toxicity related to excessive exposure are very common worldwide.

Benzene is the compound that most often appears in air and water quality–monitoring data at concentrations sufficient to cause concern. In the air, the major source of benzene is gasoline for cars. The exhaust fumes contain benzene, which is spread to water supplies via runoff from streets during rain storms. The potency of benzene as a carcinogen is known to be greater than that of most other compounds commonly encountered in the environment. Also benzene tends to be present at relatively higher concentrations in air and water pollution than those of many of these other compounds. This potency and the fact that it is often present at significant concentrations mean greater importance is attributed to benzene than to most other chemicals when calculating the risks to human health.

Bulk Raw Materials

Any type of bulk materials that can induce adverse health effects after human exposure needs careful handling to prevent accidental releases of large amounts to the environment, fires, and long-term low-level emissions. Examples of bulk materials that can cause major hazards are chlorine gas, flammable liquids and gases (oil, petrol, solvents, raw materials for plastics production, such as vinyl chloride or acrylonitrile), and cyanides used in metals extraction and finishing.

Chlorine gas is stored in large volumes at many paper pulp plants and chemical factories producing chlorinated organic compounds. The gas is heavier than air and will therefore stay close to the ground after a release. It is highly irritating and damaging to the lungs and can kill people if sufficient amounts are inhaled. Victims must be taken immediately out of exposure and given treatment to restore lung function. Regulations exist in most countries concerning the safety precautions required at a bulk chlorine storage site. These include warning devices for any leaks, availability of breathing equipment, escape routes for workers and people in the neighborhood, warning announcements to the community, and emergency treatment facilities.

Flammable gases and liquids present a fire risk as well as a risk for exposure to the toxic fumes created by any fire. The content of such fumes will depend on the chemical composition of the bulk materials, and often the fumes are more toxic than the bulk materials themselves. Because of the major economic damage caused by industrial fires, precautionary measures are generally made a part of routine management of the industry. Still, major industrial fires happen regularly in both developed and developing countries and the health impacts can be important.

Cyanides are powerful solvents for certain metal compounds and are commonly used in gold extraction and metal plating and etching. The most toxic compound, the deadly hydrogen cyanide gas, is formed when cyanides come into contact with acids. The main health risks occur among workers in the industries using cyanides, but leakage to waterways is another problem. Direct contact with these chemicals affects the skin and lungs. In the waterways, cyanides will kill fish, causing important economic hardship to people in the area. Large emergencies have occurred when tailings dams at gold mines have leaked, as happened recently in Guyana and Romania. A much more common event is worker exposure in small-scale electroplating industries, which use cyanide in corrosion protection parts for car and metal products industries. In many countries this industry first develops as a small cottage industry, often in residential areas.

Chemical Poisoning in the Community

Exposure in the home is perhaps the leading means by which children come into contact with toxic substances. Consumer education to promote awareness of the potential toxicity of common products is urgently needed. Pesticides in aerosol cans, bleaches, household cleaners, and cleaning fluids are potentially dangerous to children and must be treated as such. Another need is for facilities to collect and properly dispose of small quantities of hazardous waste. Individuals who find themselves in possession of a bottle or can of solvents, pesticides, or some unknown powder or fluid often do not understand the risk. Some decentralized system for collecting such hazardous waste from consumers is needed before it is poured on the ground, flushed down the toilet, or burned and released into the air. Such a system has been introduced in many urban areas, involving home or convenient pickup of small quantities of discarded toxic substances.

THE SOCIAL CONTEXT OF OCCUPATIONAL HEALTH AND SAFETY

The field of occupational health and safety relates to the analysis and control of hazards in particular workplaces. Occupational health primarily deals with hazards of a chemical, physical, or biological nature; occupational safety primarily addresses hazards of a mechanical nature. With increasing recognition that ergonomic factors can cause not only acute trauma but also repetitive strain injuries (e.g. occupational overuse syndrome, carpal tunnel syndrome, tendonitis, and epicondylitis), occupational health professionals must consider biomechanical factors within their realm of expertise as well. Psychosocial hazards of work (e.g., stress, burnout, harassment) are also issues that occupational health professionals must address. (The WHO and the ILO have developed many important documents in this area; the ILO's *Encyclopedia of Occupational Health and Safety [ILO, 1998]* is an excellent source of information on the issues in this field.)

Although there is a great deal of variation worldwide in the nature and severity of occupational health and safety problems and the resources available to control them, there are many more issues in common. At the beginning of development, whether historically among developed nations or currently among developing nations, occupational health and safety tend to be a low priority because of a perceived need to develop at all costs. This is unfortunate, because at this stage of development, a relatively small investment in worker protection may yield great benefits in improved worker health.

As societies become increasingly developed, the field of occupational health and safety tends to become an increasing priority. Often, a series of well-publicized accidents forces citizens to address this issue. Sometimes, trade unions force employers (and the government) to provide greater occupational safety. Occasionally, a particularly enlightened employer sets the tone and is a model for the rest of society. Historically, governments have taken the lead in controlling occupational hazards by setting permissible exposure levels and requiring periodic inspections for safe work practices.

Ideally, improving occupational health and safety is one area in which both employers and workers would perceive a common interest. After all, occupational injuries and illnesses are completely preventable and the costs that they impose on the employer, the worker, and society in general are considerable. Employers lose production time and skilled labor that must be replaced. They may, depending on the health care system in the country, have to pay directly (or indirectly, through taxes) for medical treatment. In countries where there are workers' compensations systems, their insurance premiums will go up. Workers may lose their wages, their chances for a better job, and, if permanently disabled, even their livelihood, not to mention the pain and inconvenience in daily life that an injury causes the worker and the anxiety this creates in the worker's family. Because occupational injuries are common, the cost to society as a whole is enormous. However, the financial incentive to employers to reduce occupational injuries and illnesses may be very low if their direct costs are not clear or are borne by others.

Relationships between employers and workers often affect whether and how occupational health and safety are addressed. Employers may be reluctant to make the investment to control hazards in the workplace, especially if they feel that their competitors do not. Governments may refrain from enforcing occupational health and safety standards because they are afraid that this may affect competitiveness in world markets. Workers may not cooperate with health and safety measures because they are poorly aware of hazards. Alternatively, they may feel compelled to accept high risk in order to keep their jobs.

Despite methodological difficulties, studies have shown that implementing occupational health and safety activities can save industry money, and implementing ergonomic interventions, with full worker participation, is particularly worthwhile in reducing the social and monetary costs of work-related injuries (Nosman and Wells, 2000). As wages rise, the cost to society of missed work and loss of production increases as well. Efforts to reduce the impact of occupational illness and injury will continue to take on growing importance.

There are other issues in occupational health and safety that are common worldwide. Small enterprises, all other things being equal, tend to have more dangerous working conditions than very large companies. The reason is that larger operations usually have the resources to solve their problems and can afford the protection more easily than marginal operations. Also, many very hazardous jobs are done primarily by small companies working under contract to larger ones. Some government agencies have therefore provided smaller enterprises direct assistance in the form of consultation services to help them solve their safety problems as inexpensively as possible.

The Internal Responsibility System

Many government regulatory bodies for occupational health and safety have adopted the policy of *internal responsibility* for larger enterprises. This policy holds these companies responsible for controlling hazards and ensuring compliance with occupational exposure standards. The government agency reviews their performance, audits their procedures, and occasionally inspects the premises, but does so less often than for smaller enterprises. A key feature of this system is the *joint health and safety committee*, a committee that consists of representatives from both management and workers who meet regularly to discuss occupational health and safety problems. This system works well when the worker committee members are *elected*, members are adequately *trained*, and the committee is given the *authority* to conduct inspections and play an active role in carrying out changes in the workplace. Large companies also often maintain their own occupational physicians, occupational health nurses, industrial hygienists, and other specialized occupational health and safety professionals. These professionals can help ensure that the joint committee is given the information it needs and is kept abreast of scientific innovations. While there is evidence that joint health and safety committees can play an important role in improving workplace health and safety, equally important are the regulatory environment and the structure of economic incentives (O'Grady, 2000) and workplace organizational factors (Shannon, 2000).

Workers' Compensation

Beyond a certain level of development, societies tend to introduce an insurance scheme for their workers to minimize the disruption that occupational injuries can cause and to control the costs. In particular, the cost of lawsuits associated with injuries and illnesses may rapidly grow out of control. The response to this situation may take the form of social security programs that operate as a comprehensive health care system for workers and their families. Some countries have used this to phase in more universal coverage for health services for their population. It may also take the form of *workers' compensation*, a no-fault insurance system funded by employers that compensates workers for health care and lost earnings from work-related injuries or illnesses. Some jurisdictions also provide an *impairment award*, based on measurable loss of function, regardless of whether the worker can continue working.

Workers have often had to give up their right to sue their employers in exchange for a comprehensive workers' compensation system, which is administered by an impartial board responsible to government, e.g., as in Canada. The Workers' Compensation Board (WCB), having obtained information from the employer, the worker, and the worker's attending physician, decides if the worker's health problem is work related and the extent to which it disables the worker. The system tends to work reasonably well for injuries but less well for diseases, many of which are multifactorial in origin.

Some workers are particularly disadvantaged as they have to deal with racism and sexism at work in addition to the health hazards of work. Particular problems facing women in the workplace are discussed in the next section.

Women in the Workplace

The role of women in the workforce is more complicated than that of men, in part because of social roles that women have been expected to assume, such as that of wife or mother; in part because of reproductive roles, such as childbearing and child nurturing; and in part because women have been directed into certain occupations and excluded from others. Traditional societies tend to have very different roles for men and women in society and the division of work may be determined by following cultural norms; in some tribes and countries, for example, women farm and rear children while men hunt, weave, and manufacture goods. Through the process of industrialization and urbanization these traditional roles tend to break down and women are often recruited into low wage–paying jobs in manufacturing and service industries very early in a country's economic development.

In North America and Europe, economic factors tended to push women out of the paying job market after the Industrial Revolution. Wages rose to the point that only one wage earner was needed to support most families. For social reasons, this position was considered to be the duty of the husband and father; the woman of the household was expected to stay home. Briefly during World War II, women entered the workforce in large numbers to replace men in military service. Following the war, however, the pattern of women staying at home returned. The rise of women's rights in the 1970s in North America and Europe occurred at a time when real wage rates were beginning to fall. Barriers to women returning to the workforce lessened as women entered many occupations that had previously been held nearly exclusively by men. With declining real wages, families also increasingly required two wage earners to maintain their standard of living. In addition, the number of single-parent families increased, the parent in most cases being the mother, so she was responsible for earning the family's income. The result was that what began as a movement toward social equality of opportunity became a financial necessity for many families. Currently, changes in productivity and declining real wages for workers in less skilled occupations is creating a crisis of employment and underemployment for many families that had been economically secure a few years ago. Because women generally earn less than men and are disproportionately concentrated in occupations that are made redundant by technology or subject to cutbacks, women risk being forced out of the workforce again, but this time into poverty.

In developing countries, the situation is somewhat different. Women are often the primary family wage earners, especially when they work in industries that produce goods for export, such as light manufacturing. Social barriers to women earning wages break down rapidly with urbanization and the greater availability of such jobs in many urban areas. The continued role of women in rearing children, however, places a *double burden* on women who are also wage earners in developing societies, and the risks of occupational injuries may jeopardize their ability to provide primary care to their children.

Women show some differences in physical capacity compared to men. These differences place women at a disadvantage for the relatively well-paying heavy industrial jobs in manufacturing. On average, for example, women have less upper body strength than men and perform less well on tests of strength than men. However, individual women may outperform most men on any physical tests, and may have better endurance. In any case, such physical characteristics are only meaningful in relation to a particular job specification and particular candidates;

they are irrelevant if the job is designed such that physical strength is not a factor. Women's productivity is equal to that of men or higher among employees in most jobs where the comparison can be made. Women are at comparatively less disadvantage in the rapidly growing service sector or light manufacturing, although, as discussed by Messing (1997) much more attention is needed to occupational health issues facing women.

Women workers face specific problems that arise from their reproductive and social roles and are often a disadvantage for promotion and career development. Pregnancy leave and time for child rearing is a particular problem for female workers, albeit many men face problems too if they want time off to co-parent. Many countries have legislated requirements for employers to provide pregnancy leave (or even parental leave), usually unpaid but with a guarantee of return to employment, on the grounds that the time spent nurturing young children is an investment in society and the future. Child care is often a problem for women who work out of the home. Women may have to take paid or unpaid leave to take care of members of the family; as women are usually the caregivers in the family, they may need to take care of sick or disabled children, spouses, or parents. The social division of roles between men and women often leaves women with the responsibility for the household and for food shopping, which translates into less time for relaxation after the job.

Because women usually earn less than men in the same job, their loss of earnings due to work-related injury or illness may not be protected to the same degree by social security insurance, workers' compensation, unemployment insurance, or private disability insurance. When they lose their job, these benefits may pay less than for men because they are indexed to previous income. Where such social safety nets are lacking, they may be faced with much greater difficulty earning a living if they lose their jobs. Where no work is available and the having situation is desperate, it is typical for men to resort to crime and for younger women to resort to prostitution, which carries a high risk of disease, violence, and exploitation. Inheritance and divorce laws frequently place women at a disadvantage, making single women even more dependent on their jobs.

Occupational hazards experienced by women may place others in the family at risk. Reproductive hazards may affect a pregnant woman's fetus. Some toxic exposures, such as those to lead and asbestos, may be carried home on either parent's clothing and affect children at home. An occupational injury or illness that can result in serious economic loss for a two–wage earner family may throw a single-parent household into poverty overnight.

Sensitive employers seek to understand the needs of women employees, such as the provision of child care, sensible absence policies that permit women to take time off for caregiving, and working conditions that are free of hazards that might affect the woman, the fetus in pregnancy, or children at home.

DIMENSIONS AND TYPES OF OCCUPATIONAL HEALTH PROBLEMS

The *Global Estimates for Health Situation Assessments and Projections* has suggested that there were 32.7 million occupational injuries and 146,000 occupational deaths in 1990. Among exposed populations worldwide it is estimated that the incidence of silicosis is 3.5%–43.8%; byssinosis, 5%–30%; lead poisoning, 2.6%–37%; noise-induced hearing loss, 1.7%–70%; and occupational skin diseases, 1.7%–86% (WHO, 1992e). Occupational health hazards can be classified by the nature of the hazard, as was done in Chapter 2. The main groups are chemical, physical, mechanical, biological, and psychosocial hazards. Examples of the illness and injuries they can cause are given below.

Underdiagnosis and underreporting are known to be a large problem. Thus official statistics are not reliable. In practice, the distribution of occupational diseases in developed countries is thought to be approximated by the *rule of halves*, which states that the distribution of occupational diseases in a large working population in a diversified economy tends to be divided as follows: skin disorders account for roughly half of all occupational illnesses; eye disorders, roughly half of the remainder (or 1/4); lung disorders, half of that (or 1/8); and half of the residual are systemic toxicity problems. This general approximation holds true as a rough guide for industrialized communities but may be distorted somewhat in smaller communities where a single dominant industry presents an unusual hazard, such as in coal mining. It should be noted that this analysis does not include musculoskeletal conditions, which are quite widespread.

In developing countries, where underdiagnosis and underreporting may be particularly problematic, contact with communicable diseases, toxic substances, unsafe machinery, extremes of heat and cold, and other hazards is made worse by a lack of personal protective equipment (see Chapter 4). In addition, occupational health services are lacking and standards have either not been adopted or are not enforced. Common occupational diseases include respiratory diseases caused by particulates, lead poisoning, pesticide poisoning, hearing loss, and skin diseases (Jeyaratnam, 1992; Baker and Landrigan, 1993). Health hazards in the workplace may also be exacerbated by malnutrition or chronic disease. Nonalcoholic liver disease is widespread in Africa and Asia and may make workers who suffer from it less able to detoxify the toxic substances they encounter at work (Ong et al., 1993).

Occupational Chemical Hazards

Chemical hazards are illustrated by the sections above on toxic metals, solvents, and bulk raw materials. In general, occupational exposures to these and most other hazards are much greater than exposures that occur generally in the environment. The workplace is an artificial, constructed environment that exists for an economic purpose, and its primary function is to produce a product or service. To do this, chemicals are often required as raw materials, for processes important to production, for maintenance and cleaning, and for transportation and packaging. Even in offices various chemicals are used to produce documents, maintain machines, and clean the workplace. It should not be surprising, therefore, that exposure to chemicals in the workplace is typically more intense and often more prolonged than exposure to most chemicals in the natural environment, at least for the people who work in that workplace. Much environmental pollution reflects the release of some of these same chemicals into the environment, so that control of occupational health represents one approach to controlling environmental pollution but primarily represents control of the somewhat higher exposures experienced by the people who work there. As discussed in Chapter 4, the key to controlling exposure to chemical hazards is usually to substitute less toxic chemicals for the same purpose, reduce the local concentrations through ventilation or tighter containment, or use personal protection such as respirators and gloves.

Chemical hazards may affect any organ system in the body (see Chapter 2). However, some disorders are more common than others as a result of chemical exposure in the workplace. Skin disorders are most common, particularly skin rashes caused by irritation or allergies to the chemical. Eye disorders, usually associated with irritation, are also common. Of the serious or life-threatening conditions, the most common are respiratory disorders, including asthma, irritation-induced bronchitis, and deep lung injury. The most common occupational lung diseases are discussed in Box 10.3. See ILO (1998) or an occupational lung disease text (for example, Morgan and Seaton, 1995) for further details.

BOX 10.3

Common Occupational Lung Diseases

PNEUMOCONIOSIS

The *pneumoconioses* are diseases characterized by the deposition of dust in the lungs and the pulmonary response to its presence. The degree of fibrosis (scarring) that results varies with the properties of the dust. Silica and the fibrous silicates, such as asbestos or zeolite, cause intense fibrotic reactions. Carbon black or iron oxide provokes only small and localized reactions. Even relatively benign dusts may be associated with more serious responses when combined with other exposures, such as toxic gases or carcinogens that may adsorb on the surface of particles.

Asbestosis, often called *white lung,* is a common and serious pneumoconiosis resulting from the inhalation of large quantities of asbestos fibers. The disease is a risk for shipyard workers, plumbers and pipe fitters, insulation workers, members of the building trades, and many others working where asbestos had been used heavily and without tight control. The natural history of the disease is progression of the restrictive impairment, sometimes to total disability, and a very high risk of cancer. The disease is not associated with smoking, but smoking clearly makes the symptoms worse and the management more difficult once the disease appears. Asbestos exposure also causes lung cancer and the risk of this disease increases dramatically in asbestos workers who smoke.

Silicosis is an ancient disease that continues today in numerous occupations. Silica exposure is a hazard of mining and quarrying, older techniques of sandblasting and etching, foundry work, industrial and artisan ceramics, and innumerable occupations in which finely pulverized silica flour is employed as a filler material. When combined with tuberculosis, the resulting condition of silicotuberculosis can be a devastating, swiftly progressive fibrotic process that resembles a malignancy. The complication of silicosis by tuberculosis is common and may be devastating. The impaired lung cannot contain the tuberculosis infection and the result is an accelerated fibrotic process that may require lifelong treatment with anti-tuberculosis medication to control. Individuals with silicosis are predisposed to initial infection by the

(continued)

tubercle bacillus once exposed or reactivated. They may also be vulnerable to other bacterial infections.

Coal workers pneumoconiosis (CWP), or *black lung,* is probably the best-known dust disease of the lung. This disease and other lung diseases associated with coal mining are declining in frequency as a result of dust suppression in the mines.

TOXIC INHALATION

Toxic inhalation is a general term for the serious pulmonary toxicity of a variety of gases presenting similar clinical patterns, including ozone, phosgene, chlorine, nitrogen dioxide, hydrogen fluoride, and many others. Exposure to these gases at the levels required to produce this condition is usually the result of accidental release, uncontrolled chemical reactions, or fires. Certain of these gases, particularly phosgene, chlorine, and nitrogen dioxide, are generated when plastic furnishings and interior design fixtures burn, as in a hotel fire. In such combustion situations, cyanide and carbon monoxide are also released and contribute to toxicity.

OCCUPATIONAL ASTHMA

Asthma is a complex of symptoms and signs resulting from reversible obstruction of air flow. Usually asthma presents as wheezing and shortness of breath, occurring repeatedly in isolated episodes, often immediately following exposure to a recognizable allergen. In a few cases of asthma, cough may be the major symptom. In occupational asthma, the agent may be difficult to identify and the pattern of airways obstruction may be unusual or delayed. The easiest agents to identify are those that are highly sensitizing and that trigger the familiar immediate hypersensitivity reaction. Such conventional allergic *sensitizers* include animal secretions, ethylene diamine, grain dusts, detergent enzymes, epoxy resin curing agents, and virtually any organic or small-molecular-weight compounds, including metals such as platinum salts.

A few produce reactions by mechanisms that are not typical of the common immediate hypersensitivity reaction, such as grain dust, wood dust, formaldehyde, pharmaceutical agents, and toluene diisocyanate (TDI), a particularly potent sensitizing chemical used in the production of polyurethane plastics. Isocyanates in general, and TDI in particular, are among the most common chemicals in industry, present in most paints, coatings, and finishing preparations. Isocyanate-induced asthma is particularly common in autobody shops because of the use of binders containing isocyanates in fibrous glass repair work. In such cases, the responses may be mixed with immune, irritant, and pharmacologic mechanisms playing some role. Isocyanates are both potent sensitizers and irritants, with either mechanism promoting airway reactivity.

HYPERSENSITIVITY PNEUMONITIS

Hypersensitivity pneumonitis, known in the United Kingdom as *extrinsic allergic alveolitis,* occurs when a sensitized individual inhales respirable dust containing large quantities of an antigen to which the patient mounts an immune reaction. The characteristic symptoms of hypersensitivity pneumonitis are shortness of breath, fever, chills, and cough, developing over several hours or days. Repeated exposure to the same antigen leads to an inflammatory reaction in the alveoli, a scarring reaction, and ultimately to permanent lung damage. Common antigens that produce this condition include molds, detergent enzymes, pharmaceutical agents, minute arthropods such as mites, and dust from vegetable matter such as grain or animal material such as aerosolized droppings and urine from birds. A typical situation is "farmer's lung," in which such an exposure is likely to occur when farmers handle moldy hay. This

(continued)

is an important serious lung disease to diagnose and treat. Identification and control of exposure to the offending antigen usually results in complete resolution of a potentially grave illness.

INDUSTRIAL BRONCHITIS

Workers in dusty occupations, particularly steelworkers and grain handlers, may develop a nonspecific chronic bronchitis (see Becklake, 1985; 1989). Cigarette smoking may aggravate the bronchitis.

FUME FEVERS

There are two common types of fume fever, both involving mixed pulmonary and systemic reactions to inhaled toxic agents. *Metal fume fever* results from exposure to hot metal fumes, particularly zinc, cadmium, and copper. The illness is a self-limited but highly unpleasant reaction, similar to influenza, developing an hour or so after exposure and consisting of nausea, fever and chills, malaise, myalgias, and leukocytosis. Metal fume fever lasts only 1 or 2 days and should not be confused with toxic inhalation, which may result from exposure to high concentrations of cadmium or nickel fumes or from high concentrations of volatilized mercury, or with acute lead poisoning. Metal fume fever is most often seen when inexperienced welders try to weld or cut metal that is galvanized or of mixed composition.

Polymer fume fever is a similar influenza-like reaction resulting from the pyrolysis products of Teflon and related polymers when particles settle on cigarettes and burn, and the fumes are inhaled. Polymer fume fever can be prevented by banning cigarette smoking in workplaces where products containing these polymers are fabricated. Polymer fume fever should not be confused with "meat-wrappers asthma," a problem of bronchospasm and an irritant bronchitis resulting from the inhalation of fumes generated when polyvinyl chloride film wrapping is cut using a hot wire. This used to be a common problem in supermarkets but has since been solved by adjusting the temperature of the hot wire.

Some chemicals affect the reproductive system in either men or women and can cause sterility, miscarriages, or birth defects. Table 10.1 lists agents that have been reported to adversely affect reproductive capacity. Table 10.2 summarizes known or highly suspect carcinogens in the workplace.

Neurotoxicity is another serious problem associated with both heavy metals and solvents, as described in the sections above, and with other chemicals. Likewise, liver and kidney toxicity are common responses to chemical exposure. Recently, there has been much attention given to the effect of chemical exposure on the immune system. It seems likely that research in this field will yield many insights into subtle health effects that are currently not known in detail.

Physical Hazards

Physical hazards are also very common at worksites. Noise is by far the most widespread of the occupational hazards, and the high incidence of noise-induced hearing loss worldwide demonstrates that it remains one of the most poorly controlled. (Chapter 4 provided an example of an occupational noise control pro-

TABLE 10.1

SELECTED AGENTS REPORTED TO AFFECT REPRODUCTIVE CAPACITY

ANTINEOPLASTIC AGENTS

Alkalating agents, alkaloids, antimetabolites, anti-tumor antibiotics

CENTRAL NERVOUS SYSTEM DRUGS

Alcohol, anesthetic gases/vapors

METALS AND TRACE ELEMENTS

Aluminum, arsenic, beryllium, boranes, boron, cadmium, cobalt, lead (inorganic and organic), manganese, mercury (inorganic and organic), molybdenum, nickel, selenium, silver, uranium, zinc

INSECTICIDES

Benzene hexachlorides (lindane), carbamates (carbaryl), chlorobenzene derivatives (DDT, methoxychlor), indane derivatives (aldrin, chlordane, dieldrin), phosphate esters (dichloro, hexa-methylphosphoramide), miscellaneous (chlordecone)

HERBICIDES

Chlorinated phenoxyacetic acids (2, 4-dichlorophenoxyacetic acid, 2, 4, 5-trichlorophenoxyacetic acid) quaternary ammonium compounds (diquat, paraquat)

RODENTICIDES

Metabolic inhibitors (fluoroacetate)

FUNGICIDES, FUMIGANTS, AND STERILANTS

Apholate, captan, carbon disulfide, dibromochloropropane, ethylene dibromide, ethylene oxide, thiocarbamates, triphenyltin

FOOD ADDITIVES AND CONTAMINANTS

Aflatoxins, cyclamate, diethylstilbestrol, dimethylnitrosamine, gossypol, metanil yellow, monosodium glutamate, nitrofuran derivatives

INDUSTRIAL CHEMICALS

Aniline, carbon monoxide, chlorinated hydrocarbons (hexafluoroacetone, polybromated biphenyls, polychlorinated biphenyls, tetrachloro-dibenzo-p-dioxin), ethylene oxide, formaldehyde, hydrazine, monomers (vinyl chloride, chloroprene), polycyclic aromatic hydrocarbons, solvents (benzene, carbon disulfide, glycol ethers, epichlorohydrin, hexane, thiophene, toluene, xylene), toluene diisocyanate

MISCELLANEOUS

Physical factors (heat, light, hypoxia), radiation, certain infectious agents

Source: McGuigan, 1992.

gram.) In some countries, excessively hot or cold working environments are common. There are also sources of ultraviolet irradiation outdoors and in some workplaces that have effects like those described in Chapter 11. Ionizing radiation, is a familiar type of exposure because it is common in health care settings and is a risk in the nuclear industry, as noted in Chapter 9. Although laser light (because it is so concentrated) is a serious physical hazard in some technical settings, lasers used in applications such as supermarket checkout counters are too low in energy to induce injuries.

TABLE 10.2

SELECTED KNOWN OR HIGHLY SUSPECT CARCINOGENS IN THE WORKPLACE

Substance	Where Encountered
Acrylonitrile	Plastic and textile industries
Arsenic	Very widespread
Asbestos	Very widespread, especially in construction, auto repair, shipbuilding; present in many products
Auramine and magenta	Dye manufacturing
Benzene	Very widespread in industry as solvent and chemical constituent
Benzidine	Clinical pathology laboratories; chemical dyestuffs, plastics, rubber, wood products
β-naphthylamine	Chemical, dyestuffs, and rubber industries
Bis(chloromethyl) ether (BCME)	Chemical industry, nuclear reactor fuel processing
Carbon tetrachloride	Very widespread
Chloroform	Chemical and pharmaceutical, textile, and solvent industries
Chloromethyl methyl ether (CMME)	Chemical industry
Chloroprene	Synthetic rubber industry
Chromate (hexavalent)	Electroplating, metal products, photography, textile industries
Coke oven emissions	Steel mills, coke ovens
Cutting oils	Machining, metal working trades
Ethylene dibromide	Foodstuff (fumigation), gasoline, additive industries, pesticides
Ethyleneimine	Chemical, paper, and textile industries
4,4-methylene-bis (2-chloroaniline)	Plastics manufacturing: elastomer, epoxy resins, polyurethane foam
Hydrazine	Mechanical applications, pharmaceutical industry
Ionizing radiation	Very widespread, especially medical and industrial X-ray
Leather dust	Leather goods industry
Nickel	Widespread, especially in metal products, chemicals, battery industries
N-nitrosodimethylamine	Chemical, rubber, solvent, and pesticide industries
Polychlorinated biphenyls (PCBs)	Very widespread, particularly in utilities, electric power, chemical and wood products industries
3,3-dichlorobenzidine	Pigment manufacturing, polyurethane production
Trichlorethylene	Previously very widespread use as solvent and degreasing agent, now withdrawn from use
Ultraviolet light	Ubiquitous
Uranium and radon	Underground mining
Vinyl chloride	Petrochemical, plastics, and rubber industries
Wood dust	Hard wood industries

For more information on carcinogens as classified by various organizations, see www.esh.bnl.gov/cms/carcinogens.

Mechanical Hazards

Mechanical hazards may be of two general types: unsafe working conditions and ergonomic hazards. The science of *ergonomics* generally includes the control of hazards that may result in acute injury as well as chronic disorders usually of the musculoskeletal system, as noted in Chapter 2. Unsafe working conditions are those that may allow a sudden release of energy (such as an overly pressurized gas cylinder) that can cause injury or that place the worker at risk of injury, such as a fall, laceration, or a sprain. The key to controlling unsafe working conditions is to reduce the amount of energy that could be released and to build in guards, barriers, and other devices that protect the worker.

Ergonomic hazards result from a mismatch between the worker's body and the design of the workstation. The result is a disproportionate strain that is placed on an intrinsically weak part of the body—e.g., a chair fails to support the back properly or a work station is designed in such a way that the worker must stretch to perform a common task. The usual result is an injury that results from the cumulative effect of the strain, not a single injury event. Repetitive strain injuries among typists and keyboard operators, assembly line workers using vibrating tools for prolonged periods, or supermarket checkout clerks who handle items with repetitive motion at the wrist are examples of ergonomic hazards (see Yassi, 1997; 2000 for a review of this topic).

Biological Hazards

Biological hazards are most obvious in health care and agriculture but may occur in many other industries. Infection with one or more viruses that cause hepatitis is another major concern. *Tuberculosis* (TB) is a serious problem among hospital workers. Infection with the *human immunodeficiency virus* (HIV) (the AIDS virus), or with the hepatitis B virus can occur from needlestick injuries or blood contact and, understandably, is widely feared. *Leptospirosis*, a bacterial infection spread by contact with rat urine, occurs in some occupations and is a risk in the sugar cane industry. *Brucellosis* is another disease of farmers and slaughterhouse workers and is caused by contact with cows, pigs, and goats. Sewage workers are at risk for some of these infectious diseases (although not TB or AIDS; see Box 10.4).

Problems associated with allergies and reactions to organic products are common in agriculture. Encounters with poisonous or otherwise hazardous species can occur in clearing brush and working in remote areas, especially in the tropics. These problems tend to be highly specific to particular areas and so it is difficult to generalize about them.

Psychological Hazards

As discussed in Chapter 2, it is now generally accepted that stress at work is associated with lack of control over the working environment and with high workplace demands. Such stress-producing circumstances, however, are precisely what has been created in the workplace as a result of economic restructuring. In this vein, expectations of behavior in the workplace that show commitment and a drive for increased productivity may be seen as positive to managers and stressful by workers. The psychological stress from being unemployed can also be severe. Generally, it is difficult to separate out stress at work from stress in daily life.

INDUSTRIAL ENVIRONMENTAL ACCIDENTS

Table 10.3 lists examples of the major environmental disease outbreaks that resulted in a substantial number of reported deaths or severe illness. Numerous other incidents have been reported with fewer reported cases of illness, often because of effective management of the mishap. The accidents listed in the table include only chemical poisoning outbreaks in the community around an industry or in the community consuming certain contaminated food products. Some of these have been due to sudden accidental releases of chemicals, such as the Bhopal case, and others have involved long-term low-level pollution that finally reached danger levels, such as the Toyama case. These major poisoning

TABLE 10.3

SELECTED MAJOR "ENVIRONMENTAL DISEASE" OUTBREAKS DUE TO
NONRADIOACTIVE CHEMICALS

Location and Year	Environmental Hazard	Type of Disease	Number Affected
Toyama, Japan, 1950s	Cadmium in rice	Kidney and bone disease ('Itai-itai disease')	200 with severe disease, many more with slight effects
Minamata, Japan, 1950s	Methylmercury in fish	Neurological disease ('Minamata disease')	200 with severe disease, 2000 suspected with disease
Fukuoka, Japan, 1968	Polychlorinated biphenyls in food oil	Skin disease, general weakness	Several thousands
Iraq, 1972	Methylmercury in seed grains	Neurological disease	500 deaths, 6500 hospitalized
Madrid, Spain, 1981	Anilin or other toxin in food oil	Various symptoms	340 deaths, 20,000 cases
Bhopal, India, 1984	Methylisocyanate	Acute lung disease	2000 deaths, 200,000 poisoned

outbreaks of an epidemic type are those that receive the most attention and become known as classic environmental diseases. However, it should not be forgotten that long-term pollution situations, such as the high level of particulate pollution in many major cities of developing countries, leads to a much greater public health impact than the dramatic outbreaks. If these dramatic outbreaks serve as warnings of what can happen if proper prevention is not applied, their negative consequences can perhaps be balanced by improved prevention in the future.

As mentioned in previous sections, major accidents due to fires in industries are not uncommon. Injuries can be dramatic, and both the burning materials themselves and the smoke may contain very toxic compounds. The water and foam spread on fires by firefighters can, of course, contain the fire, but they can also spread the pollution of chemicals burning or chemicals stored on the burning premises. Depending on the type of chemicals involved, the current advice to firefighters is to let the fire burn out, and to use water and foam only to cool surrounding buildings so that they do not catch fire. Radioactive contamination from fires in nuclear power stations or other nuclear installations a particularly dangerous problem. The fire in the Chernobyl power station in 1986 is the most dramatic accident of this type (WHO, 1995c).

Apart from fires, major natural disasters, including earthquakes, landslides, floods, and storms, can lead to damage to industrial installations and accidental release of environmental hazards. Prevention of serious injury involves careful planning of the siting of installations, so that they are protected from these natural hazards to the extent possible. In addition, emergency plans and drills involving workers and the community should be established.

APPROACHES TO PREVENTION

Applying a Prevention Framework

The principles of managing risks and controlling hazards were introduced in Chapter 4. Prevention of injuries and diseases from occupational health hazards is based on two basic concepts: (1) the work environment and the production technology itself should be designed so that health risks are reduced to a minimum, and (2) the worker should be educated and encouraged to behave safely and use protective equipment. In the former case, the main responsibility for ensuring a safe and healthy workplace lies with the employer; in the latter case, a major part of this responsibility is shifted to the employee. In most situations both concepts apply, but it has been shown in many countries that focusing on improving the work environment and avoiding the use of dangerous processes rather than merely telling workers to be careful is the most effective preventive approach.

Human errors do occur in all of life's situations, but the impact of such errors can be reduced by building health and safety into the work environment. Countries that have developed policies for a healthy work environment in collaboration with employer and worker organizations have been particularly effective in reducing occupational injuries and diseases.

Creating a healthy work environment involves a series of decisions, including the following:

1. Can the process be designed so that the raw materials are as safe as possible?

For instance, if the paints used in painting the products use less toxic solvents (the least toxic is water), the workers will be at less risk of poisoning. The UNEP has coined the term *cleaner production* for this type of choice.

2. Can the production machinery be contained so that noise, chemicals, and dangerous machinery parts are kept away from the workers?

For instance, if paper production machines or printing presses are encapsulated at all times when they are in operation, the workers at the machine can be protected from loud noise, leakage of chemicals, and physical injuries. Modern video and computer equipment make it possible to monitor the functioning of the different parts of the machinery without workers directly observing or handling the parts when they are in operation.

3. Can levels of hazards in the work environment be reduced so that adverse health effects are prevented?

To give guidance on the maximum exposure levels that can be accepted, whether for noise, radiation, chemicals, or biological hazards, most countries have developed lists of *occupational standards*. These appear under different names, depending on the country; e.g., *maximum allowable concentrations* (MACs), *threshold limit values* (TLVs), standards, and guidance values. In some countries these are legally binding levels. In others they are aims that industry should strive for, but exceeding the guidance limits does not involve penalties. The derivation of occupational exposure standards is discussed further in the next section.

4. What type of personal protective equipment is needed for individual protection of workers?

For emergency operations and certain maintenance operations, it is clear that special protective equipment is needed. Preferably, the need for such equipment in continuous daily work situations should be reduced, because almost all equipment of this type causes difficulties for the wearer. Comfort and ease of use are just as important as the equipment's protective efficiency. A variety of products are available worldwide, and improvements and innovations in equipment design should be sought and encouraged.

5. What types of encouragement and training do workers need to ensure safe operation of the process and appropriate use of protective equipment?

All people working in industry—employers and supervisors, as well as workers—need to have a strong health and safety attitude and commitment. Encouragement for workers is best provided by industry leaders who invest in a safe working environment and participate in a dialogue about how health can be protected within the industry. Collaborative decision making in health and safety committees, combined with targeted training for all has been successful in many countries. Training for employers and supervisors is equally important.

6. What type of monitoring, evaluation, and reporting will contribute best to the encouragement of a strong health and safety attitude?

Measurement of the levels of the different hazards in the work environment, monitoring of injuries and other health damage, epidemiological analysis, eval-

TABLE 10.4
PRINCIPLES OF TESTS OF WORKERS IN OCCUPATIONAL HEALTH SURVEILLANCE

The information obtained must be of demonstrable importance to the health or safety of the worker being tested.

The test should not be a substitute for eliminating or controlling the hazard.

The test results should be applied for the purpose of improving the health and safety situation at the worksite and maintaining or improving the health of the individual tested.

The test should be specific for that substance or the family of substances being studied.

If the test is to anticipate an effect, it should detect signs at an early stage.

The workers' baseline status (i.e., before exposure in the workplace) should be known to permit later comparison and interpretation.

The test must be acceptable to the workers; a test that is painful (beyond drawing blood), very uncomfortable, or inconvenient must be clearly justified and agreed upon by the workers subjected to it.

The advantages of using a particular method to identify cases should be greater than the advantages of using alternative measures.

Each worker should be informed of his or her individual and group test results as well as the meaning and health implications of the results.

---

uation in relation to standards, and regular reporting to all workers creates confidence and ownership of the prevention process. Each report should include conclusions for further preventive actions and timetables for their implementation and should be based on joint discussions between employers and employees.

The principles of controlling hazards were introduced in Chapter 4; Table 10.4 expands on the principles of surveillance programs as they apply to the workplace. Controlling industrial hazards, whether to prevent occupational injuries and illness or environmental exposures that could have a negative impact on the community, requires an interdisciplinary approach with all members of the environmental health team working together.

Occupational Exposure Standards

Different countries set their occupational exposure standards in different ways. Most industrialized countries use *occupational exposure levels* (OELs, also called *permissible exposure levels* in the United States and *maximum allowable concentrations* in Europe), which are either peak or average concentrations that must not be exceeded in the workplace over a particular period of time. The usual times are either 8 hr or 15 min, depending on the rapidity with which health effects can occur.

The 8-hr OELs are average concentrations over this time period. A system of averaging called the *time-weighted average* (TWA) simplifies calculation; an 8-hr TWA is the average of each measured concentration weighted by the length of time it lasted during the work shift. The 8-hr TWA is fine for a standard 8-hr working shift but it may not provide sufficient protection for workers who work overtime or on longer shifts, especially against chemicals such as organic solvents that are retained in the body. Sometimes toxic effects can occur with short exposures to high concentrations, regardless of the overall average. In such cases, 15-min *short-term exposure levels* (STELs) or instantaneous ceiling levels are used as absolute maximum concentrations that cannot be exceeded under any circumstances.

The appropriate levels of standards are widely discussed and debated around the world. Although individual countries often adapt standards to fit local conditions, there is a strong tendency for countries, as they develop, to adopt a consistent international set of standards. The European Community harmonized the conflicting standards of its member states to ensure uniformity and consistency, both for worker protection and to prevent unfair economic advantages for countries that did not enforce safe workplaces.

The most influential single body in recommending and promoting these levels has been the *American Congress of Governmental Industrial Hygienists* (ACGIH), which, despite its name, is international in its membership, has no relationship to Congress or the U.S. government, and includes many occupational health professionals who are not hygienists. The ACGIH, through its committees, establishes *threshold limit values* (TLVs), which are recommended occupational exposure levels set to protect all or most workers (excepting those with particular susceptibility) and are based on the best available evidence in the scientific medical and hygiene literature. The ACGIH also establishes *biological exposure indices* (BEIs), which are special tests that detect a chemical or its metabolite in the blood, urine, or expired air of a worker and that can be used together with, or instead of, workplace measurements. The TLVs are often adopted, without change, by governments around the world as the basis for their OELs.

Despite its prestige and authority, the ACGIH has been heavily criticized for setting TLVs on the basis of inadequate evidence and being influenced by economic issues. In particular, it has been accused of allowing a conflict of interest by having industry representatives on its TLV committees. Its BEIs have also been criticized as being efforts to make workers "guinea pigs," blaming them for the exposure rather than controlling exposure in the workplace. The ACGIH can be defended on the grounds that its recommendations take into consideration what was practical at the time and that any effort to set standards without the participation of industry would be doomed to failure. The BEIs are also highly sensitive and protect workers' health because they measure all the exposure that the worker has actually experienced, not just what may be in the particular area of the workplace where a monitor is set up.

Lists comparing standards in different countries have been published by the ILO and the UNEP/IRPTC (see website irptc.unep.ch/irptc). The WHO has prepared health-based maximum exposure limits for a selection of chemicals and produces jointly with the ILO and the UNEP a series of *Environmental Health Criteria* that provide guidance on the exposure levels that may affect health (see website www.who.int/pcs/). Similarly, the WHO continues to work jointly with the International Atomic Energy Association, the Industrial Radiation Protection Association, and other international agencies to produce guidance on safe exposure levels to various radiation hazards.

1. Consider the ethical issues that may arise in occupational health, particularly with respect to the competing interests of employers and workers. As an official or consultant attempting to solve a problem related to an occupational hazard, how would you deal with these ethical issues?

2. Consider the situation for women in the workplace in you country. Is it likely that their health is affected differently from men's health by the conditions discussed in this section? If so, how?

3. Consider the differences between industry-related (i.e., occupational and environmental) health problems in developed countries compared to those in developing countries. How do these differences influence the programs that must be developed to manage these problems? Consider the role of the various professionals involved in assessing and managing industrial pollution.

11

TRANSBOUNDARY AND GLOBAL HEALTH CONCERNS

LEARNING OBJECTIVES

After studying this chapter you will be able to do the following:

- describe the relationship between global ecological change and health
- summarize the evidence and the debates regarding these global health threats
- identify the obstacles to resolving these problems and be able to formulate strategies that encourage people to think globally and act locally

We live in a time of rapid change on a global scale. Many of these changes hold the promise of positive developments in quality of life and international cooperation. Improved communication, rapidly expanding trade, and new technologies that conserve energy and resources are just a few of the changes that have a worldwide impact on society and may make tomorrow's world better than today's. However, not all global developments are likely to be positive. *Global ecological changes*, including those related to stratospheric ozone depletion, the greenhouse effect, deforestation and desertification, loss of biodiversity, interregional transport of pollution, and large-scale resource depletion, are having a major impact on communities worldwide. The implications of environmental trends for weather, human habitation, and food supply suggest serious trouble ahead. To these environmental hazards, which are largely due to industrial development or economic pressures on agriculture, must be added the environmental consequences of intentional destruction from war. Willful destruction for military or political advantage has become one of the major issues in global ecological change.

In the past, most of these environmental hazards and the effects of environmental pollution were treated as local issues and were generally handled on a local level by public health authorities. In recent years, however, the scope of environmental issues has broadened considerably and there is no clear dividing line between problems that used to be considered public health problems and those that involve large-scale ecological change. The degradation of the environment has become a major global problem, outstripping its local public health dimensions and becoming a serious threat, perhaps even to human survival. We begin this chapter by examining the intentional destruction that occurs in warfare, both because of its own damaging effects and because it interferes with the international and regional cooperation needed to solve the other problems.

The general outline of the global ecological crisis is clear: rapid technological development in the developed world introduces new potential hazards in a society in which environmental degradation is historically severe but coming under relative control. Rapid population growth and industrial development, based largely on obsolete technologies in the developing world, accelerates existing environmental degradation. This is aggravated by poverty, urbanization without adequate infrastructure, rural development policies that do not strengthen local economies, and a limited economic base that is too often dependent on commodity prices. The problem of environmental degradation has become global in three distinct senses:

1. There is now imbalance on the level of entire global systems, such as climate.

2. The distribution of familiar environmental problems, such as air pollution, has become much more widespread and regionalized until these problems are encountered worldwide and not just in areas of development and urban growth.

3. The economic and political systems that operate to create and sustain these problems (but that might also hold the key to some of the solutions) have become global to the extent that the world is rapidly becoming one large market economy, beyond the capacity of governments to regulate effectively. Much of this change deals with drastic increases in consumption levels of resources and consumer goods, and rising expectations for consumption among developing societies.

The most destructive human activity is warfare. As noted by Garfield and Neugut (1997), the 1960s expression "war is not healthy for children and other living things" is so understated that one hesitates to attempt to define how unhealthy war is. Not only is war intentionally destructive between the sides engaged in fighting, but when modern warfare is practiced, the environment is another casualty. The first and most tragic consequence of war is the *direct casualties*, the soldiers and civilians who die or are maimed in the fighting, and their loved ones who must carry on. Table 11.1, with all the limitations and inaccuracies in data collection of this sort, indicate that mortality rates from war rose dramatically in the twentieth century. This was largely attributable to large increases in mortality during World Wars I and II. Prior to World War II, more war-related deaths occurred due to disease than to battlefield deaths.

The need to support a war effort and the care required by those who are wounded but survive place a burden on the society supporting the fighting. Modern warfare also strikes directly at the economic and logistical ability of the society to make war, often by targeting the environment directly. Garfield and Neugut (1997) suggest that civilian deaths compose 90% of all deaths in twentieth-century wars.

In *War and Public Health* (Levy and Sidel, 1997), the impact of war on public health is documented and suggestions of what health professionals could do to prevent war and minimize its consequences are offered. With respect to the Gulf War, for example, studies have shown that the war and trade sanctions caused a threefold increase in mortality among Iraqi children under 5 years of age (Ascherio et al., 1992). The suggestion that by using high-precision weapons with strategic targets the Allied forces were producing only limited damage to the civilian population was shown to be false, confirming that the casualties of war still extend far beyond those caused directly by warfare.

Modern Conventional Warfare

The primary purpose of modern warfare is to defeat or debilitate the enemy's society and support systems to control a strategic resource and thereby impose or avoid political domination. This is in contrast to warfare in earlier societies, when battles tended to be fought by smaller armies with limited force and the fighting

TABLE 11.1

ESTIMATED AVERAGE ANNUAL MILITARY DEATHS IN WARS, WORLDWIDE, BY CENTURY

Century	Average Annual Military Deaths	World Mid-Century Population in Millions	Average Annual Military Deaths per Million Population
17th	9500	500	19.0
18th	15,000	800	18.8
19th	13,000	1200	10.8
20th	458,000	2500	183.2

Source: Levy and Sidel, 1997.

was confined to soldiers or warriors. Sometimes, such battles were really only rituals, hurting only a small fraction of the population, and the losers were taken as hostages for ransom. Although there are many examples in history of horrific wars undertaken with crude weapons that led to great suffering, such as the Hundred Year's War in Europe, for the most part, the damage that could be done was limited.

In the eighteenth century the so-called art of war changed and by the time of Napoleon, new tactics and artillery had greatly increased the damage that one army could cause. *Scorched-earth strategies* of intentional widespread destruction were used by Russia to stop Napoleon and by General Sherman against the rebels in the American Civil War. By the time of World War I, the world had had extensive experience with a type of warfare that made all civilians targets. Such warfare did not hesitate to destroy the environment for the sake of depriving the other side of food and shelter, and it aimed at shredding the fabric of civil society to demoralize and confuse the enemy. The emphasis in modern warfare became disruption of the economy and civil society, not merely the defeat of troops and the destruction of military targets.

Displacing civilians by warfare and making them *refugees* is often part of the enemy's strategy to occupy the conquered territory (*ethnic cleansing* was the term used for this in the former Yugoslavia). Large movements of dispossessed people reflect profound human tragedy, create problems for public health and primary health care services, and add to crowding and overpopulation in the camps and communities that receive them (see Box 11.1 for environmental health management issues in refugee camps). Children of refugees may be denied education or health services and may face growing up in an unstable, hostile, and unfamiliar society. Scavenging for food and firewood may cause local ecological damage.

As tragic as scorched-earth strategies and refugee movements are, given the opportunity, people rebuild and carry on with their lives and the land usually recovers. However, following chemical, biological, or nuclear warfare, land could be contaminated for generations to come. These acts of warfare at least have a military purpose in seeking to defeat the enemy. Armies intent on winning a war are not generally interested in their environmental impact. In addition to this largely intentional devastation, the arbitrary destruction and confusion that occurs incidental to war leads to ecological damage from air and water pollution, road building through sensitive environments, and troop movements.

Chemical Warfare

Chemical warfare, introduced on a large scale in World War I, involves the controlled release of toxic chemicals, usually nerve toxins or intensely irritating agents. When used in the field, these poisons are indiscriminate in their actions and may affect civilians or troops on either side, as well as wildlife and domestic animals. These agents can cause considerable local damage and may wipe out entire villages. As a consequence, they are often considered to be weapons of terror and civilian intimidation rather than effective military measures. The agents that have actually been used in recent years do not seem to be very persistent in the environment, perhaps because armed forces that use them know that they may have to enter and occupy the same area later. The storage of chemicals used for chem-

BOX 11.1

Environmental Health Management of Refugee/Displaced Persons Camps

People who are suddenly displaced by the events of war and forced to migrate usually take their belongings with them. Such refugees are forced to depend on foster assistance to meet their most basic needs, such as food, shelter, medical care, and water. In assessing what public health measures are appropriate, officials in refugee/displaced person camps must consider the following: the types of make-shift shelters being used, the physical environment, the demographic profile of the people in the camp, and the extent and type of disease circulating in the population. The goal of the resulting public health measures should be primarily to prevent the occurrence and spread of the diseases favored by this situation. The process of identifying needs and setting priorities requires an immediate assessment of the population's health and nutritional status, as well as a rapid environmental health assessment of the available accommodation. A monitoring and reporting system should be established to assess the effectiveness of the measures, and to ensure the timely detection of newly developed risks. Environmental health measures taken should include the following:

SELECTION OF SITE AND ACCOMMODATION

- The site should be selected according to the facilities needed to provide hygienic and healthy conditions. Flood areas and natural foci of infection must be avoided.
- The accommodation site should afford an adequate protection against inclement weather conditions.
- Overcrowding should be avoided.

WATER SUPPLY

- Ensure that water is adequate in quantity and quality (consider access to water treatment and cooking facilities), and protect the source of water and water supply facilities from pollution.

REFUSE DISPOSAL

- Build hygienic field toilets according to the planned length of stay.
- Provide waste water drainage, solid waste collection and disposal, and incineration of medical wastes.

FOOD WHOLESOMENESS AND FOOD HYGIENE

- Distribute dried and preserved foods. Prepare food individually. Place storerooms (if they exist) and community feeding facilities under health surveillance, and provide hygienic food preparation courses.

INSECT AND RODENT CONTROL

- Controls should be based on prevention.

In addition, provisions must be made for child immunization, health education, patient treatment, drug supply, medical personnel, and a health service scheme, including a system for referrals to inpatient facilities.

Provided by Krunoslav Capak, Croatian National Institute of Public Health.

ical warfare has sometimes created a hazard, particularly over many years when the containers begin to disintegrate. Although chemical weapons have been outlawed for a very long time by an international agreement known as the *Hague Declaration*, there have been many documented instances of their use and many more suspected incidents in which absolute proof has been lacking or controversial.

Biological Warfare

Biological warfare, which is even more difficult to control, involves targeted release of pathogens such as viruses and bacteria. In the few instances in which it has been tried, there have been limited outbreaks of disease involving local residents and wildlife. The effects of biological weapons are short term and unpredictable, but certain agents, are transmissible and could cause widespread epidemics. Because the weapons perform poorly in the battlefield and are unreliable against civilians, biological warfare has been used only rarely, although it has been often alleged. In recent years, world concern over biological weapons has focused chiefly on the testing and development of these weapons and the use of biological agents in laboratories released into the environment during studies to develop protective measures. These weapons have been outlawed by the *Geneva Protocol* since 1925. This was strengthened by a further Convention in 1972, to which 100 countries subscribe. In recent years there have been fears that terrorist groups would use biological agents.

Nuclear Warfare

The ultimate extension of ecological warfare is, of course, nuclear war, where the target is both the people and the region. The massive destructive power of nuclear weapons led to an impasse that dominated the latter half of this century: both sides held such massive military power that any attempt by either side to use nuclear weapons assured their mutual destruction. This climate of fear is thought to guarantee that neither side would use these weapons, a terrifying basis for peace but, to many, an effective one. Since the collapse of the Soviet Union, there is little immediate prospect of total nuclear war, but the proliferation of nuclear weapons to other countries carries a grave risk that they will be used in regional conflicts. Should a nuclear exchange ever occur, the regional devastation it would bring would be inconceivable: sudden death, fire, massive destruction, and slow death by radiation sickness for those survivors at the periphery. However, this would be only part of the impact. Release of radiation, potentially carried many miles by wind and water, disruption and contamination of food supplies, shortages of medical services and supplies, and the susceptibility to infection of malnourished and irradiated survivors would result in massive casualties well beyond the initial blast zone. It is also possible that a massive exchange would propel huge quantities of debris into the atmosphere, creating dust clouds that would block sunlight and cause a prolonged cooling of the earth's surface called *nuclear winter* (see Robock, 1991).

The testing and production of nuclear weapons continue to pose a threat of accidental release and local contamination. The sites of several nuclear weapons plants are reported to be seriously contaminated and radionuclides have been detected in groundwater downstream from at least one plant in the United States, although the details are usually military secrets. Test sites in the South Pacific used by the United States after World War II have shown high levels of residual radiation and radionuclide contamination decades after the test, which is not surprising considering the long half-lives of some decay products of uranium and plutonium.

Release to the atmosphere and across long distances was a serious concern for above-ground nuclear testing and venting from below-ground testing, and low levels of radionuclides such as strontium-90 were well documented to have migrated with prevailing winds from test sites in the 1950s and 1960s, before bilateral test ban treaties were negotiated between the United States and the Soviet Union. In the current complicated world situation, there is somewhat more concern over accidental release from deteriorating stockpiles or handling accidents involving nuclear weapons.

Guerrilla Warfare, Terrorism, and Deliberate Environmental Destruction

In the twentieth century, there have been a number of regional conflicts involving *guerrilla warfare*, where one side avoids direct engagement with the enemy and instead attacks periodically and without warning, often by ambush, and seeks to escape into the surrounding countryside before an effective retaliation can be launched. Guerrilla warfare is usually undertaken by a weaker, poorly armed indigenous force against an occupying or dominant power with conventional military resources. This form of warfare rapidly escalates into environmental destruction because the dominant force finds it difficult to engage the insurrectionary force directly and so responds by destroying the villages and countryside where the insurrectionary force is concealed and supported. Indeed, destruction of the environment is often a military strategy to inflict damage on the other side in a guerrilla war. In particular, the dominant forces have sprayed tropical forests with herbicide, burned off vegetation, and employed carpet bombing of large areas, leaving craters and many unexploded bombs, and both sides have commonly planted land mines. The result has been devastated forest growth and the creation of deadly hazards that last well beyond peace or a cease-fire. In many areas of the world today, buried *land mines* are a serious hazard, particularly for people working in agriculture. It is thought that there are 100 million land mines, planted in some 64 countries. About 26,000 people, mostly civilians, are killed or injured by mines each year (see Stover et al., 1997).

Terrorism is an increasingly serious concern for the world community. The public health impact of terrorism is relatively small, in the sense that terrorist attacks create only a small number of casualties compared to the much greater number of deaths and cases of disability caused by more traditional hazards. Terrorism creates a climate of fear and depends on a collective state of anxiety to achieve its ends. There are signs, however, that terrorism may become more of a direct threat to health. The 1995 terrorist attack on the Tokyo subway, with the nerve gas sarin, caused over a dozen deaths and over a thousand casualties, making it one of the most devastating such incidents on record. The same group had also attempted attacks with biological agents. The apparently increasing capacity of some terrorist groups using explosives, biological and chemical agents and the potential access of terrorists to biological or nuclear weapons raise grave concerns about the future. The fear raised by the threat of attack adds to stress and interferes with civil society, sometimes provoking a political reaction that restricts human rights.

In recent years, a new type of environmental destruction has emerged that has no apparent military purpose. This is the practice of *ecological vandalism*, where a combatant, usually on the losing side, creates widespread ecological destruction as an act of revenge. The most familiar example of this was the oil field fires set by Iraqi troops in Kuwait during their defeat in the Gulf War. Huge clouds of smoke created a massive air pollution event that took many weeks to bring under control.

OZONE DEPLETION AND ULTRAVIOLET RADIATION

In the *stratosphere,* the upper, relatively dense layer of the atmosphere, ozone molecules tend to accumulate through the action of ultraviolet (UV) radiation on oxygen molecules. The energy quanta in UV radiation disrupt the oxygen molecule, which forms ozone (O_3). Ozone has accumulated over time in the stratosphere, where it tends to absorb UV radiation and act as a partial screen that protects the surface of the earth from higher levels of exposure. Reduction of the concentration of ozone in the stratosphere reduces the absorption of UV radiation and allows more to get through. *Ozone depletion* therefore increases exposure to UV radiation at the earth's surface. (Many excellent publications now exist on this subject; see, for example, Mungall and McLaren, 1990; WHO, 1990b; Chivian et al., 1993; McMichael, 1993; McMichael et al., 1996; UNEP, 2000).

Ultraviolet Radiation

Ultraviolet radiation carries much energy and causes tissue damage in human beings and animals (see Chapter 2, Physical Hazards). There are three types of UV radiation, all of which differ in wavelength (see Fig. 11.1). The longest wavelength, UV-C, carries the most energy but is almost completely absorbed by the upper atmosphere so it does not reach the earth's surface; UV-C will not be discussed further here. Ozone in the stratosphere in particular absorbs UV radiation completely in the UV-C range (200–290 nm) and a large proportion in the UV-B range (290–320 nm). This serves as a shield, reducing exposure at the earth's surface below the ozone layer. UV-A carries relatively low energy and is less harmful. UV-B carries somewhat more energy and causes skin damage and tanning in lighter-skinned people.

Stratospheric Ozone Depletion

Stratospheric ozone depletion is not to be confused with *tropospheric* (lower atmospheric) *ozone accumulation*. Although the same molecule is involved, both types of ozone have different health effects. Ozone in the lower troposphere is an air pollutant and throughout the troposphere it is a greenhouse gas, but in the stratosphere it provides a vital protective shield against potentially harmful UV-B irradiation. Stratospheric ozone is regenerated by splitting and recombination of oxygen when it absorbs energy from UV radiation (a process called *photolysis*). Stratospheric ozone is only minimally affected by migration of tropo-spheric ozone upward into the stratosphere.

At ground level UV irradiation is easy to measure at a single point in time but trends are difficult to interpret. Attenuation of UV radiation may occur from

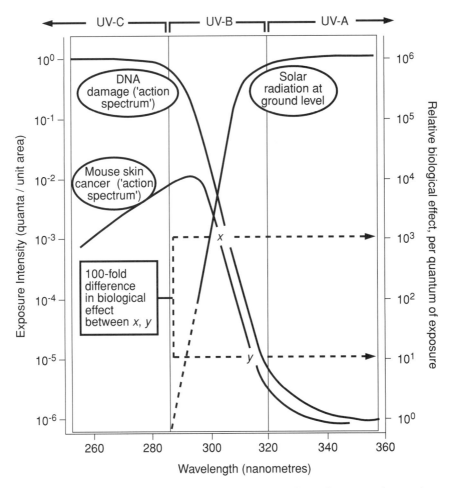

Figure 11.1 Wavelength composition of solar ultraviolet radiation at the Earth's surface, and relative biological effect. From McMichael, 1993, with permission.

dust in the atmosphere, so that at any one location there may be considerable variability in measurements from moment to moment and from year to year. Carbon dioxide accumulation and increased cloud cover tend to offset ozone depletion, introducing another set of variables that are poorly understood. Ozone depletion may not be the only significant factor to take into account in projecting future UV-B radiation at ground level. All of these factors complicate the projections that scientists make regarding future trends.

Despite these technical problems the overall pattern is clear. Ozone levels in the stratosphere are decreasing at several locations, most particularly at the North and South Poles, and UV irradiation at the earth's surface appears to be increasing in the areas beneath the thinning ozone ("ozone holes") (National Academy of Sciences, 1992). This interpretation fits with the facts as we now know them. There are early suggestions of a consistent increase in ground-level UV-B irradiation in readings in the Alps, although the areas of maximal increase are over the Poles and particularly the southern oceans where regular reduction in stratospheric ozone seems to have been most marked. It is expected that the first evidence of substantial increases in surface UV-B radiation will be seen in New Zealand, Australia, and the southern part of South America.

The stratospheric ozone layer was observed to be thinning over Antarctica about 20 years ago. Repeated observations have confirmed the attenuation and charted its progress. In 1956–76, the first 20 years of observations from space, the ozone layer was stable; since then, it has declined in thickness over Antarctica from about 300 to between 125 and 200 Dobson units (units of concentration in a vertical atmospheric column under standard conditions). The cause is the release into the atmosphere, and gradual diffusion into the stratosphere, of chemicals that destroy ozone by catalytic action, particularly the chlorofluorocarbons (CFCs).

The CFCs release chlorine by photolysis in the atmosphere; this free chlorine scavenges ozone and destroys it. One CFC molecule may destroy as many as 10,000 ozone molecules. Release of CFCs into the atmosphere occurs through industrial activity, leaks, or the decommissioning of old refrigeration and air conditioning units, as well as by use of aerosol cans that use the compounds as propellants. Substantial progress on curbing CFC generation and release on a national level has already been made with the *Montreal Protocol,* an international treaty calling for reductions in CFC production and emissions. However, given the long half-lives of the CFCs (75 years or more), the emissions already released are expected to persist in their ozone-depleting activity at significant levels well into the 22nd century (National Academy of Sciences, 1992).

Human Health Effects of Ozone Depletion

Intracellularly, UV absorption results in breakage of covalent bonds in critical macromolecules and may eventually lead to carcinogenesis, accelerated aging, and cataracts. Those at greatest risk for direct effects of UV exposure on skin are people with fair skin who sunburn easily. The human health effects of increased UV irradiation due to ozone depletion include higher risks of *non-melanoma skin cancer*, particularly squamous cell carcinoma and actinic keratitis, a premalignant condition; *malignant melanoma, cataract*, and *retinal degeneration*; and possibly impaired *immunological* responses (Jones, 1987; Rundel and Nachtwey, 1983; WHO, 1994a). Relatively minor but cosmetically significant effects may include *accelerated aging* of skin and perhaps increased frequency of *pterygia*, small wedge-shaped tissue webs on the whites of the eye. Of these conditions, the effects on immune status and the propensity for inducing skin cancer are potentially the most serious (Moan et al., 1989; Morrison, 1989). Figure 11.2 shows an estimate of the increase in skin cancer during 1979–1993 and the ozone depletion during that period.

The use of protective clothing, sunscreens, and eyeglasses (both tinted and clear) may reduce the risk of individual exposure to UV light, as may changing fashions in sunbathing and outdoor recreation. Measures taken by people to protect themselves against higher levels of UV radiation are likely to be less effective as commercial sunscreens may be effective against UV-induced sunburn if they have a high enough sun protection factor for the exposure period, but their effectiveness against UV-induced cancer is unproven. Other measures include dark or reflective clothing, parasols, truly protective sunglasses, and hats. Increased shade will be more difficult to ensure in deforested rural areas or dry areas.

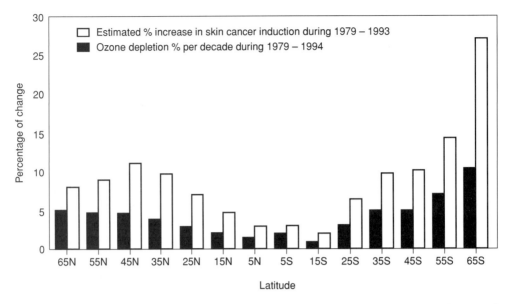

Figure 11.2 Estimated relationship between increases in stratospheric ozone depletion and skin cancer induction by latitude. From McMichael et al., 1996, with permission.

CLIMATE CHANGE AND THE GREENHOUSE EFFECT

Global climate change will occur as a result of changes in the balance of heat taken on and retained by the planet. An increase in heat may lead to global warming and chaotic weather conditions, and a decrease in heat may lead to cooling, longer winters, and an increase in water trapped in the polar ice caps. Human activity, primarily reflecting changes in industry and agriculture, causes an increase in the amount of heat retained by the planet. This leads to an average warming of the earth's surface but with a great deal of local variation, which makes it difficult to predict changes for local areas. Changes in climate of the magnitude that is predicted may lead to many health problems related to heat stress, natural weather disasters, changes in the distribution of vectors causing human and animal diseases, new infectious disease patterns, unreliable crop production, local food shortages, and flooding. Many of the health problems are likely to be indirect, resulting from the social and economic consequences of these effects (Leaf, 1989; Mungall and McLaren, 1990; Chivian et al., 1993; McMichael et al., 1996; UNEP, 2000). The *Intergovernmental Panel on Climate Change* (IPCC), which represents the concensus of the international scientific community (WRI, 1998), estimates that current emission patterns are likely to increase the average temperature 1°C to 3.5°C by 2100, and raise sea levels 15–19 centimeters (IPCC, 1996). The effects could be devastating.

The Greenhouse Effect

The term *greenhouse effect* is used to describe how the earth's atmosphere acts like the panes of glass in a greenhouse where plants are grown (see Fig. 11.3). Carbon dioxide, water vapor, and other gases in the atmosphere act like the glass in the greenhouse. The glass in the windowpane is transparent to infrared radia-

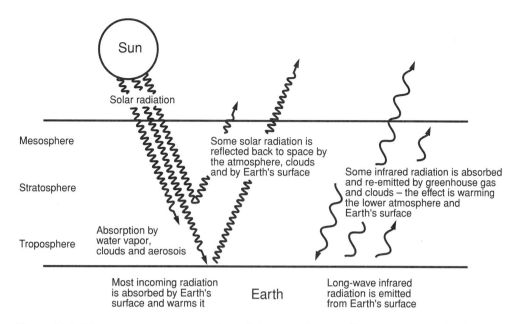

Figure 11.3 Diagrammatic representation of the greenhouse effect. From McMichael et al., 1996, with permission.

tion in sunlight, so the radiation passes through and warms the plants and interior of the greenhouse. However, the glass also insulates the greenhouse, trapping the heat that is created when the infrared radiation is absorbed Likewise, infrared radiation from the sun passes through the earth's atmosphere, but the carbon dioxide and some other gases in the atmosphere tend to insulate the earth, trapping heat. The greenhouse effect normally contributes to stability of the world's temperature and maintains the biosphere within a temperature range conducive to life—the earth absorbs a certain amount of heat and loses the same amount by radiation; the carbon dioxide and water vapor in the atmosphere keep the average temperature higher than it otherwise would have been.

Until recently, the earth's heat budget was said to be in balance, i.e., its average temperature remained stable. However, in recent years there has been an accumulation of gases in the atmosphere that upset this balance. Certain atmospheric gases trap too much heat from infrared radiation, so global temperature rises. The exaggerated greenhouse effect and resultant global warming may result in changes in regional climate and weather patterns. The accumulation of greenhouse gases appears to have raised average global temperature by an estimated $1/2$ to $1°$ Celsius from 1930 to 1990. These changes in average temperature have occurred more rapidly in the last 10 years than in any earlier period. A warming trend has been apparent since 1980, and 1998 was the warmest year ever recorded up to that time. Rises of several degrees more are predicted in the coming century. In fact, an overall global temperature rise of $3°–4°C$ degrees in the next 50 years is predicted by some experts. This increase may seem small, but on a global scale this average masks marked extremes of temperature and that has substantial implications (Mungall and McLaren, 1990; WHO, 1992a; Chivian et al., 1993; McMichael, 1993; McMichael et al., 1996). These changes are happening much faster than ever before, even considering the rapid changes at periods of transition at the end of the Ice Ages (Mungall and McLaren, 1990).

Global Warming

Global warming is likely to produce exaggerations in existing trends in weather and to make extreme weather conditions more frequent. There is no simple prediction as to what effect atmospheric changes will have on climate, except that there will not be a uniform, stable trend of rising temperature. No one weather pattern will predominate or envelop the planet.

Regional predictions are much more difficult than global predictions about average temperature and are greatly confounded by local factors of land contour, prevailing weather patterns (which may be disrupted), and proximity to the ocean. The rise in average temperature is likely to be less at the equator and in high latitudes, and greatest in mid-range latitudes where winters may be colder and the summers considerably warmer than at present (Hansen et al., 1989; WHO, 1992a; McMichael et al, 1996). Figure 11.4 shows how estimated global temperature has increased during the last 140 years.

Effects of Global Warming

Changes in climate of the magnitude that is anticipated are likely to lead to certain important outcomes: health problems related to heat stress, natural weather

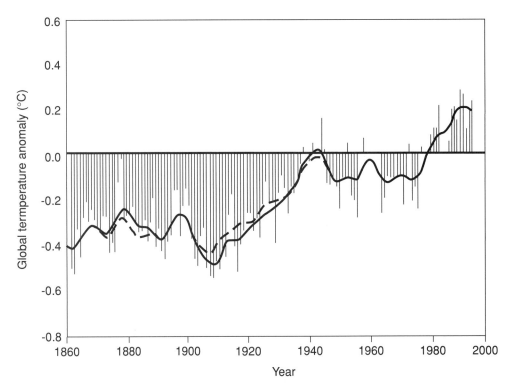

Figure 11.4 Combined land and sea temperatures, 1861–1994. From McMichael et al., 1996, with permission.

disasters, changes in vector distribution and, consequently, infectious disease patterns, unreliable crop production, and flooding (McMichael et al., 1996). Many of the health problems are likely to be indirect. Unlike previous periods of rapid change in climate, humankind is now dependent on an intricate system of agriculture, trade, and communication that threatens to be disrupted. Social disruptions leading to violent behavior may also be a factor in situations of food shortage or prolonged heat stress. Violent behavior has been shown to increase in frequency in hot weather, leading to the possibility of increased incidents of civil disturbance (Last, 1992; Chivian et al., 1993).

Major cities of the world may have increased numbers of very hot days each year, and the heat waves may last longer. The effect of this on mortality is likely to be diffuse, affecting all causes of death and not just cardiovascular causes. An estimate of the likely effect of an increase in summer temperatures of only 2°C can be derived from a surveillance study of heat-related fatalities in the major cities in the state of Missouri from 1979 to 1987. In July 1980, a prolonged heat wave of this magnitude occurred; the temperature exceeded the normal daily maximum of 31°C for 21 days and exceeded 38°C on several occasions. Approximately 1 in every 4000 residents developed heat stroke and 1 in every 1400 developed a heat-related illness that was either fatal or required hospitalization. An excess of approximately 300 deaths from heat-related conditions was observed, somewhat under half due to heat stroke (Jones et al., 1982; see Fig. 11.5).

Global warming may disrupt ocean currents and establish anomalous flows of air, comparable to the trade winds and jet streams. As well as causing more prolonged droughts, global warming may increase the frequency of severe precipitation, especially in the tropics. The result may be an increase in the frequency and severity of violent weather disturbances such as hurricanes, tornadoes, typhoons, floods, and blizzards. In 1988, North America experienced a major

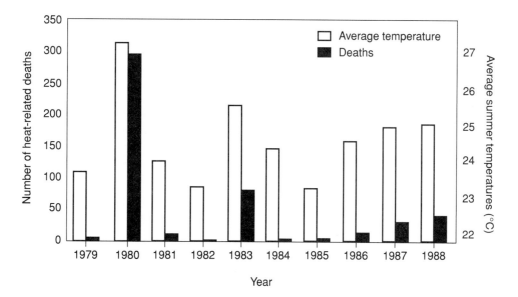

Figure 11.5 Annual fluctuations in average summer temperature and heat-related health in Missouri, USA, 1979–88. From McMichael, 1993, with permission.

drought associated with the previous year's *El Niño,* which is a periodic mid-ocean upswelling in the southeastern Pacific. The high-pressure area displaced the jet stream (a current in the atmosphere) northward and diverted rain-carrying weather systems away from their usual region of precipitation. Whether this episode was influenced by a global warming trend is unclear. The conditions that were set up, however, appear to be very similar to those that would occur with increasing ocean temperatures (Schneider, 1987; Mungall and McLaren, 1990).

Agriculture may also be significantly affected by global warming. A combination of effects of global warming could lead to food shortages. The negative effects on productivity of increased temperature and aridity on crop yields and growing ranges are likely to counteract the increase in growing yields predicted for many crops as a result of increased availability of carbon dioxide. An unpredictable consequence of climate change is the impact it may have on the distribution of major pests affecting crop yields, and the subsequent effect on food spoilage.

Global warming may cause a rise of about a meter in sea level over the next 50–100 years. Exaggerated tides may threaten low-lying cities and coastal zones. Many cities and populated regions are built in low-lying coastal areas for historical reasons usually related to shipping access. Examples include Shanghai, London, Bangkok, New York City, Tokyo, Osaka, Vancouver, Rio de Janeiro, Bombay, Saint Petersburg, Dar es Salaam, New Orleans, almost all of Bangladesh, and most of The Netherlands. These population centers face significant flooding threats due to global warming (Last, 1992; Chivian et al., 1993).

Through the impact of climate on temperature and geochemistry of the world's oceans, the functional relationships within marine food webs may be altered. Thus one finds increasing evidence of coastal eutrophication and altered phytoplankton biomass and species dominance. Paralytic, diarrheal, neurologic, and amnesic *shellfish poisoning* as well as ciguatera, pufferfish, and scromboid fish poisoning, all related to algal biotoxins, appear to be spreading in a global epidemic of coastal algal blooms (Anderson 1992; Smayda and Shimizu, 1993). These effects, along with the changing environments from many other stresses, have direct consequences for human health and nutrition (Rapport 1995a, 1995b, 1997; see Box 11.2).

The distribution of vegetation would also change drastically in a short period of time, relative to the past rate of change on earth, if global warming occurs on a massive scale. One likely consequence of this redistribution of vegetation ranges is expansion in the geographical range of insect vectors of human disease, including that of *anophelene* and *colicine mosquitoes.* The arthropod-borne virus diseases may extend their range, including viral hemorrhagic fevers such as yellow fever, dengue, and different types of viral encephalitis. Malaria may also extend its range. In fact, evidence suggests that this has already been occurring (see Box 11.3).

Box 11.4 illustrates how tick-borne diseases, such as *typhus* and *Lyme disease,* may change in distribution because of the change in range of the ticks' mammalian host species. *Schistosomiasis,* which is caused by a tropical and subtropical waterborne parasite that depends on a snail host, is also likely to spread as the range of its host expands, particularly with more damming for water con-

BOX 11.2

Emerging Diseases Related to Changes in Marine
Environment Source

Coastal marine environments are being altered as a result of excessive loading of
wastes and nutrients, as well as physical restructuring (e.g., reclamation of wetlands,
building of harbours), overharvesting of fish, and other stresses. These changes coupled with local rises in sea temperatures have led to the emergence of new diseases
and the resurgence of old ones. A few examples are illustrative of changes over the
past decade:

EMERGENCE OF *PFIESTERIA PISCIDA:* THE "AMBUSH PREDATOR"

This species is responsible for major fish kills in Maryland, North Carolina and off
the Florida coast.

ASSOCIATION OF PERIODIC OUTBREAKS OF VIBRIOS WITH ALGAL BLOOMS

In Asia, there has long been an association between the seasonal appearance of
cholera and the yearly blooms of algae, zooplankton, and sea plants in coastal waters. Recently discovered is the nonculturable form of *V. cholerae* in a wide range of
marine life (research by International Center for Diarrheal Diseases Research,
Bangladesh). In unfavorable conditions, *V. cholerae* assumes spore-like, quiescent
forms; with proper nutrients, pH, and temperature, the bacteria revert to a readily
transmissible and infectious state. *V. cholerae* and *V. vulnificus* are present in coastal
waters of the United States. The latter is associated with a 67% case-fatality rate
among those with preexisting liver disease.

INCREASED PREVALENCE OF BACTERIAL AND VIRAL DISEASES

Both viral and bacterial diseases from the marine environment are on the increase.
Hepatitis A and bacterial diseases such as salmonella and campylobacter infections
continue to be major health problems throughout the world. A recent multistate
outbreak of viral gastroenteritis was related to the consumption of oysters from a
few U.S. states.

Contributed by D. Rapport. See also Epstein and Rapport, 1996.

servation in arid regions. The endemic zones of diseases currently limited to the
tropics are likely to extend into currently temperate zones. It is also possible that
such diseases will extend their ranges vertically to higher altitudes, especially in
the tropics (WHO, 1990b; Chivian et al., 1993; McMichael et al., 1996; WRI,
1996).

Causes of the Problem

The reasons for this projected change in climate are complex, but all relate to
the release of increasing amounts of greenhouse gases, such as carbon dioxide

and water vapor, into the earth's atmosphere. The increase in the release of these
gases exaggerates the greenhouse effect (see section The Greenhouse Effect), but
the underlying reason for this increase is intensive industrial and agricultural development and increasing consumption of fossil fuels. The rapid rise in concentration of these greenhouse gases is occurring in the troposphere. Carbon dioxide is increasing at 0.4% per year, methane at about 1% per year, CFCs until
recently at about 5% per year, and oxides of nitrogen at 0.3% per year; the concentration of ozone and a miscellaneous group of other gases is also on the rise.
This increase is mostly the result of industrial and transport development, especially the use of internal combustion engines and coal-burning electric power
generators. Methane also comes from agriculture, landfills, and other sources,
such as the decomposition of rotting vegetation and from the digestive tracts of
plant-eating animals like cattle. Water vapor, another important greenhouse gas,
has not been increased as much by human activity and does not seem to be rising (Mungall and McLaren, 1990; National Academy of Sciences, 1992).

Of these greenhouse gases, carbon dioxide is the most important, accounting
for half of the effect. It is also particularly difficult to control, because it is generated by any form of combustion and is inevitable in the burning of fossil fuels. By contrast, the CFCs are no longer increasing in concentration. A worldwide moratorium on their manufacture and distribution in new products was
negotiated when they were identified as the principal cause of stratospheric ozone
depletion (see section Stratospheric Ozone Depletion, above).

Climate Change and Tick-borne Diseases

Ticks belonging to the Ixodidae family have a wide geographical distribution range, including parts of the subarctic regions. These ticks are vectors for several diseases, such as Lyme disease and tick-borne encephalitis (TBE). Several animals, such as birds, rodents, and deer, act as hosts for the tick. They may be infected with the pathogen and can pass it on to humans through a blood-sucking tick. Ticks as well as their host animals and habitat are all dependent on changes in local weather conditions. A future climatic change would affect the complicated ecological interactions associated with the transmission of tick-borne diseases. As a result, tick-borne diseases may spread into new areas that are located at higher northern latitudes and altitudes than present endemic regions.

Contributed by E. Lindgren, Sweden.

Support for these projections of greenhouse gas accumulation comes from a variety of sources. Among the most useful are studies of trapped air in glacier ice and lake sediment. Carbon dioxide concentrations in the atmosphere today are thought to be the highest in 160,000 years, as judged from trapped bubbles in Antarctic glacier ice. Methane levels are also much increased in more recent ice core samples. A close association throughout this period between carbon dioxide levels and estimated global average temperature at the time (as indicated by fossil biota and carbon isotope concentrations) is discernible in most of these studies (Mungall and McLaren, 1990; WHO, 1992a).

Carbon dioxide is absorbed by plant life and is thereby removed from the atmosphere through natural growth and agriculture. A mechanism for relatively unlimited removal of a chemical from the environment is called a *sink*. The most significant sinks for carbon dioxide appear to be in the Amazon rain forest and the temperate zones of the Northern Hemisphere, where widespread destruction of the forests has occurred. The boreal forests in Canada and Siberia may also of great concern. Deforestation reduces the capacity of the biosphere to remove carbon dioxide and to act as a stabilizing mechanism to climate change. Thus, there is a direct link between global climate change and changes in land use patterns such as deforestation, as discussed below.

Solutions to the Problem

The solution to the problem of climatic change is deceptively simple but difficult to achieve: reduce the generation of greenhouse gases, particularly of carbon dioxide, and increase the capacity of the sink for carbon dioxide by stopping deforestation and increasing forest growth (see Fig. 11.6). Although what needs to be done may seem obvious, it is very difficult in practice to reduce the combustion of fossil fuels and to increase forest growth.

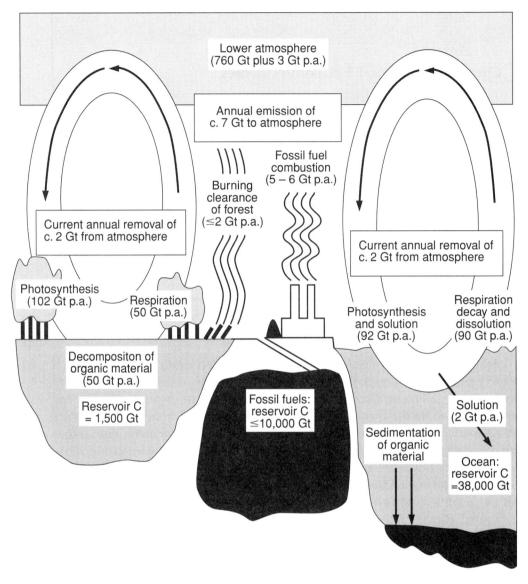

Figure 11.6 The carbon cycle. From McMichael, 1993, with permission.

Economic growth in modern industrial societies is based on relatively inexpensive energy supplies. Regional economies, such as the Middle East, Western Africa, and North America, are highly dependent on the sale of petroleum and petroleum products for their stability. Virtually the entire developed world is dependent on oil imports for transportation and energy needs. A reduction in the dependence on fossil fuels would require extensive energy conservation, creating economic hardship in many parts of the world. Many rapidly developing countries are understandably reluctant to agree to limits on the production of carbon dioxide that would restrict their own economic growth, especially since they see themselves as needing to catch up with the developed countries that caused the problem in the first place. At the same time, oil supplies are limited worldwide, so extensive conservation would have the effect of expediting by one generation or so the inevitable depletion of petroleum reserves. However, many nations are counting on revenue from oil in the short term to build the infrastructure of a stable economy that will continue after the oil runs out. Thus progress toward a negotiated reduction in greenhouse gas emissions has been much slower than that for controlling CFCs (WHO, 1992a).

DEFORESTATION AND DESERTIFICATION

Human activity has changed the face of the earth considerably. Only remnants now remain of the huge forests that once covered Europe, the Middle East, and China. Central Europe was once a dense forest and in Roman times the cedar groves of Lebanon were famous. North America used to be much more heavily forested along the East Coast than it is today, although the forest is coming back in many areas of the East Coast. Large tracts of forest remain in protected areas in North America, in the mountains of the West, along the Pacific Northwest, and in the far North. Southeast Asia, South America, and Africa still have vast expanses of rain forest but through the clearing of huge areas for agriculture and industrial development, the total area of forest coverage has been rapidly reduced.

Clearance is usually undertaken on a piecemeal basis for agriculture. Often, as in the Amazon Basin and Indonesia, woodlands are cleared by fire. Sometimes, as in northern Africa and China, forests are consumed for firewood. The resulting depletion of forests can result in serious ecological consequences.

Forest Ecosystem Changes

Woodlands protect the soil on which they stand in many ways. Root systems and ground cover slow down the passage of water through the ground and keep soil in place. Forest debris and ground cover recycle nutrients and provide food for wildlife. Trees and fallen trees provide shelter and habitat for wildlife and reduce the impact of strong winds.

In general, forests tend to be cooler and more humid than arid country and provide a much greater diversity of ecological niches in which wildlife may flourish. This is particularly true at the edge between forests and open land and between forests and wetlands, where the complicated interface supports great diversity. In tropical rain forests, soils tend to be acidic and relatively poor in nutrients but the forest and its debris support many forms of life. In northern or boreal forests, growth tends to be very slow because of the cold weather, and the less diverse wildlife tends to experience great cycles of population growth and decline.

When woodlands are cut down and cleared, these complicated natural systems are lost and are replaced by a much simpler, artificial environment that is much less stable ecologically and much less productive biologically, although there may be short-term economic gain. In arid regions and when the destruction of the forest is too extensive, the ability of the forest to recover is lost. In some places, the cleared forest may return to scrub brush whereas in other places soil changes and loss of ground cover may create a desert where forest existed before. This latter process is called *desertification* and it has been a particular problem recently in northern Africa. Desertification happened long ago in many parts of the Middle East and areas that are now very dry were once wet and heavily forested.

Erosion by wind and water is much more severe when woodland and brush cover are removed. Unprotected soils are carried into streams and rivers, where silt affects fish stocks and clogs small channels. Soils newly available for agriculture can be rapidly depleted once the forest cover is removed; this is a particular problem in the tropics where certain types of soil become hard when the ground cover is removed. Nutrients in the soil can also be leached out by the rapid passage of water through the topsoil. Wind may be much harsher in human settlements without the protection of a woodland windbreak and there may be local climate changes when the moderating effect of the forest is removed. Habitat for wildlife is destroyed and along with it the stability of the local ecosystem. This leads to the degradation of lands that could attract mixed uses, such as grazing, hunting, tourism, and wood harvesting. Biodiversity is much reduced (as described below) and with it, much of the economic potential for the region. Agriculture introduced into areas of deforestation may lead to a single-crop economy and dependence on world or regional commodity markets.

Forest Ecosystems and Global Change

Forests also play a critical role in the removal, storage, and release of carbon dioxide from the atmosphere, as discussed earlier. Throughout history, at least since the last Ice Age, it would appear that the global sinks for carbon dioxide have had sufficient capacity to absorb any excess caused by volcanic eruption or forest fires. As a result, the content of carbon dioxide in the atmosphere remained relatively stable. Today, however, production of carbon dioxide exceeds the capacity of the global sinks, and the concentration of the gas in the atmosphere is steadily increasing, leading ultimately to the exaggerated greenhouse effect described above (see McMichael et al., 1996).

Deforestation reduces the capacity of the world's forests to serve as a carbon dioxide sink. Burning forested areas aggravates the global accumulation of carbon dioxide in the atmosphere. When forests are cut down for firewood or catch on fire, the stored carbon in the wood and brush is released into the atmosphere again. Even when wood is used for building construction and other purposes, some carbon dioxide is eventually released. Another, and quite unexpected, consequence of deforestation is mercury contamination, as described in Box 11.5.

Reforestation, on the other hand, takes carbon dioxide out of the atmosphere and traps it in biomass. That is why one response to the challenge of global climate change has been to encourage the planting of trees and the reforestation of forests.

As mentioned in the section Solutions to the Problem, the most significant sinks for carbon dioxide appear to be in the Amazon rain forest and the temperate zones of the northern hemisphere. Large-scale destruction of the Amazonian forests and, potentially, the boreal forest in Canada and Siberia will reduce the capacity of the biosphere to remove carbon dioxide and act as a

Mercury Contamination in the Amazon: Effects of Gold Mining and Deforestation

Gold mining in the Amazon, originally thought to be the only cause of the mercury pollution of some of the rivers, began approximately three decades ago when thousands of impoverished miners, known as *garimpeiros,* swept into the jungle to mine gold using a mercury mining method they use to this day (see Chapter 10). About half of the approximately 130 tons of mercury per year used is emitted into the air while the other half seeps into the water, contaminating fish.

The team of Canadian and Brazilian scientists investigating the mercury contamination and its health effects on the villagers (see Lebel et al., 1995) began to suspect that there was too much methylmercury in the Amazon to be the result solely of *garimpeiros* activities. Everywhere they collected river sediment samples they recorded 1.5 to 3 times more mercury than there had been 40 years ago, even 400 kilometers downstream from the gold mining. They soon found that deforestation was the other source. When impoverished people from northern Brazil colonize the Amazon jungle they usually clear the forest in a 10 to 20 kilometer area on both sides of a river and burn the remaining rubble. Following deforestation, heavy rains wash out nutrients from the soil into the waterways. As the Amazon basin has considerable natural mercury in its soil, mercury released into the water contaminates the fish to cause mercury poisoning in people consuming large quantities of fish.

The Canadian team had a particular interest in mercury because in the northern area of two Canadian provinces, high mercury exposure occurred in the aboriginal community from a similar process: hydroelectric dams and reservoirs raised water levels, the water inundated ancient soils, which then degraded and released their naturally occurring mercury.

Although Brazil has officially banned the use of mercury for mining, this technique is still occurring. Moreover, the reforms instituted have not added the problem of landless settlers burning trees and destroying the soil, thereby releasing mercury into the Amazon. In the meanwhile, in discussing the results with the community, it was advised that they vary their diet so as to eat more "fish that do not eat other fish."

Contributed by D. Mergler

stabilizing mechanism to climate change. Thus much attention has been given to the development of the Amazon Basin and concern expressed over the clearing of rain forests in South America and the northern hemisphere (Canada and Siberia). Not surprisingly, the few countries with large forested areas remaining have been singled out for criticism, notably Brazil. This issue has led to a conflict over the right of a particular country to pursue its short-term development strategy and the right of the world as a whole to be protected from massive change in the long term that will affect everyone. Forests in many parts of the world, such as Brazil, are being cleared in remote areas for agriculture and economic development by people who have limited economic opportunities and are not easily policed by their governments. Although it seems clear that deforestation may be a poor economic strategy in the long term, it provides needed jobs and agricultural productivity in the short term for local residents. There has been little success in changing deforestation practices on a local level because of the lack of alternatives available to these people.

Reducing deforestation and increasing forest growth are difficult to achieve. Some countries have had success in preserving their forests while increasing economic opportunities through so-called debt-for-equity swaps. In these deals, countries with large debts may have some of the debt forgiven or refinanced at a lower rate in exchange for restricting access to and development of ecologically critical areas like forests. The problem with such programs is that the country loses some control over its economic future, although it does reduce its accumulated debt. Other countries, such as China, have had success with massive reforestation programs to restore woodlands in areas that have been badly depleted.

BIODIVERSITY

Biodiversity refers to the multiplicity of species of plants and animals in a biological community and the many ecological niches that they may occupy. It is a fundamental principle of ecology that diversity in animal and plant species leads to greater stability of the ecosystem. The ecosystem functions more efficiently, with different species occupying more niches and extracting full benefit from the energy and nutrients available. More complicated systems have greater adaptability in the face of environmental changes and the ecological niches occupied by different species may partly overlap and allow substitutions if one or more are lost. Loss of biodiversity therefore means a less stable, less adaptable, less self-restoring ecosystem (Chivian et al., 1993).

Biological Significance of Biodiversity

Biodiversity is also a means of preserving genetic diversity. Each species and subspecies contain within their genes the result of hundreds of thousands, even millions of years of evolution. This genetic constitution is written onto DNA, the molecule that conserves the genetic code. It constitutes a library of 'blueprints' for living beings and for biological adaptation. For all groups of organisms recognized as species, there is a basic genetic constitution consisting of characteristics common to all members of the species, and a set of variations that have been introduced by mutations, random changes in the gene pool introduced by mistakes in replication of DNA or the effect of ionizing radiation on DNA. Most of such mutations are harmful and do not survive; a few confer new traits that may or may not be useful to the individual that carries them. The variation in genetically determined traits among individual members of any species or subspecies is what drives evolution: natural selection favors some variants and not others, so that some traits survive and others do not. Many of the variants represent traits that survived because they were useful; the individuals who carried the traits could adapt to new conditions or exploit new ecological niches. Loss of biodiversity means that even if the species as a whole survives, the variation within the species is reduced, making it less adaptable and, in effect, stopping its evolution (Chivian et al., 1993).

Economic Aspects of Biodiversity

Much of the diversity among species and subspecies and many of the variations among individuals within a species have direct practical uses to human society. They have been the basis for developing all agricultural crops and breeding all livestock, for example. Biodiversity is reduced in agriculture in the long run as certain strains are chosen for their greater productivity, resistance to pests, or ability to grow with less water, for example, and these strains are selected or hybridized to existing strains. The new strains are then planted as a *monoculture*, a uniform stand or herd of genetically similar or even identical organisms. This monoculture tends to be very susceptible to new pests or diseases to which it is vulnerable. Once it is infected, the entire stand or herd is at risk because there is no native resistance. The monoculture is also bred for a particular environment and when the environment changes, as, for example, during a drought, it is unlikely to adapt. Sometimes, genetic traits that would have conferred resistance or that would have allowed adaptation to a changing environment were present in the wild strain but have been lost through selective breeding for other characteristics. For this reason, scientists try to maintain biodiversity in the laboratory by keeping seed stocks and cultivating representatives of genetically unusual plants to ensure that they are not lost.

Among the many forms of biodiversity is the variation among species and subspecies in synthesizing unusual chemicals. Snake venoms, pheromones that attract insect mates, squid ink, and the light-producing chemicals of fireflies are just a few examples. Plants, especially, produce a wide variety of novel chemicals for special purposes, such as to protect themselves against insect pests. Many of these chemicals have unusual properties that may or may not be related to the advantages they confer on the plant or animal. Medical researchers take advantage of this diversity by identifying chemicals produced by plants and animals that have a biological effect and turning them into useful drugs. With loss of biodiversity, a huge reservoir of potentially useful chemicals may be lost that could be found in no other way (Chivian et al., 1993).

The search for economically useful biological products that become available because of biodiversity has been called *bioprospecting*. One of the more important methods of bioprospecting has been to use the knowledge of indigenous peoples who have used herbal remedies and natural products for millennia and who have accumulated over time a deep understanding of their effects through experience. The ethics and economics of sharing the benefits of bioprospecting and production with the indigenous peoples who passed on the knowledge have become major issues in recent years. The future economic development of many of these peoples, and their control over their own culture and development, may rest on how this issue is resolved.

In biotechnology, methods of genetic engineering are being used to select genes directly for new product development. Because of biodiversity, biotechnologists have an essentially unlimited library of genes from which to construct new materials. However, genetic engineering may also accelerate the process of developing monocultures, by allowing agricultural scientists to be even more se-lective in choosing the specific traits they want while overlooking seemingly less important traits (WHO, 1992a).

Loss of Biodiversity

Ecosystems can lose biodiversity in many ways. Individual species may become extinct through hunting, habitat loss, or reduction in the species that they de-pend on for food. Entire ecosystems or large areas of larger ecosystems may be changed or lost by urbanization and agricultural clearance. Particular habitats of individual species with limited ranges may be lost in the same way: the essen-tial area lost might relate to feeding requirements, territoriality, or breeding. Sometimes foreign species are introduced into a stable ecosystem, preying on and reducing the numbers of the local species that give the ecosystem stability. Of-ten all of these mechanisms occur at the same time (Chivian et al., 1993).

Even ecosystems that appear to be healthy may suffer loss of biodiversity. Old-growth forests, for example, are forests that have not been cut down and that maintain a much richer diversity of species and considerably more stable ecosystems than new-growth forests, which arise by ecological succession after earlier forests have been cut down. Even though the forest may look the same, appearances can be very deceiving.

Loss of biodiversity is an important indicator of the magnitude of these trends. It shows the extent to which the ecosystem is being simplified. Because the sta-bility of ecosystems depends on complexity and variability, simplification is nec-essarily environmental degradation, regardless of what else is happening in the environment. That is why it is a mistake to concentrate too narrowly on the eco-logical or economic importance of a particular species when it comes to local is-sues of conservation and ecosystem protection. The loss of a particular species or subspecies is important in and of itself, but it is also another thread that is cut in the ecological web and reflects a trend toward an increasingly simplified and unstable ecosystem. Biodiversity is a critical part of the network of ecological re-lationships that supports human society. Loss of biodiversity is both a serious problem in its own right and a sensitive sign of the deterioration of the envi-ronment as a whole.

ACID PRECIPITATION

Acid precipitation (acid rain) occurs when rainwater, snow, and other forms of precipitation have a lower than natural pH as a result of dissolved acidic chem-icals that occur from air pollution. This is caused by increased production of acid-ifying emissions from industrial sources, principally sulfates and nitrates, and air-borne transport of these pollutants. Often, these pollutants are carried very long distances and fall as acid precipitation hundreds or even thousands of kilometers away from the original site of production. When the precipitation reaches the ground, it can change the pH of small lakes and the soil, causing ecological dam-age. This is particularly a problem in areas where there is little natural buffering capacity in the soil or water (WHO, 1992a).

In recent years, surveys of soil and water acidity in the Northern Hemisphere have shown increased acidity (or, more accurately, reduced acid neutralizing capacity) and presumably irreversible changes in pH in soils. The problem has been most severe and most heavily documented in Canada (largely as a result of emissions from the U.S. Midwest) and Scandinavia (from emissions arising in Germany and Britain). The situation in Russia and Eastern Europe is still being assessed. Similar processes are probably occurring in China, India, and Central Asia. The result has been extensive changes in the biology of small bodies of water. Acid precipitation is highly detrimental to delicate aquatic ecosystems, marine biota, and some terrestrial species of plants and trees. It is blamed for severe and widespread effects on forests in Scandinavia and Germany in particular (Berdén et al., 1987; Mungall and McLaren 1990; WHO, 1992a; Chivian et al., 1993).

Direct effects of acid precipitation on humans have been difficult to study. Transregional transportation of pollution, as with acid deposition and the long-range transport of air toxins, may result in increased airway reactivity and asthma. Asthma has been observed as a result of increased levels of acidic chemicals, such as sulfates, in the air in southern Canada (Franklin et al., 1985). Some authors have speculated that if metals are leached into groundwater at excessive concentrations, there may be toxic effects, but this is not yet proven (Goyer et al.,1985).

The obvious control strategy for acid precipitation is to reduce the generation of air pollutants at the source. A particularly important step would be to reduce the consumption of fossil fuels in producing energy. Not every country agrees with the scientific analysis of the problem nor is every country willing to curtail its own economic development by imposing regulation or decreasing production. A major technical problem is the consideration of control strategies for acid precipitation without having a clear understanding of loading capacities, i.e., the maximum emissions that an ecosystem can absorb before its capacity to neutralize, transform, or dilute the pollutant is exceeded. Such information has been estimated for regions in northern Europe but is not available for most parts of the world (Berdén et al., 1987).

TRANSBOUNDARY MOVEMENT OF HAZARDOUS WASTE

Toxic and hazardous chemicals are increasingly mobile in today's world. Not only are they being shipped around the world as commodities for various purposes in production but also chemical and radioactive wastes are being moved about as concern grows about proper storage and handling. In the developed world, it is becoming increasingly unacceptable to local residents to permit the storage or disposal of hazardous waste. In many developed countries, the options for getting rid of such wastes are disappearing. Hazardous waste disposal sites are closing because of community opposition, and chemical treatment facilities are becoming increasingly costly because of ever more stringent measures to protect the environment. It has been estimated that approximately 400 million tons per year of hazardous waste cross international boundaries, much of it being illegally moved to unauthorized disposal sites. The result is that unscrupulous parties are often tempted to ship hazardous material to countries where environmental regulations are more relaxed and enforcement is not as strong. The receiving coun-

TABLE 11.2

PROVISIONS OF THE BASEL CONVENTION

1. The generation and movement of wastes should be reduced to the minimum required and the wastes disposed of as close as possible to the site of origin.
2. Every country has the right to ban importation of hazardous wastes, and signatory countries shall not allow transboundary movement of hazardous waste to any country that has banned its importation, whether a signatory or not. Also, signatory countries will not allow the export of hazardous wastes if there is a reason to believe that they will not be disposed of in an appropriate and environmentally safe manner.
3. Signatory countries will not allow hazardous wastes to be imported from or exported to nonsignatory countries unless their movement is governed by agreements that are at least as strict as the Basel Convention.
4. The exporting country will not allow the hazardous waste to leave until it has written confirmation of consent on the part of the importing country and any country of transit, reflecting a decision based on knowledge of what the shipment contains.
5. When the hazardous waste cannot be safely transported or handled, the exporting country has a duty to take it back.
6. Anything that does not conform to these principles is considered illegal traffic, to be punished by criminal sanctions that each signatory country must develop and legislate.

tries are often willing partners because of the money the importation of hazardous waste brings in the form of fees, facilities, and, sometimes, bribes. However, these countries usually have no effective means of controlling hazardous waste once it arrives. In some cases, the waste is simply dumped where it may pollute groundwater, the oceans, or land. In a few cases, the wastes may be chemically treated and disposed of in a manner that is similar to good practices in the developed world but without the stringent supervision and monitoring that is needed to ensure that the material does not pollute the environment.

Such practices are not confined to the developing world. Some of the worst incidents documented recently have involved the former East Germany and the former Soviet Union. Developing countries are particularly vulnerable to this form of "toxic blackmail." Since 1989 an international protocol on the movement of hazardous waste, the *Basel Convention*, has governed the transboundary movement of hazardous wastes, on the basis of the six principles paraphrased in Table 11.2.

DISASTERS

By definition, disasters involve many casualties occurring in a short period of time, following an unusual event. They may be natural or the result of human activity. The emphasis in modern times in responding to disasters is on disaster planning and preparation. A complete discussion of disaster preparation is beyond the scope of this text.

Emergency Actions

Depending on the magnitude of the disaster and its extent, disasters can overwhelm the health care system in the area and disrupt the operations of fire, transportation, and rescue services. In the first few hours following a disaster, the first priorities are to identify and provide medical care to the injured, locate and rescue missing persons, and identify and control physical hazards, such as ruptured gas lines. In the case of chemical or radiation incidents, decontamination is a high and urgent priority to prevent further exposure. Subsequently, the provision of basic services, including shelter, food, potable water, sanitary facilities such as latrines, and psychological intervention become an urgent priority if the disaster has disrupted services in the community. Burial of the dead, provision of warm clothing, and evacuation of the injured or vulnerable may become health priorities, depending on circumstances. The risk of infectious disease increases in the days following the disaster, as water supplies may be interrupted and sanitation becomes an increasing problem. Over the long term, rehabilitation and reconstruction become increasingly important as the community comes to terms with the devastation.

Natural and Technological Disasters

Disasters are of two general types, and the responses of communities tend to differ with each type. *Natural disasters* occur as a result of the action of natural forces and tend to be accepted as unfortunate but inevitable. *Technological disasters* occur as the result of some human activity and tend to be deeply disturbing to a community, leading to the blaming of culprits and a sense of shame in the community. Chapter 4 discussed factors that affect risk perception; similarly, the responses to natural disasters tend to be very different from those to technological disasters (see Table 11.3). Each are discussed in detail, below.

Natural disasters result from natural forces of climate and geology. Although there is often a history of such disasters in a given area, natural disasters are usually unpredictable in the short term. The circumstances preceding the actual event may make the disaster much worse than it had to be. For example, extensive building on an earthquake fault or on an exposed shoreline subject to storms may greatly increase the casualty rate from an otherwise moderate event. Building with inadequate materials and failing to provide access to evacuation or emergency services routes may greatly complicate the rescue effort. The rescue effort may be inadequate or poorly organized; if it is delayed by more than a few hours in a major disaster, the responsible agency often comes under heavy criticism. The reconstruction effort may be prolonged, poorly coordinated, and complicated by bureaucracy, often leading to great public dissatisfaction, even if the immediate response to the disaster was received with gratitude.

Natural disasters that result from climate, such as hurricanes, tornadoes, and flooding due to prolonged rains, tend to cause more property damage than deaths.

TABLE 11.3

PERCEIVED DIFFERENCES BETWEEN NATURAL AND TECHNOLOGICAL DISASTERS

	Natural Disasters	*Technological Disasters*
Nature of disaster	Clean, unavoidable	Dirty, contaminated
Responsibility	No agent	Culpable party
Objective magnitude of loss	Often great	Usually less
Perceived magnitude of loss	Usually minimized	Usually maximized
Community support for those affected	Nonjudgmental	Highly judgmental, ambiguous

They are profoundly demoralizing to the people displaced from their homes, but the community affected tends to respond quickly, and the long-term consequences are often less than one would expect. These are relatively familiar hazards, are easily understood, and are often common enough in the area affected to be thought of as a fact of life. Disruption of sanitary facilities and transportation tends to be less severe than in other types of natural disasters, except in the case of flooding. A severe storm is clearly terrifying and threatening, but communities tend to handle this type of disaster more easily than other types.

Natural disasters that result from geological activity, such as earthquakes, volcano eruptions, mud slides, *tsunamis* (seismic tidal waves), and flash floods (involving sudden rainfall in terrain that funnels it into swiftly flowing channels), tend to result in more casualties than those due to climate and may severely disrupt the ability of the community to take care of its own needs in the hours and days following the event. Forest fires share many of these characteristics. In both kinds of disasters, there are often many missing persons and trapped victims who require rescue. The type of injury is usually more severe, reflecting the risk of collapsing buildings and the massive forces involved, and may lead to serious public health problems even when adequately treated. Psychological stresses associated with the event appear to be greater than for disasters related to climate, and affect both victims and rescuers.

Technological disasters result from some human activity such as explosions, the release of toxic chemicals or radioactive material, bridge or building collapse, fires, and crashes. Technological disasters tend to involve many more casualties than natural disasters of the same magnitude of energy release. They are also much more difficult for the community to deal with and for victims to accept. The psychological factors that influence perception of technological disasters are very different from those for natural disasters. In technological disasters, there are issues of blame involved and the community spends much time discussing who was responsible and what mistakes were made. Often there are complicated lawsuits, investigations and claims for disability involved. If there was previously a feeling that the owners of the facility responsible were abusing the community or making excessive profits, this adds to the fury of the community's response. Sometimes victims are shunned by their neighbors, who feel that they are exploiting the situation for personal gain or who are fearful that the response to the incident will cause economic loss to the community. As a result, technological disasters tend to divide the community and to cause long-lasting psychological trauma to local residents as well as to victims. Examples of major technological disasters in recent times include the release of toxic methyl isocyanate gas in Bhopal, India in 1984 and the explosion and release of radiation from the Chernobyl nuclear reactor in the Ukraine in 1986. Incidents on a much smaller scale are not rare but do not get as much attention.

An important exception to the generalizations made about natural and technological disasters above is *drought*. Drought is related to climate and is relatively slow to develop. The primary public health consequence of drought in less developed regions, where food cannot be easily imported, is famine. Casualties from starvation may be very high, as in the prolonged drought in Sub-Saharan (Sahelian) Africa where around 1970 over 200 million people were estimated to have been affected. In addition, drought and famine may cause extensive, long-lasting social tensions because they act to deepen poverty very suddenly and divide society between those who can afford to get food at any price and those who cannot. Drought and famine are also associated with large population movements that complicate the task of providing medical care, food, and water to the affected communities. Thus, the combination of drought and famine is one type of natural disaster related to climate that has many of the worst characteristics of technological disasters.

Psychological Effects of Disasters on Survivors

Psychological symptoms following disasters tend to be similar among children, but among adults they are somewhat more complicated and variable. Children are often fearful and show disproportionate anxiety over separation from their friends or parents. They may lose motivation, act in rebellious ways, and begin to do poorly in school. Children often respond well to immediate mental health interventions aimed at helping them to express their feelings and fears about the event. Adults are often able to cope reasonably well during the event but may fall apart afterward; a small minority will become incapable of acting during the stress of a crisis and will have to be forced to move. Adults who survive a disaster may experience a range of adverse effects, such as nightmares, uncontrollable thoughts that involve reliving the events, trouble sleeping, no emotion, and a sense of detachment from the other people in their lives and the world in general. In adults these symptoms are characteristic of post-traumatic stress syndrome. Adults may also be helped by mental health professionals who discuss with them as a group what happened and what their reactions are, a process known as *critical incident debriefing.* Part of what is helpful about this process is the reassurance that these feelings are natural and that those affected are not mentally ill. Rescue personnel often have the same symptoms and feelings as survivors and victims, and may also benefit from critical incident debriefing. While there is some questioning of the value of psychological debriefings in preventing posttraumatic stress disorder (Bisson et al., 1997), most authorities do recommend it when appropriate (Mitchell and Evans, 1999).

Mutual assistance and disaster intervention programs may significantly limit the impact of a disaster on the community. International assistance is difficult to manage and coordinate but may make a decisive difference in the outcome, especially in countries and areas with very limited resources.

GLOBAL CHEMICAL CONTAMINATION

The problem of global chemical contamination due to ozone layer depletion was described earlier in the section Ozone Depletion and Ultraviolet Radiation. In this case, the offending chemicals, the CFCs, have no direct impact on human health occurring during their use, but they are very persistent, dispersing into the atmosphere, and eventually reaching the stratospheric ozone layer, where they react chemically with ozone. The resultant reduction in ozone concentration reduces the blocking effect on UV radiation of the ozone layer and increases the UV radiation that reaches the surface of the globe. As already discussed, the increased UV exposure at ground level effects both humans and ecosystems, some of these effects are extremely important for agricultural and fisheries productivity.

Another issue that has been given increasing attention is the use of chemicals that persist for long periods of time in the environment; the possibility exists that a buildup of these chemicals may eventually affect human and ecosystem health. A well-known warning about this problem was sounded already in the 1960s in the book *Silent Spring* (Carson, 1962). At that time, one of the main concerns was about the effects of DDT and other chlorinated hydrocarbon pesticides. Adverse effects on birds had been clearly demonstrated, but those on humans at the relatively low exposures occurring in the general environment were not demonstrated. Recently it has been shown that some of these pesticides have estrogen-like effects on experimental animals, and links have been made to human breast cancer and sperm damage, possibly leading to male infertility (see Chapter 2). DDT is now banned from use in all developed countries, but some developing countries still produce and use this pesticide, as it is the cheapest and most cost-effective means of killing certain important insects, such as malaria-bearing mosquitoes and locusts. There is evidence that DDT and other persistent organic pollutants (POPs) evaporate into the air in the tropical countries where they are used, get transported via winds to the colder latitudes, and eventually get deposited in these colder countries via rainfall. This transfer of pollutants may create a situation in which the eventual buildup of these chemicals is highest in the colder countries where they are not used directly.

Study Questions

1. Your health minister has been invited to attend a special cabinet meeting to discuss your country's response to recent reports regarding climate change. She has been told that there are no major health impacts in your jurisdiction, therefore it is not necessary for her to prepare a detailed report. She has asked you if you think that she ought to attend. Formulate a memo of no more than two pages offering her advice. Discuss how global warming could affect health in your country.

2. What are the most serious global health concerns? Prioritize and justify your list.

3. Summarize the areas of greatest debate and state why these debates exist.

4. What are the obstacles to overcome in addressing global health problems?

5. What strategies exist to address these obstacles?

12

ACTION TO PROTECT HEALTH AND THE ENVIRONMENT

LEARNING OBJECTIVES

After studying this chapter you will be able to do the following:
- describe the actions that can be taken by environmental health professionals to address environmental health problems
- apply the notion *"think globally and act locally"* to a specific situation
- understand the important ethical principles involved when taking action on environmental health issues

FROM KNOWLEDGE TO ACTION

It is often difficult to reach agreement on the root causes of environmental problems because different cultures and individuals often hold very different opinions regarding the causes of these problems. One society may see the problems as arising from technological arrogance, the attitude that human beings can do all things without fear of consequences. Another society may see the problems as representing a moral failure on the part of government and society and a desire by individuals to live easily without hard work. Yet another society may see these problems as inevitable, as part of the costs that must be paid to achieve a decent lifestyle and to get out of poverty. These ideas about cause are not necessarily right or wrong, but they cannot be proven and provide little practical guide for action. It is usually more productive to concentrate on what the problems are today and what actions are needed to keep them from getting worse.

What is not so clear is what to do about them. Many individuals and many political groups have their own ideas about radical changes that would correct specific problems at what they perceive to be their root causes. However, the root cause for some people (for example, overpopulation) may be seen as a secondary phenomenon by others (as, for example, the lack of education and empowerment of women). Radical solutions are easy to conceive but very difficult to implement. It is clear that the world does not have much more time to debate these issues before the damage to the environment will be permanent, irreversible, and sufficiently advanced to constrain the life choices and freedoms of the next generation. Regardless of their view of the causes of the problems, however, many thoughtful and conscientious people are arriving at a common point of view regarding the most urgent changes that are needed to give society and the environment breathing room. At least the outline of a consensus is emerging in countries around the world on the minimal steps necessary to deal with the issues. These are summarized in Table 12.1, not necessarily in any order of fundamental importance.

If there is an emerging consensus on the minimum that must be done, the next question is who should do it. Clearly, many of these actions have a practical, technical component that must be handled by trained professionals. However, these professionals cannot act in isolation. There must be support from the people who are directly affected, from national leaders, from institutions, and from leaders at the lo-

TABLE 12.1

COMPONENTS TO ADDRESSING ENVIRONMENTAL HEALTH CONCERNS

Pollution control, to prevent the release of pollution into the environment in the first place, and the economic and regulatory structures that support vigilance in pollution control

Remediation, to clean up polluted areas and to restore them to the extent feasible to their natural or at least an acceptable state

Resource conservation, including recycling and reuse, to reduce the amount of raw materials needed by industry and increase the efficiency of use of these resources

Ecosystem conservation, to ensure that habitats for the world's species will be preserved in full productivity and that appropriate human uses can be sustained

Commitment to end extreme poverty and support of national efforts to achieve a sustainable economy, to provide for most of the world's peoples at least a comparable level of economic security and personal wealth to that in the developed world today

Technology transfer, to allow the developing world to industrialize with the advantage of the more efficient, less hazardous, and less polluting technologies

Sustainable economic systems that base their economic productivity on what can be extracted from the environment without permanent damage over the long term

Control of population growth, with a concomitant commitment to improved quality of family life and individual security

Acceptance of some degree of risk as part of daily life, along with a commitment by society to moderate the effects of risk on its citizens through education, regulation, and economic incentives so that the hazards of life are not constant preoccupations

Prevention of conventional and nuclear war to the fullest extent that human institutions can manage, and the redirection of funds spent for armaments for peaceful purposes, including environmental reconstruction

cal level who are perhaps most influential of all in determining whether reforms can be incorporated into the daily life of commerce and social interaction. Forming alliances with community leaders, elders, or traditional healers is essential. For this reason, among others, environmental health professionals cannot be just technical experts. They must also serve as agents of change within their society, educating people about the importance of these issues and mobilizing others into effective action.

ETHICAL PRINCIPLES THAT GUIDE ACTION ON ENVIRONMENTAL HEALTH

The environmental health professional must make many decisions in daily work that involve not only technical-scientific issues but also issues of ethics. The basic ethical principles in environmental health work follow the same ethical principles as have been developed for other health work, except that these guidelines ask environmental health professionals to pay even greater attention to the broader social consequences of their work. Table 12.2 provides the ethical guidelines that have been developed for environmental epidemiologists. They apply to other members of the environmental health team as well.

At the personal level the application of ethical principles involves how one's own lifestyle and resource consumption reflect the environmental health concerns that have been outlined in this book. Ultimately, every environmental health professional must strike a balance between his or her own convictions and personal commitment and what is required to be professional. Some useful guidelines are shown in Table 12.3.

In the broader global context, the environmental health professional also has responsibilities in promoting and facilitating community application of a precautionary environmental health approach. As a member of an interdisciplinary team, strengthening one's specialized knowledge in one's own profession will help contribute to the solution of environmental health problems. The following section outlines these roles more specifically.

ROLE OF ENVIRONMENTAL HEALTH PROFESSIONALS

Environmental health professionals are the repository of technical expertise in a society and the first resource consulted for technical advice on how to deal with environmental health problems. Such professionals must adopt different roles in interacting with different groups and in different situations; one approach will not work all the time or in all situations. This means that environmental health professionals must understand their various roles thoroughly and achieve the skills required to be effective in these different roles.

Technical Expertise

The first and most obvious role of the environmental health professional is to master the technical details and context of environmental problems. In order to solve a problem, it is usually necessary to understand what caused it, and it is always necessary to understand what perpetuates it. This textbook will help achieve this level of mastery, but it is not sufficient in and of itself. Further de-

TABLE 12.2
ETHICAL GUIDELINES FOR ENVIRONMENTAL EPIDEMIOLOGISTS

OBLIGATIONS TO RESEARCH PARTICIPANTS

Respect the rights and personal autonomy of all
Advise of both individual and collective benefits and harms from proposed research
Protect their welfare
Obtain informed consent whenever feasible
Protect privacy/maintain confidentiality
Use data and specimens for only the purpose(s) that consent was provided

OBLIGATIONS TO SOCIETY

Avoid partiality
Distinguish one's role as scientist from that of advocate
The public interest always takes precedence over any other interest
Be objective in disseminating research findings and be understandable in public discussions
Involve communities being proposed for study throughout all stages of the research and its reporting
Engage with other disciplines to advance and maximize the public utility of environmental epidemiology
Consider the broader social consequences, including psychosocial and physical health outcomes
Consider both equity and remediation in the allocation of resources applied to environmental epidemiology research across the different areas of research, social strata, and jurisdictions
Environmental epidemiology findings are based on uncertainty and as such must be used appropriately in their application to, for example, the development of risk analyses, policy, and interventions
Be diligent in executing professional responsibilities

OBLIGATIONS TO SPONSORS AND EMPLOYERS

Ensure that both researcher and sponsor/employer are apprised of one another's respective responsibilities and expectations
Emphasize obligations to other parties
Protect privileged information, but release research methods, procedures and results

OBLIGATIONS TO COLLEAGUES

Promote rigor in research design and neutrality in the execution of research
Report and publish methods and results in the peer reviewed literature of all studies, regardless of whether the findings are positive or negative or have no effect
Confront unacceptable behavior and conditions
Communicate ethical requirements

OBLIGATIONS ACROSS ALL THE ABOVE-NAMED GROUPS

Consult with stakeholders, including community members
Avoid conflicting interests and partiality
Pursue responsibilities with due diligence
Communicate findings in publicly understandable ways

Source: Soskolne and Light, 1996.

velopment of knowledge and skills will be required. In fact, the learning process continues throughout one's professional life. This process will be more effective if every problem faced is seen as an opportunity to understand better how to solve the next problem. To become an effective professional in this field, one needs to keep up-to-date with the technical-scientific knowledge, as well as de-

TABLE 12.3

ETHICAL PRINCIPLES TO GUIDE ENVIRONMENTAL HEALTH PRACTITIONERS IN THEIR DAILY LIVES

Avoid obvious contradictions between your lifestyle and your professional role, such as owning big and heavily polluting automobiles.

Keep your home as clean as feasible and avoid creating obvious pollution.

When pollution cannot be avoided, keep it to a minimum, do it openly, and use the opportunity as an object lesson to demonstrate that this must be changed.

Never try to conceal something in your life that looks like a contradiction with your role as an environmental health professional; it will someday be used for embarrassment.

Participate visibly and personally in community efforts to improve the environment and do so outside of working hours to demonstrate personal commitment.

Concentrate on living a lifestyle that has less environmental impact than the lifestyle of those around you.

Do not try to be perfect or completely nonpolluting because this is impossible.

velop skills to do things and skills in working as a team member with other professionals and the community.

The in-service learning process can be greatly facilitated by structured discussions and reviews of experiences in handling environmental health problems. If a program for such discussions does not exist in your workplace, consider taking the initiative to get it started. The program could include regular reviews of particularly interesting cases you and your colleagues have dealt with. It could include all colleagues reading selected articles in scientific or professional journals or chapters in selected textbooks, and discussing their content and the implications for your work.

Formal higher-level training in environmental health topics is another way to develop one's knowledge and skills. The availability of such training varies from country to country. National professional societies in the field usually maintain information about these types of courses. Courses promoted at the international level can be found, for instance, in the inventories and databases provided by the WHO.

The environmental health professional who wishes to be truly effective must be committed to a lifelong effort of reading, thinking, and analysis to understand the problems and the possible solutions. Above all, a capacity for sound judgment is needed to know what will work in the real world, what will not work, and how to achieve a workable solution in an imperfect world.

Professional Practice

Closely related to the role of environmental health professionals as technical expert is the skill that they show as practitioners. Professional practice as an environmental health practitioner depends on the job and the setting but typically requires mastery of a certain number of health indicators and standardized laboratory tests (for example, to determine water quality) and an ability to interpret the results and draw conclusions about the problem. These are basic skills in technical proficiency, and environmental health professionals are expected to be highly skillful and accurate in the performance of these duties. The professional must also have the necessary judgment for knowing what tests are needed, when they should be implemented, and how the pieces of the puzzle fit into the big picture in defining the problem. The environmental health professional must then decide on appropriate solutions and may have to convince others that one approach is better than another or that any action is necessary at all. This means that skills in communicating are just as important as technical skills.

An important aid to maintaining quality in professional practice is to support and to work within associations and professional societies. These provide a forum for discussing new developments and for sharing educational materials. They also create a network among professionals that tends to reinforce appropriate standards of performance and expectations about appropriate practice.

Public Education and Capacity Building

One of the most important functions of an environmental health professional is to educate the public. It is most useful for environmental health professionals to think in terms of creating opportunities for learning rather than to think of themselves as conduits of information. Because learning takes place in many ways, it is useful for the environmental health professional to understand these different modes of education.

The most effective educational encounters are usually those that take place on a case-by-case basis, when an opportunity arises to explain something. Often this occurs when the environmental health professional is consulted on a problem that the learner wants to have resolved. In this situation, the learner is motivated and receptive, and learns quickly and usually completely with respect to specific, concrete details. The learner may initially seem impatient with extraneous detail and may not fully comprehend the context of the problem. The educator must resist the temptation to be incomplete and must ensure that the learner does not leave with a distorted idea of what the problem is about. In addition, this reductionist approach to science has been blamed for the state of the environment, which requires a more holistic approach to formulating and implementing feasible and sustainable solutions. Thus, when providing the technical information to address a specific problem, effort should be made to put the problem into an overall context. How this is best done depends, of course, on the setting.

Teaching in school is perhaps the most familiar type of education. In this setting, education is usually focused on teaching the background to a problem and on understanding it thoroughly. The usual format is that of a teacher speaking to a large group of people and the content is usually structured to explain the problem from its beginnings or to outline how something works. The problem with teaching working adults in this way, as noted above, is that adults are usually motivated by problems rather than by a desire to understand everything there is to know about a topic. As adult learners tend to be results oriented, it is generally most useful to provide frequent opportunities for them to ask questions, and one must make the presentation as concrete and practical as possible. Often, teaching by exploring details of a case study is much more effective than giving a lecture on the same topic.

In any case, some basic principles of effective teaching need to be appreciated

TABLE 12.4

COMPARISON OF EFFECTIVE TEACHING METHODS FOR ADULTS, CHILDREN, AND YOUNG STUDENTS

	Children and Young Students	*Adults*
Teaching methods	Lectures, seminars, games, and simulations	Problem-solving exercises, special projects
Teaching approach	Systematic instructions, theory, history	Start with learner's own interests and problems, emphasize case studies
How to handle fundamentals	Build from basics, provide theory first	Draw out basics from an exploration of practical matters, introduce theory as needed
Theory and practice	Emphasize firm grasp of theory that learner can apply as needed	Emphasize practical applications that help learner to grasp theory
Setting	Classrooms, regular sessions	"Real-life" settings such as workplaces, community halls

by environmental health professionals in conducting this aspect of their tasks. Educators generally believe that teaching working adults requires teaching methods that are different from those used for teaching children or full-time students. Some expert educators note, however, that many of the methods developed for teaching working adults also have a major role to play in traditional teaching settings. Effective teaching methods that have been successfully applied in each of these groups are shown in Table 12.4.

Community presentations are usually given in response to specific problems. Residents of the community want the problem explained to them and want to hear about how it affects them. They usually want to know what will be done about the problem and can be very persistent in holding the authorities responsible for solving the problem. Community residents may be less interested in detailed explanations of the background to a problem and many not want to hear elaborate discussions of the implications of the problem beyond the effect on their own lives and their own community. There may also be individuals who come to these meetings with a specific agenda of their own and will use this as an opportunity to ask questions or make statements that are designed to change community attitudes or to commit the authorities to a course of action that may not be in the best interest of the community as a whole. The environmental health professional needs to be prepared for this situation.

In making community presentations, it is very important for the environmental health professional to maintain an appropriate attitude and demeanor. Presentations in which professionals appear to be too proud, too distant, and too busy to concern themselves with the residents own situations are doomed to failure and may cause great hostility in the crowd. Presentations in which professionals appear sympathetic, caring, accessible to the people, honest, and knowledgeable but not overbearing work best. Chapter 4 reviewed the key elements in risk perception and risk communication. These should always be borne in mind when preparing community presentations.

Education may also take place through the media. Environmental health professionals must often speak to journalists. Journalists control what they write and editors control how it appears, whether in newspapers or on television or radio. Journalists take great pride in their writing and do not like to be manipulated in their preparation of a story. As a result, it is very difficult for the environmental health professional to control how a story will appear in the media and any effort to control the story will usually be resisted by the journalist who is interviewing the professional. Efforts to distort or to downplay a story are very likely to lead to vigorous efforts by the journalist to investigate further in the hope of showing that there has been a cover-up. Most environmental stories are complicated and require detailed explanations to understand the situation thoroughly. Journalists usually do not have enough time to investigate routine stories prior to their deadlines and they rarely have the specialized training in science needed to understand the details. This places environmental health professionals at a big disadvantage when they are interviewed. Usually the best approach is to be open and honest, to keep the language about the problem simple, and to disclose freely and quickly any reservations, unknowns, and difficulties one may face in dealing with the problem. Otherwise, they are likely to come out anyway and will embarrass the environmental health professional and the agency that he or she represents. Once a problem is admitted, however, it ceases to be as newsworthy. It often helps to prepare a short and simple press release before meeting with the media, so that the details can be kept straight. Sometimes, it helps to practice describing the problem in short, vivid sentences that can be quoted directly. However, misquotes are inevitable. All practicing environmental health professionals have had some bad experiences with the media but there is no better way to educate large numbers of people in the community. Tips for working with the media were provided in Chapter 4. These should be reviewed before press conferences.

A good approach to handling community education and media requests for information is to create an information service or speakers corps within a professional association. Community organizations and media can be informed that if they would like to get an explanation of a particular problem or hear a speaker on a particular topic, they can contact the organization and a qualified speaker will be assigned.

Personal Example

Personal lifestyle was discussed in the section Ethical Principles That Guide Action on Environmental Health, in the context of being ethically consistent. One of the most powerful ways through which environmental health professionals can influence other people is by setting a good example in their own lives. Living in a way that is conserving of resources, nonpolluting (or at least minimally polluting), respectful of others, and that does not involve conspicuous overconsumption is one way to demonstrate to others that a lifestyle that is environmentally responsible can also be satisfying.

Expectations on the part of the public place a heavy responsibility on environmental health professionals. People are quick to see discrepancies between what one says and what one does. On the other hand, it is difficult to be effective as a professional when one cannot use the same tools and systems as other professionals, particularly in societies that are wasteful of resources and that value displays of wealth as symbols of power and authority. For example, bicycles are effective and nonpolluting means of transportation at the local level, but it is difficult to be effective as a national authority on environmental health if one cannot fly in airplanes or drive an automobile to get from one place to another. Wearing second-hand clothes made from local materials may be a very responsible and practical way to demonstrate concern at a local level, but this practice is likely to be counterproductive when one is talking to a business person about pollution-limiting measures or trying to persuade a national politician to change a policy that has implications for the economy.

Another opportunity to demonstrate commitment to environmental quality is to make one's own agency or workplace as environmentally sound as possible. Depending on the setting, this may mean encouraging recycling or reusing materials in the office, arranging work schedules of employees to make it easier to use less polluting public transportation, conserving energy in the building, and trying to influence the ministry, agency, or institution of which one is a part to reduce pollution, conserve energy, and recycle materials. For example, some hospitals have formed *green teams* to review their procedures to reduce waste, improve efficiency, and promote recycling and other environmentally sound measures.

Advocacy

A critically important role of environmental health professionals is to serve as advocates for environmentally sound policies and practices, much akin to the role of physician as the patient's advocate. This role overlaps the responsibilities mentioned earlier for public education and implies attempting to influence decision makers to adopt enlightened policies.

Within the environmental health professional's role as a technical expert, it is appropriate to advocate a preferred or scientifically rational solution to resolving a question after presenting an overview of the potential solutions and their implications. It generally works best if the pro's and con's of each potential solution are spelled out and a justification is given as to why one option is superior to the others. For narrowly technical problems, this is usually enough. The analysis by the experts will decide the matter. However, most major decisions are complicated by issues of cost, local history, public perception, political acceptability, and interrelation with other problems in the community. For better or for worse, it is up to the political decision-making bodies to decide on the best course of action that takes all of these factors into account.

Although the decision as to how far to go in attempting to influence decision makers is a personal issue for each environmental health professional, it is part of the professional's role to guide society in seeking the most appropriate solution. Depending on the country and political system, this may or may not be easy to do. One approach is to form or join professional associations and societies and to work within them to develop recommendations and policies that will influence decision makers. Often a statement on an issue prepared by a large organization carries much more weight than the opinion of an expert. It also shows that the problem was discussed in detail and thought through. For issues that are extremely urgent or serious, coalitions can be created among different organizations. These coalitions may issue statements, take positions, and express opinions in the name of all the member organizations. Politicians usually take these coalitions very seriously because they represent many different interests among their memberships and show that there is a broad consensus supporting the position. However, coalitions generally only work for specific issues and only then for a limited time. They tend to be unstable over the long term because the interests of each member organization will limit the degree of cooperation that can be obtained.

Networking

A very effective way for environmental health professionals to enhance their role and to increase their contribution to society is to network, by forming relationships between themselves and their organizations. Networks can be formal or informal, personal or institutionalized. They are created whenever colleagues keep in touch and share ideas and resources. A professional in a network is in a much stronger position than a professional in isolation.

Networks expand the range of options for dealing with a problem because they enable professionals to get good ideas, share or loan needed resources, learn about and adapt good ideas or innovative methods, and continuously stay educated about developments in the field and in the region. Interdisciplinary networks can also be effective in keeping the various members aware of new developments in their fields of expertise. The simplest network is the set of colleagues and friends in the field that environmental health professionals may have and the organizations to which they belong. More sophisticated networks may include WHO initiatives such as the Global Environmental Epidemiology Network (GEENET) and the Global Environment and Health Libraries Network (GELNET), which provide access to educational and practical tools by mail and electronic mail.

Although national and international networks are very useful and important, local or community networks may be exceptionally powerful when one needs to solve a local environmental problem. It is very helpful to be able to draw on community leaders, business representatives, scientists, and engineers as needed to solve a particular problem, and because they know the community that they live in, the solutions are likely to be more practical and feasible than solutions proposed by colleagues who do not live there. There is also likely to be greater support for proposed solutions.

Research and Documentation

A major responsibility of environmental health professionals is to document problems in their communities and, where appropriate, to conduct research to understand them. This may mean original laboratory research for those specially trained and with access to facilities, but more often it means a thorough investigation and consultation of references to determine how the problem started, why it continues, and what alternatives there are for solving the problem.

Documentation may be invaluable by providing hard evidence that something needs to be done and is often the key to motivating action. It also provides a benchmark against which subsequent improvement or deterioration can be evaluated. Original research to investigate the nature of environmental problems is difficult and often expensive. It requires special training and is often highly technical. However, most of our understanding of environmental issues has come from this difficult process and from the commitment of dedicated investigators who contributed facts, ideas, and analysis.

Although it is not always practical for an individual environmental health professional to conduct research personally, it is always possible to support good research. This can be done by encouraging talented students in the community to follow careers in environmental science, raising funds for such work, providing investigators with access to data, talking about the need for research in the community, and advocating support of research by government and professional societies.

The roles of professional societies in supporting good research cannot be overstated. Not only do they often raise money for research themselves but they provide the networks for investigators to organize their studies, a forum for judging the quality of research (sometimes just by providing an opportunity for it to be discussed), and meetings at which research findings can be presented. They also usually influence government and the private sector in supporting good-quality research.

Study Questions

Assuming that you agree that professionals should get involved, in the issues they study, what can you do with respect to each of the categories discussed in the section Role of Environmental Health Profession? Be as concrete as possible, with specific examples of actions that you might take.

REFERENCES

Following are abbreviations for the institutional organizations cited:

ACOHOS   Advisory Committee on Occupational Health and Occupational Safety (Canada)
ATSDR   Agency for Toxic Substances and Diseases Registry (U.S.)
CEMP   Center for Environmental Management and Planning
FAO   Food and Agriculture Organization of the United Nations
GEMS   Global Environment Monitoring System
HC   Health Canada
HWC   Health and Welfare, Canada
ILO   International Labour Organization
JBMC   James Bay Mercury Committee (Canada)
NCIPC   National Committee for Injury Prevention and Control (U.S.)
NILU   Norwegian Institute for Air Research
NIOSH   National Institute for Occupational Safety and Health (U.S.)
NRC   National Research Council (U.S.)
OECD   Organization for Economic Cooperation and Development
OTA   Office of Technology Assessment (U.S.)
UN   United Nations
UNDP   United Nations Development Program
UNEP   United Nations Environment Program
UNICEF   United Nations Childrens Fund
USEPA   U.S. Environmental Protection Agency
WCE   Watt Committee on Energy (U.K.)
WCED   World Commission on Environment and Development
WHO   World Health Organization
WRI   World Resources Institute

ACOHOS. (1983) *Principles and Procedures for the Interpretation of Epidemiological Studies.* Advisory Memorandum 82-V to the Minister of Labor, Toronto, Ontario, Canada.

Ad Hoc Population Dose Assessment Group. (1979) *Population Dose and Health Impact of the Accident at Three Mile Island Nuclear Station.* Washington, DC: U.S. Environmental Protection, and National Research Council.

Ajzen I. (1991) The theory of planned behaviour. *Organ Behav Hum Decision Processes* 50: 179–211.

Ames BN, Gold LS. (1990). Dietary carcinogens, environmental pollution, and cancer: some misconceptions. *Med Oncol Tumor Pharmacother* 7(2–3):69–85.

Anderson DM. (1992) The fifth international conference on toxic marine phytoplankton: a personal perspective. *Harmful Algae News* (Suppl. to *Int Marine Sci* 62:6–7).

Ascherio A, Chase R, Cote T, Dehaes G, Hoskins E, Laaquej J, Passey M, Qaderi S, Shuqaider S, Smith MC, Zaidi S. (1992) Effect of the Gulf War on infant and child mortality in Iraq. *N Engl J Med* 327:931–936.

Ashton SR, Fowler SW. (1985) Mercury in the open Mediterranean: evidence of contamination? *Sci Total Environ* 43(1–2):13–26.

ATSDR. (1992) *Public Health Assessment Guidance Manual.* MI: Lewis Publishers.

Baker D, Landrigan P. (1993) Occupational exposures and human health. In: *Critical Condition: Human Health and the Environment.* Chivian E, McCally M, Hu R, Haines A. (eds). Cambridge, MA: MIT Press.

Baker SP, O'Neill B, Karpf FS. (1984) *The Injury Fact Book.* Lexington: D.C. Health.

Bearer C. (1995) How are children different from adults?" *Environ Health Perspect* 103, (Suppl 6: 7–12).

Beaglehole R, Bonita R, Kjellström T. (1993) *Basic Epidemiology.* Geneva: World Health Organization.

Becklake MR. (1985) Chronic airflow limitation: its relationship to work in dusty occupations. *Chest* 4:608–617.

Becklake MR. (1989) Occupational exposures: evidence for a causal association with chronic obstructive pulmonary disease. *Am Rev Respir Dis* 140:S85–S91.

Beneson AS (ed). (1995) *Control of Communicable Diseases Manual.* United Book Press Inc., Baltimore, MD.

Berdén M, Nilsson SI, Rosén K, Tyler G. (1987) *Soil Acidification: Extent, Causes, and Consequences.* Solna, Sweden: National Swedish Environment Protection Board.

Bisson JI, Jenkins PL, Alexander J, Bannister C. (1997) Randomised controlled trial of psychological debriefing for victims for acute burn trauma. *Br J Psychiatry* 171:78–81.

Bosnir J, Puntaric D, Smit Z, Capuder Z. (1999) Fish as an indicator of eco-system contamination with mercury. *Croat Med J* 40(4):546–549.

Briggs D, Corvalan C, Nurminen M. (1996) *Linkage Methods for Environment and Health Analysis.* General Guidelines, Document WHO/EHG/95.26. Geneva: World Health Organization.

Brooks S, Gochfeld M, Herzstein J, Jackson R, Schenker MB. (1995) *Environmental Medicine.* St Louis: C.M. Mosby.

Bryan FL. (1989) *HACCP: Hazard Analysis Critical Control Point Manual.* Washington, DC: Food Marketing Institute.

Bryan FL. (1992) *Hazard Analysis Criticial Control Point Evaluations.* Geneva: World Health Organization.

Capuder Z. (1999) Fish as an indicator of eco-system contamination with mercury. *Croat Med J* 40(4):546–549.

Carson R. (1962) *Silent Spring.* Boston: Houghton Mifflin.

Cameco. (1996) *McArthur River Mining Development Environmental Impact Statement.* Saskatoon: Cameco Corporation.

Chivian E, McCally M, Hu R, Haines A. (1993) *Human Health and the Environment.* Cambridge, MA: MIT Press.

Clarkson TW, Friberg L, Nordberg GF, Sager PR (eds). (1988) *Biological Monitoring of Toxic Metals.* New York: Plenum Press.

Clatworthy S, Stevens H. (1987) *An Overview of the Housing Conditions in Registered Indians in Canada.* Ottawa: Department of Indian Affairs and Northern Development.

Codex Alimentarius Commission, Joint FAO/WHO, Food Standard Programme. (1989).

Colborn T, Dumanoski D, Peterson Myers J. (1996) *Our Stolen Future.* New York: Penguin.

Corvalán C, Kjellström T. (1995) Health and environment analysis for decision making. *World Health Stat Q* 49(2):71–77.

Corvalán C, Nurminen M, Pastides H. (1997) *Linkage Methods for Environment and Health Analysis.* Technical Guidelines, Document. WHO/EHG/ 97.11. Geneva: World Health Organization.

Covello VT. (1989) Informing people about risks from chemicals, radiation, and other toxic substances: a review of obstacles to public understanding and effective risk communication. In: *Prospects and Problems in Risk Communication.* Leiss W (ed). Canada: University of Waterloo Press, Waterloo.

Covello VT, Allen FW. (1988) *Seven Cardinal Rules of Risk Communication.* Washington, DC: U.S. Environmental Protection Agency.

Davies DL, Bradlow HL, Wolff M, Woodruff T, Hoel DG, Anton-Culver H. (1995) Medical hypothesis: xenoestrogens as preventable cause of breast cancer. *Environ Health Perspect* 101:372–377.

Dean K, Hancock T. (1992) *Supportive Environments for Health.* Copenhagen: World Health Organization.

Dejoy DM. (1984) A report on the status of research on the cardiovascular effects of noise. *Noise Control Engineering J* 23:32–39.

de Koning HW. (1987) *Setting Environmental Standards. Guidelines for Decision-Making.* Geneva: World Health Organization.

Dhara R, Dhara VR. (1995) Bhopal—a case study of international disaster. *Int J Occup Environ Health* 1(1):58–69.

Dunser HJ, Howells H, Templeton WL. (1959) District surveys following windscale incident in October 1959. In: *Proceedings of the Second United Nations International Conference on the Peaceful Uses of Atomic Energy* (Sept. 1–13, 1958). Geneva: United Nations.

Elinder CG, Friberg L, Kjellström T, Nordberg G, Oberdoerster G. (1994) *Biological Monitoring of Metals.* WHO Document WHO/EHG/94.2. Geneva: World Health Organization.

Environmental Agency (1975). *Studies on the Health Effects of Alkylmercury in Japan.* Tokyo, Japan: Environmental Agency.

Environment Canada. (1976) *Criteria for Air Quality Objectives.* Report for the Federal/Provincial Committee on Air Pollution. Ottawa: Environment Canada.

Environment Canada. (1987) The Great Lakes: An Environmental Atlas and Resource Book. Toronto, Ont: Environment Canada, in collaboration with US Environmental Protection Agency, Chicago, Illinois, as cited in Environment Canada (1991) State of the Environment Report. Ministry, Supply and Services, Ottawa, Canada.

Epstein PR, Rapport DJ. (1996) Changing coastal marine environments and human health. *Ecosystem Health* 2(3):166–176.

Ewetz L, Camner P (eds). (1983) *Motor Vehicles and Cleaner Air: Health Risks Resulting from Exposure to Motor Vehicle Exhaust.* A report to the Swedish Government Committee of Automotive Air Pollution Stockholm National Institute of Environmental Medicine. Stockholm, Sweden.

Falk H, Heath C. (1986) Vinyl chloride and cancer. In: *Teaching Epidemiology in Occupational Health.* Atlanta: U.S. National Institute for Occupational Safety and Health and World Health Organization.

FAO/WHO. (1994) *Codex Alimentarius.* Rome and Geneva: Food and Agricultural Organization/World Health Organization.

Federspiel JF. (1983) *The Ballad of Typhoid Mary.* New York: E.P. Dutton.

Fernández N, Tate RB, Bonet M, Cañizares M, Mas P, Yassi A. (2000) Health-risk perception in the inner city community of Centro Habana, Cuba. *Int J Occup Environ Health* 6(1):34–43.

Fletcher RG, Fletcher SW, Wagner EH. (1982) *Clinical Epidemiology—The Essentials.* Baltimore: Williams & Wilkins.

Foley G. (1992) Renewable energy in third world energy assistance. *Energy Policy* 20(4):335–361.

Folinsbee LJ. (1992) Human health effects of air pollution. *Environ Health Perspect* 100:45–56.

Franklin CA, Burnett RT, Paolini RJ, Raizenne ME. (1985) Health risks from acid rain: a Canadian perspective. *Environ Health Perspect* 63:155–68.

Garfield M, Neugut A (1997) The human consequences of war. In: *War and Public Health.* Levy BS, Sidel VW (eds). New York: Oxford University Press, pp. 27–38.

Goldman LR. (1995) Children—unique and vulnerable: Environmental risks facing children and recommendations for response. *Environ Health Perspect* 103(Suppl 6):13–18.

Goyer RA, Bachmann J, Clarkson TW, Ferris BG, Graham J, Mushak P, Perl DP, Schlesinger R, Sharpe W. (1985) Potential human health effects of acid rain: report of workshop. *Environ Health Perspect* 60:355–368.

Green LW, Kreuter M. (1999) *Health Promotion Planning: An Educational and Ecological Approach* (3rd ed). Mountain View, CA: Mayfield.

Gregory K. (1992) The earth summit: opportunity for energy reform. *Energy Policy* 20(6):547.

Guidotti TL. (1986) Managing incidents involving hazardous substances. *Am J Prev Med* 2(3):148–154.

Guidotti TL. (1995) Perspective on the health of urban ecosystems. *Ecosystem Health* 1(3): 141–149.

Guyer B, Gallagher SS. (1985) An approach to the epidemiology of childhood injuries. *Pediatr Clin North Am* 32:5–16.

Haddon W. (1980) Advances in epidemiology of injuries as a basis for public policy. *Public Health Reports* 95(5):411–421.

Haglund BJA, Pettersson B, Finer D, Tillgren P. (1992) *The Sundsvall Handbook: "We Can Do It!"* 3rd International Conference on Health Promotion, Sundsvall, Sweden. June 10–15, 1991 Karolinska Institute, Stockholm.

Hallenbeck WH. (1993) *Quantitative Risk Assessment for Environmental and Occupational Health.* Western Springs, MI: Lewis Publishers.

Hammond GW, Rutherford BE, Malazdrewicz R, MacFarlane N. (1988) *Haemophilus influenzae* meningitis in Manitoba and the Keewatin District NWT: potential for mass vaccination. *Can Med Assoc J* 139:743–747.

Hancock T. (1996) Planning and creating healthy and sustainable cities: the challenge for the 21st century. In C. Price and A. Tsouros (eds.) *Our Cities, Our Future: Policies and Action for Health and Sustainable Development.* Copenhagen: WHO Healthy Cities Project Office.

Hancock T. *Urban Ecosystems and Human Health.* A paper prepared for the seminar on CIID-IDRC and urban development in Latin America, Montevideo, Uruguay, Apr 6–7, 2000.

Hansen J, et al. (1989) Regional greenhouse climate effects. In: *Coping with Climate Change* (Proceedings of the Second North American Conference on Preparing for Climate Change, 6–8 December 1988). Washington, DC: Climate Institute.

Havlicek P. (1997) The Czech Republic: First steps toward a cleaner future. *Environment* 39(3):38–39.

HC. (1992) *Guidelines for Canadian Recreational Water Quality,* Health Canada, Ottawa, Canada.

HC. (1993) *Investigating Human Exposure to Contaminants in the Environment: A Handbook for Exposure Calculations* (draft). Ottawa: Great Lakes Health Effects Division, Health Protection Branch, Health Canada.

HC. (1995). *Health and Environment: A Handbook for Health Professionals.* Ottawa and Toronto: The Great Lakes Health Effects Program, Health Canada and The Environmental Health and Toxicology Unit, Ontario Ministry of Health.

Hertzman C, Frank J, Evans RG. (1994) Heterogeneities in health status and the determinants of population health. In: Evans R, Barer, ML, Marmor, TR. (eds) *Why Are Some People Healthy and Others Not?* New York: Aldine de Gruyter pp. 67–92.

Hespanol I, Helmer R. (1993) The importance of water pollution control for sustainable development. Presented at WHO Symposium on Water Use and Conservation, Amman, Jordan.

Howe GR, Nair RC, Newcombe HB, Miller AB, Abbatt JD. (1986) Lung cancer mortality (1950–80) in relation to radon daughter exposure in a cohort of workers at the Eldorado Beaverlodge uranium mine. *J Nat Cancer Inst* 77:357–362.

Howe GR, Nair RC, Newcombe HB, Miller AB, Burch JD, Abbatt JD. (1987) Lung cancer mortality (1950–80) in relation to radon daughter exposure in a cohort of workers at the Eldorado Port Radium Uranium Mine: Possible modification of risk by exposure rate. *J Natl Cancer Inst* 79:1255–1260.

Huq A, Colwell RR. (1996) Vibrios in the marine and estuarine environment: tracking vibrio cholerae. *Ecosystem Health* 2(3):198–214.

HWC. (1990) *Nutrition Recommended, The Report of the Scientific Review Committee.* Ottawa: Health and Welfare, Canada.

ILO. (1998) *Encyclopaedia of Occupational Health and Safety,* 4th ed. Stellman JM (ed). Geneva: International Labor Organization.

Inhaber H. (1979) Risk with energy from conventional and nonconventional sources. *Science* 23;203(4382):718–723.

Intergovernmental Panel on Climate Change. (1996). *Climate Change 1995: The Science of Climate Change* Cambridge, U.K.: Cambridge University Press, p. 4.

Jacob M. (1989) *Safe Food Handling: A Training Guide for Managers of Food Service Establishments.* Geneva: World Health Organization.

JBMC. (1995) *Report of Activities 1994–1995.* Montreal: James Bay Mercury Committee.

Jedrychowski W, Krzyzanowski M (eds). (1995) *Host Factors in Environmental Epidemiology.* Proceedings of the Conference and Workshop, Cracow, June 11–14, 1995. Central and Eastern European Chapter of ISEE/ISEA, WHO

Jeyaratnam J (ed.) (1992) *Occupational Health in Developing Countries.* Oxford: Oxford University Press.

Jones RR. (1987) Ozone depletion and cancer risk. *Lancet* 11:443–445.

Jones TS, Liang AP, Kilbourne EM, Griffin MR, Patriarca PA, Wassilak SG, Mullan RJ, Herrick RF, Donnell HD Jr., Choik Thacker SB. (1982) Morbidity and mortality associated with the July 1980 heat wave in St. Louis and Kansas City, Mo. *JAMA* 247:3327–3331.

Kaferstein FK, Miyagishima K, Miyagawa S, Motarjemi Y, Moy G. (1995) What is food quality and safety? In: *Proceedings of Food Session, 39th EOQ Annual Congress.* Hochschulverlag.

Kalimo R, El-Batawi MA, Cooper CL (eds). (1987) *Psychosocial Factors at Work and Their Relation to Health.* Geneva: World Health Organization.

Kawachi I. (1999) Social capital and community effects on population and individual health. *Ann N Y Acad Sci* 896:120–30.

Kjellström T, (1986a) Itai-itai disease. In: *Cadmium and Health,* Vol. 2. Friberg L, Elinder CG, Kjellstrom T, Nordberg G. et al. (eds). Boca Raton, FL: CRC Press

Kjellström T. (1986b) Critical organs, critical concentrations, and whole body dose–response relationships. In: *Cadmium and Health,* Vol. 2. Friberg L, Elinder CG, Kjellstrom T, Nordberg G (eds). Boca Raton, FL: CRC Press.

Kjellström T, Hicks N. (1991) Atmospheric fog in greater London. In: *Problem-Based Training Exercises for Environmental Epidemiology.* WHO Document WHO/PEP/92.05-A. Geneva: World Health Organization.

Kjellström T, Rosenstock L. (1990) The role of environmental and occupational hazards in the adult health transition. *World Health Stat Q* 43:188–196.

Kjellström T, Yassi A. (1998) Linkages between environmental and occupational health. In: *Encyclopaedia of Occupational and Safety,* 4th ed. Stellman JM (ed). Geneva: International Labour Organization, pp. 532–534.

Kleinman MT, Phalen RF, Mautz WJ, Mannix RC, McClure TR, Crocker TT. (1989) Health effects of acid aerosols formed by atmospheric mixtures. *Environ Health Perspect* 79:137–145.

Kraus JF, Robertson LS. (1992) Injuries and the public health. In: *Public Health and Preventive Medicine,* 13th ed. Last JM, Norwalk (eds). New York: Appleton-Century-Crofts.

Kusiac RA, Ritchie AC, Muller J, Springer J. (1993) Mortality from lung cancer in Ontario uranium miners. *Br J Ind Med* 50(10):920–928.

Last JM. (1992) Global environment, health, and health services. In: *Public Health and Preventive Medicine,* 13th ed. Last JM, Norwalk (eds). New York: Appleton-Century-Crofts.

Last JM (ed). (1995) *A Dictionary of Epidemiology,* 3rd ed. New York: Oxford University Press.

Leaf A. (1989) Potential health effects of global climatic and environmental changes. *N Engl J Med* 321:1577–1583.

Lebel J, Mergler D, Lucotte M, Amorim M, Dolbec J, Miranda D, Arantes G, Rheault I, Pichet P. (1996) Evidence of early nervous system dysfunction in Amazonian populations exposed to low levels of methylmercury. *Neurotoxicology* 17:157–168.

Lemeshov S, Hosmer DW, Klar J, Lwange SK. (1990) *Adequacy of Sample Size in Health Studies.* New York: John Wiley & Sons.

Levy BS, Sidel VW (eds). (1997) *War and Public Health.* New York: Oxford University Press.

Levy BS, Wegman DH (eds). (1988) *Occupational Health: Recognising and Preventing Work-Related Disease,* 2nd ed. Boston/Toronto: Little, Brown and Company.

Letourneau EG, Krewski D, Zielinski JM, McGregor RG. Cost-effectiveness of radon mitigation in Canada. *Radiat Protection Dosimetry* suppl 1–4:593–598.

Lovelock J. (1988) *The Ages of Gaia. A Biography of our Living Earth.* London: Norton.

Mage DT, Zali O. (1992) *Motor Vehicle Air Pollution: Public Health Impact and Control Measures.* WHO Document WHO/PEP/92.4. Geneva: World Health Organization.

Manitoba Labour. (1991) *Guidelines for Work in Hot Environments.* Manitoba Government, Winnipeg, Canada.

Marrett LD, King WD. (1995) *Great Lakes Basin Cancer Risk Assessment: A Case–Control Study of Cancers of the Bladder, Colon and Rectum.* Ottawa: Laboratory Centre for Disease Control, Health Canada.

McGuigan MA. (1992) Teratogenesis and reproductive toxicology. In: *Hazardous Materials Toxicology: Clinical Principles of Environmental Health.* Sullivan JB Jr, Krieger GR (eds). Baltimore: Williams & Wilkins, pp. 179–189.

McMichael AJ. (1993) *Planetary Overload: Global Environmental Change and The Health of the Human Species.* Cambridge, UK: Cambridge University Press.

McMichael AJ, Haines A, Slooff R, Kovats S. (1996) *Climate Change and Human Health.* WHO Document WHO/EHG/96.7. Geneva: World Health Organization.

Meinhardt PL, Casemore DP, Miller KB. (1996) Epidemiologic aspects of human cryptosporidiosis and the role of waterborne transmission. *Epidemiol Rev* 18:118–136.

Michaels D, Barrera C, Gacharna MG (1985) Economic development and occupational health in Latin America: new directions for public health in less developed countries. *Am J Public Health* 75:536–542.

Mitchell JT, Everly GS Jr. (1999) As cited from—*Critical Incident Stress Debriefing: An Operations Manual for the Prevention of Traumatic Stress Among Emergency Services and Disaster Workers.* Ellicott City, MD: Chevron Publishing Corp.

Moan J, Dahlback A, Larsen S, Henriksen T, Stamnes K (1989) Ozone depletion and its consequences for the influence of carcinogenic sunlight. *Cancer Res* 49:4247–4250.

Morgan WKC, Seaton A (eds). (1995) *Occupational Lung Diseases,* 3rd ed. Toronto: W.B. Saunders.

Morrison WL. (1989) Effects of ultraviolet radiation on the immune system in humans. *Photochem Photobiol* 50:515–524.

Mungall C, McLaren D (eds). (1990) *Planet Under Stress: The Challenge of Global Change.* Toronto: Oxford University Press/Royal Society of Canada.

Murray CJL, Lopez AD. (1996) The Global Burden of Disease: Volume 1. Geneva: World Health Organization, Harvard School of Public Health, and The World Bank.

Murray CJL, Yang G, Qiao X (1992) Adult mortality: levels, patterns and causes. In: *The Health of Adults in the Developing World.* Feachem RGA, Kjellström T, Murray CJL, Over M (eds). Oxford: Oxford University Press.

Nafis S. (1990) *Investing in Women: The Focus of the '90's.* New York: United Nations Population Fund.

National Academy of Sciences. (1992) *Ozone Depletion, Greenhouse Gases, and Climate Change.* Washington, DC: National Academy Press.

NCIPC. (1989) The National Committee for Injury Prevention and Control. Introduction: a history of injury prevention. *Am J Prev Med* 5:4–18.

Nell J, Stewart K. (1994) *Death in Transition: The Rise in the Death Rate in Russia Since 1992.* Florence: United Nations Children's Fund International Child Development Center.

Newman LS. (1992) Pulmonary toxicology. In: *Hazardous Materials Toxicology: Clinical Principles of Environmental Health.* Sullivan JB Jr, Krieger GR (eds). Baltimore: Williams & Wilkins, pp. 124–144.

Niesink, et al. (1996) *General Toxicology, Principles and Applications.* Boca Raton, FL: CRC Press.

NIOSH. (1988) *Proposed National Strategy for the Prevention of Disorders of Reproduction.* Cincinnati: National Institute for Occupational Safety and Health.

NIOSH. (1995) *Cumulative Trauma Disorders in the Workplace: Bibliography.* Cincinnati: National Institute for Occupational Safety and Health.

Noguiera DP. (1987) Prevention of accidents and injuries in Brazil. *Ergonomics* 30:387–393.

Norman R, Wells R. (2000) Ergonomic interventions for reducing musculoskeletal disorders. In: Sullivan T (ed). *Injury and the New World,* Vancouver, UBC Press, pp. 115–139.

NRC. (1991) *Human Exposure Assessment for Airborne Pollutants.* Washington, DC: National Research Council.

NRC. (1999) Biological Effects of Ionizing Radiation (BEIR) VI Report. The Health Affects of Exposure to Indoor Radon. NRC. National Academy of Sciences: 28 May 1999. (http://www.ruderserv.com/discussion).

OECD. (1991) *State of the Environment Report.* Paris: Organization for Economic Cooperation and Development.

O'Grady J. (2000) Joint Health and Safety Committees: finding a balance. In: Sullivan T (ed). *Injury and the New World,* Vancouver, UBC Press, pp. 162–197.

Ong CN, Jeyaratnam J, Koh D. (1993) Factors influencing the assessment and control of occupational hazards in developing countries. *Environ Res* 60:112–123.

Ostro B. (1996) *A Methodology for Estimating Air Pollution Health Effects.* WHO Document WHO/EHG/96.5 Geneva: World Health Organization.

OTA. (1992) *Fueling Development: Energy Technology for Developing Countries.* Washington, DC: Office of Technology Assessment.

Pandey MR. (1984) Domestic smoke pollution and chronic bronchitis in a rural community of the hill region of Nepal. *Thorax* 39:339–339.

Pandey MR, Boleij JS, Smith KR, Wafula EM. (1989) Indoor air pollution in developing countries and acute respiratory infection in children. *Lancet* 25;(8635):427–429.

Pisaniello DL, McMichael AJ, Woodward A. (1993) *Guidelines on Planning Education and Training for the Control of Environmental Health Hazards: A Contribution to Capacity-Building at National and Sub-National Levels.* Geneva: World Health Organization.

Pless M. (1994) Editorial. Unintentional childhood injury—where the buck should stop. *Am J Public Health* 84:537–539.

Polanyi M, Frank J, Shannon H, Sullivan T, Lavis J. (2000) Promoting the determinants of good health in the workplace. In: Poland B, Green L, Rootman I. (eds.). *Settings for Health Promotion: Linking Theory and Practice.* Newbury Park, CA: Sage, pp. 138–160.

Putnam RD. (1993) *Making Democracy Work.* New Jersey: Princeton University Press.

Rapport DJ. (1995a) Ecosystem health: exploring the territory. *Ecosystem Health* 1:5–13.

Rapport DJ. (1995b) Ecosystem health: an emerging integrative science. In: *Evaluating and Monitoring the Health of Large-Scale Ecosystems.* Rapport DJ, Gaudet CL, Calow P (eds). NATO ASI Series 1. Global Environmental Change Vol 28 Springer-Verlag, Berlin, Germany.

Rapport DJ. (1998) Editorial: ecosystem health as an ecotone. *Ecosystem Health,* 4(1):1–2.

Rapport DJ. (1997) The dependency of human health on ecosystem health. *Ecosystem Health* 3:4:195–196.

Rees W, Wackengel M. (1992) *Our Ecological Footprint: Reducing Human Input on the Earth.* Gabriola Island, B.C., Canada: New Society Publishers.

Robock A. (1991) Nuclear winter: global horrendous death. In: *Horrendous Death, Health, and Well-Being.* Leviton D (ed). New York: Hemisphere Publishing.

Royal Commission (on the Health and Safety of Workers in Mines). (1976) *Report of the Royal Commission on the Health and Safety of Workers in Mines.* Toronto: Government of Ontario.

Rundel RD, Nachtwey DS. (1983) Projections of increase non-melanoma skin cancer incidence due to ozone depletion. *Photochem Photobiol* 38:577–591.

Rutten AAJJ. (1997) Adverse Effects of Nutrients. In: deVries J (ed) *Food Safety and Toxicity.* Boca Raton, FL: CR Press, pp 163–171.

Rylander R. (1992) Effects on humans of environmental noise particularly from road traffic. In: *Motor Vehicle Air Pollution: Public Health Impact and Control Measures.* Mage DT, Zali O (eds). Geneva: Ecotoxicology Service and Canton of Geneva and World Health Organization, pp. 63–83.

Samet JM, Utell MJ. (1990) The risk of nitrogen dioxide: what have we learned from epidemiological and clinical studies. *Toxicol Indust Health* 26:247–262.

Sandman P. (1986) *Explaining Environmental Risk.* Washington, DC: U.S. Environmental Protection Agency, Office of Toxic Substances.

Schaefer M. (1991) *Combating Environmental Pollution: National Capabilities for Health Protection.* WHO Document WHO/PEP/91.14. Geneva: World Health Organization.

SCHEP. (1983) *The Swedish-Coal-Health-Environment Project.* Stockholm: The Swedish State Power Board.

Schneider SH. (1987) Climate modeling. *Sci Am* 256(5):72–80.

Schultz TJ, Galloway WJ, Beland D, Hirtle PW. (1976) Recommendations for changes in HUD's noise policy standards. Washington, DC: Department of Housing and Urban Development.

Shah CP. (1994) *Public Health and Preventive Medicine in Canada.* Toronto: University of Toronto Press.

Shannon, H. (2000) Firm-level organizational practices and work injury. In: Sullivan T (ed.) *Injury and the New World.* UBC Press pp. 140–161.

Sharpe RM, Skakkeback NE. (1993) Are oestrogens involved in the falling sperm counts and disorders of the male reproductive system. *Lancet* 341:1392–1395.

Shiklomanov IA. (1993) World Fresh Water Resources. In Gliek H. (ed) *Water in Crisis.* New York: Oxford University Press, pp 1–25.

Sims J. (1994) *Women, Health and the Environment. An Anthology.* WHO Document WHO/EHG/94.11. Geneva: World Health Organization.

Smayda TJ, Shimizu Y. (1993) *Toxic Phytoplankton Blooms in the Sea.* Oxford: Elsevier.

Smith KR. (1987) *Biofuels, Air Pollution and Health: A Global Review.* New York: Plenum Press.

Smith KR. (1991) *Biomass Cookstoves in Global Perspective: Energy, Health and Global Warming.* Geneva: World Health Organization.

Somerville MA, Rapport D. (2000) *Transdisciplinarity: Recreating Integrated Knowledge.* EOLLS Publishers, Oxford, UK, 272 pp.

Soskolne CL, Light A. (1996) Towards ethics guidelines for environmental epidemiologists. In: *The Science of the Total Environment.* pp. 137–147.

Sparks PJ, Daniell WM, Black DW, Kipen WM, Altman LC, Simon GE, Terr AI (1994) Multiple chemical sensitivity syndrome: a clinical perspective. *J Occup Med* 36:718–737.

Sparks PJ. (2000) Multiple chemical sensitivity and idopathic environmental intolerance. *Occ Med: State of the Art Reviews* 15(3):497–675.

Spiegel JM. (2000) A comparison of economic valuation methods for environmental health risk reduction: Assessing residential radon mitigation in Manitoba. Winnipeg, MB. PhD Thesis University of Manitoba, Dept of Community Health Sciences.

Spiegel J, Yassi A. (1991) Occupational disease surveillance in Canada: a framework for considering options and opportunities. *Can J Public Health* 82:294–299.

Spiegal J, Bonet M, Yassi A, Molina E, Concepcion M, Mas P. (2001) Developing ecosystem health indicators in Centro Habana: a community based approach. *Ecosystem Health* forthcoming.

Statistics Canada. (1994) *Human Activity and the Environment 1994.* Ottawa: Minister of Supply & Services.

Stephens B, et al. (1985) Health and low-cost housing. *World Health Forum* 6:59–62.

Stephens C, Akerman M, Borlina Maia P. (1995) Health and Environment in Sao Paulo, Brazil: Methods of data linkage and questions of policy. *World Health Stat Q* 48(2):95–107.

Stover E, Cobey JC, Fine J. (1997) The public health effects of land mines: long-term consequences for civilians. In: *War and Public Health.* Levy BS, Sidel VW (eds). New York: Oxford University Press, pp. 137–146.

Sullivan T, Frank J. (2000) Restating Disability or Disabling the State: Four Challenges. Introduction in Injury and the New World of Work, Vancouver, UBC Press, pp. 3–24.

Tengs TO, Adams ME, Pliskis JS, Safron DG, Siegel JC, Weinstein MC, Graham JD. (1995) Five hundred life-saving interventions and their cost-effectiveness. *Risk Anal* 15(3):369–390.

Thomas L. (1984) Scientific and national frontiers: a look ahead. *Foreign Affairs* 62(4): 966–994.

Turco RP, et al. (1990) Climate and smoke: an appraisal of nuclear winter. *Science* 247:166–176.

Turkenburg W. (2000) Renewable energy technologies. In: *World Energy Assessment*. New York: United Nations Development Program, Chapter 7.

UN. (1948) *Universal Declaration of Human Rights.* New York: United Nations.

UN. (1993) *Agenda 21: The United Nations Programme of Action from Rio.* New York: United Nations.

UN. (1996). *World Population Prospects 1950–2050* (The 1996 Revision). On diskette (U.N. Population Division, New York).

UN. (1997) Population Division. (1997) *World Urbanization Prospects: The 1996 Revision, Annex Tables* New York: U.N. Population Division, pp. 66–71.

UNDP. (1995) *Human Development Report.* New York: Oxford University Press, United Nations Development Program.

UNDP. (1997). *Human Development Report 1997* New York: Oxford University Press, pp. 3–4.

United Nations Educational, Scientific and Cultural Organization (UNESCO). (1996). *Statistical Yearbook 1996.* Paris: UNESCO, pp. 2–9.

UNEP. (1992a) *Saving Our Planet: The State of the Environment (1972–1992).* Nairobi: United Nations Environment Program.

UNEP. (1992b) *Chemical Pollution: A Global Overview.* Nairobi: United Nations Environment Program.

UNEP. (1993) *Environmental Data Report.* Nairobi: United Nations Environment Program.

UNEP/GEMS. (1992) *Contamination of Food.* Geneva: United Nations Environment Program and Global Environmental Monitoring System.

UNEP/ILO/WHO. (1993) *How to Use the IPCS Health and Safety Guides.* Nairobi and Geneva: United Nations Environment Program, International Labor Office, and the World Health Organization.

UNEP/WHO. (1984) *Urban Air Pollution 1973–1980.* Nairobi and Geneva: United Nations Environment Program and World Health Organization.

UNEP/WHO. (1987a) *Improving Environmental Health Conditions in Low-Income Settlements.* Nairobi and Geneva: United Nations Environment Program and the World Health Organization.

UNEP/WHO. (1987b) *Global Pollution and Health, Results of Health-Related Environmental Monitoring.* London: United Nations Environment Program and World Health Organization.

UNEP/WHO. (1992a) *Introductory Guide to Human Exposure Field Studies: Survey Methods and Statistical Sampling.* Nairobi and Geneva: United Nations Environment Program and the World Health Organization.

UNEP/WHO. (1992b) *Human Exposure to Pollutants.* Nairobi and Geneva: United Nations Environment Program and the World Health Organization.

UNEP/WHO. (1992c) *Urban Air Pollution in Megacities of the World.* Oxford: Blackwell, United Nations Environment Program and the World Health Organization.

UNEP/WHO. (1993) *Guidance on Survey Design for Human Exposure Assessment Locations (HEAL) Studies.* Nairobi: United Nations Environment Program and World Health Organization.

UNICEF. (1994) *State of the World's Children.* New York: Oxford University Press.

United Nations Environment Programme (UNEP). (2000) GEO-200 Global Environment Outlook. (http://www-cger.nies.go.jp/geo2000/index.htm) (www.grida.no/geo2000).

UNICEF. (1997) *The Progress of Nations 1997* New York: UNICEF.

USEPA. (1973) *Public Health and Welfare Criteria for Noise.* Washington, DC: U.S. Environmental Protection Agency.

USEPA. (1997) *1997 Declaration of the Environment Leaders of the Fight on Children's Environmental Health* (Miami, Florida). Washington, DC: U.S. Environmental Protection Agency.

Utell MJ, Samet JM. (1993) Particulate air pollution and health. New evidence on an old problem. *Am Rev Respir Dis* 147:1334–1335.

Van Wijnen JH. (1990) Health risk assessment of soil contamination. PhD Thesis, University of Amsterdam, Rodopi, Amsterdam, The Netherlands.

Vincent JH. (1993) Perspectives on international standards for health related sampling of airborne contaminants. *Appl Occup Environ Hygiene* 8:233–238.

Waldram D, Herring DA, Young TK. (1995) *Aboriginal Health in Canada: Historical, Cultural, and Epidemiological Perspectives.* Toronto: University of Toronto Press.

Waller JA. (1986) Prevention of premature death and disability due to injury. In: *Public Health and Preventive Medicine,* 12th ed. Last JM, Norwalk (eds). New York: Appleton-Century-Crofts, World Health Organization.

WCE. (1990) *Risk and the Energy Industries.* Watt Committee on Energy 27th Consultative Conference, University of Birmingham, U.K.

WCED. (1987) *Our Common Future.* Report of the World Commission on Environment and Development. Oxford: Oxford University Press.

WHO. (1948) *Constitution of the World Health Organization.* Geneva: World Health Organization.

WHO. (1980a) *Noise: Environmental Health Criteria No. 12.* Geneva: World Health Organization.

WHO. (1980b) *Health Guidelines for the Use of Wastewater in Agriculture and Aguaculture.* Geneva: World Health Organization.

WHO. (1982) *The Epidemiology of Accident Traumas and Resulting Disabilities.* WHO Document ICP/ADR 051(1). Copenhagen: World Health Organization.

WHO. (1985) *Environmental Health Impact Assessment of Urban Development Projects: Guidelines and Recommendations.* Copenhagen: WHO Regional Office for Europe.

WHO. (1986) *The Ottawa Charter for Health Promotion.* Copenhagen: WHO Europe.

WHO. (1986) *Health and Safety Component of Environmental Impact Assessment.* Copenhagen: WHO Regional Office for Europe.

WHO. (1987a) *Air Quality Guidelines for Europe.* WHO European Series No. 23. Copenhagen: World Health Organization.

WHO. (1987b) *Agrochemical Report.* Geneva: World Health Organization.

WHO. (1988) *Food Irradiation.* Geneva: World Health Organization.

WHO. (1989) *Health Principles of Housing.* Geneva: World Health Organization.

WHO. (1990a) *Public Health Impact of Pesticides Used in Agriculture.* Geneva: World Health Organization.

WHO. (1990b) *Potential Health Effects of Climatic Change: Report of a WHO Task Group.* WHO Document WHO/PEP/90.10. Geneva: World Health Organization.

WHO (1990c) Third Meeting of the WHO Scientific Committee for the Toxic Oil Syndrome. Report EUR/SPA/PCS/010/B. Copenhagen: World Health Organization.

WHO. (1991a) *Investigating Environmental Disease Outbreaks: A Training Manual.* WHO Document WHO/PEP/91.35. Geneva: World Health Organization.

WHO. (1991b) *Indoor Air Pollution from Biomass Fuel.* Geneva: World Health Organization.

WHO. (1992a) *Our Planet, Our Health.* Geneva: World Health Organization.

WHO. (1992b) *Panel Report on Food and Agriculture.* Geneva: World Health Organization.

WHO. (1992c) *Panel Report on Urbanisation.* Geneva: World Health Organization.

WHO. (1992d) *Report of the Panel on Energy.* WHO Document WHO/EHE/92.3. Geneva: World Health Organization.

WHO. (1992e) *Report of Panel on Industry.* WHO Document WHO/EHE/92.4. Geneva: World Health Organization.

WHO. (1992f) *Cadmium: Environmental Health Criteria No 134.* Geneva: World Health Organization.

WHO. (1993a) *Global Strategy: Health, Environment and Development: Approaches to Drafting Country-Level Strategies for Human Well-Being Under Agenda 21.* WHO Document WHO/EHE/93.1. Geneva: World Health Organization.

WHO. (1993b) *The Urban Health Crisis: Strategies for Health for All in the Face of Rapid Urbanisation.* Report of the Technical Discussions at the Forty-fourth World Health Assembly. Geneva: World Health Organization.

WHO. (1993c) *Air Quality Guidelines for Europe.* WHO European Series No. 23. Copenhagen: World Health Organization.

WHO. (1993d) *Guidelines for Drinking Water Quality.* Geneva: World Health Organization.

WHO. (1994a) *Ultraviolet Radiation: Environmental Health Criteria.* No. Geneva: World Health Organization.

WHO. (1994b) *Nuclear Power and Health: The Implications for Health of Nuclear Power Pro-*

duction. WHO Regional Publications European Series #51. Geneva: World Health Organization.

WHO. (1995a) *World Health Report 1995: Bridging the Gap.* Geneva: World Health Organization.

WHO. (1995b) *Twenty Steps for Developing a Health Cities Project.* WHO Document ICP/HSC 644(2). Copenhagen: WHO Regional Office for Europe.

WHO. (1995c) *Health Consequences of the Chernobyl Accident.* Geneva: World Health Organization.

WHO. (1996) *Bovine Spongiform Encephalopathy (BSE) Fact Sheet N113.* Geneva: World Health Organization.

WHO. (1997) *Health and Environment in Sustainable Development: Five Years After the Earth Summit* Geneva: WHO.

WHO. (1998a) *The World Health Report. Life in the 21st Century. A Vision for All.* Geneva: World Health Organization.

WHO. (1998b) *Problem-Based Training Exercises For Environmental Epidemiology.* Document WHO/EHG/98.2. Geneva: World Health Organization.

WHO. (1999) *Air Quality Guidelines for Europe, World Health Organization, Regional Office for Europe.* Copenhagen. (www.who.int/peh/air/Airqualitygd.htm).

WHO/CEMP. (1992) *Environmental Impact Assessment of Development Projects. A Handbook for Practitioners.* London: Elsevier Applied Science, World Health Organization and Center for Environmental Management and Planning.

WHO/NILU (1996) *Quantification of Health Effects Related to SO_2, NO_2, O_3 and Particulate Matter Exposure.* WHO Document EUR/ICP/EHAZ 94 04/DT01. Copenhagen: WHO Regional Office for Europe and Norwegian Institute for Air Research.

WHO/UNEP. (1989) *Global Freshwater Quality: A First Assessment.* Geneva and Nairobi: World Health Organization Global Environmental Monitoring Program.

WHO/UNEP. (1991) *An Introductory Guide to Human Exposure Field Studies Survey Methods and Statistical Sampling.* Nairobi and Geneva: World Health Organization and United Nations Environment Program.

Will RG, Ironside JW, Zeidler M, Cousens SN, Estibeiro K, Alperovitch A, Poser S, Pocchiari M, Hofman A, Smith PG. (1996) A new variant of Creutzfeldt-Jakob disease in the UK. *Lancet* 347(9006):921–925.

Wilson R, Crouch EA. (1987) Risk assessment and comparisons: an introduction. *Science* 236(4799):267–270.

World Bank. (1990) *World Development Report.* Washington, DC: World Bank.

World Bank. (1993) *World Development Report.* Washington, DC: World Bank.

WRI. (1992) *World Resources (1992–93).* Washington, DC: World Resources Institute.

WRI. (1994) *World Resources (1994–95).* Washington, DC: World Resources Institute.

WRI. (1996) In collaboration with the United Nations Environment Programme, the United Nations Development Programme, and the World Bank. *World Resources Report 1996–97* New York: Oxford University Press.

WRI. (1998) in collaboration with the United Nations Environment Programme, the United Nations Development Programme, and the World Bank. *World Resources Report 1998–99* New York: Oxford University Press.

Yassi A. (1997) Repetitive strain injuries. *Lancet* 349:943–947.

Yassi A. (2000) Work-related musculoskeletal disorders. *Curr Opin Rheumatol* 12:124–130.

Yassi A, Cheang M, Tennebein M, Bawden G, Spiegel J, Redekop T. (1991) An analysis of occupational blood lead trends in Manitoba, 1979 through 1987. *Am J Public Health* 81:736–740.

Yassi A, McLean D. (2001) Assault and abuse in healthcare facilities. *Clin Occupational Environ Med.* 1(2): in press.

Yassi A, Mas P, Bonet M, Tate RB, Fernandez N, Spiegel J, Perez M. (1999) Applying an ecosystem approach to the determinants of health in centro Habana. *Ecosystem Health* 5(1):3–19.

Yassi A, Redekop T, Alberg N, Cheang M. (1996) Occupational blood lead trends in Manitoba, 1979–1994: assessing the effectiveness of regulation and surveillance. In: *Lead in the Americas: A Call for Action.* Howson CP, Hernandez-Avila M, Rall DP (eds).

INDEX

Page numbers followed by b, f and t indicate boxes, figures and tables, respectively

chemical hazards, 75–79, 77t
  chronic, 77t, 78
  in experimental animals, 75–79
  genotoxic short-term, 79
  in humans, 79
  reproductive studies, 77t, 78
  specialized studies, 77t, 78–79
  structure–activity relationships, 79
  subchronic, 77t, 78
Toxicologist, 50
Toxicology, developmental, 27
Toxins, natural, in food, 249, 260–61
Trace elements, health effects, 191t, 198
Transportation, energy needs, 314
Trichinellosis, foodborne transmission, 252b, 253f
Trickling filters and towers, 235
Trihalomethanes, cancer and, 229b
Tropical parasitic disease, 57
Tuberculosis
  among hospital workers, 361
  housing conditions and, 289–90
  resurgence, HIV/AIDS and, 60
Tumor, primary, 74
Turkey, Lower Seyhan Irrigation Project
  environmental impact assessment, 141b
  malaria and, 323–24
Typhoid, transmission, 212–13, 251

Ultraviolet radiation (UVR), 87–89
  carcinogenicity, 76b, 88
  health effects, 88–89, 377, 378f
  ozone depletion and, 375–77, 378f
  protection against, 377
  sources, 88
  types, 375, 376f
Uncertainty, sources of, 106, 107t
Uncertainty factors, dose–response
    relationship, 123, 125–27, 125t, 127f
United Kingdom, industrial development, 11–12
United Nations
  Agenda 21, 7
  Universal Declaration of Human Rights, 8
United Nations Conference on Human
    Settlements, 237
United Nations Environmental Program
    (UNEP)
  Global Environmental Project, 18
  International Register of Potentially Toxic
    Chemicals, 61–62
United States, air quality standards, 202, 203t
United States Environmental Protection
    Agency (EPA), risk communication
    rules, 150t
Universal Declaration of Human Rights, 8
Unsaturated aliphatic hydrocarbons, 63
Upflow anaerobic sludge blanket reactors, 235

Uranium
  mining, health hazards, 326
  for nuclear energy, 325, 326
Urban areas
  air pollution, 201, 202, 202t, 298–300, 299f, 300f, 301b, 331
  energy needs, 314
  "Healthy Cities" approach, 306–10, 307b
  poverty, 297, 298f
  psychosocial hazards, 102–3
  sanitation, 231, 233, 233t
  water supply, 233t
Urban ecosystem
  basic health requirements, 282, 285–86
  DPSEEA framework, 282, 283b–285b
  sustainable, 282
Urbanization, 297–306
  factors affecting, 294–95, 294t
  infrastructural requirements, 297–98
  trends, 293, 293f, 294t
UVR. *See* Ultraviolet radiation (UVR)

Valuation methods
  contingent, 173, 175
  cost-of-illness approach, 175
Vanadium exposure, health effects, 198
Vapor, 186
Vasculitis, vibration, 85
Vector-borne disease
  environmental management, 324
  global warming and, 382, 384b
  spread, 57, 59
Vegetable matter, combustion, indoor air
    pollution from, 315
Vehicles
  motor. *See* Motor vehicles
  nonmotorized, 301b
Ventilated improved pituitary latrine, 231, 232, 232b
Ventilation
  general (dilution), control at source by, 152b, 153
  local exhaust, control along the path by, 154, 155f
Vibration
  arm and hand, 85
  health effects, 82–83, 85
Vibrio cholerae outbreaks, 382, 383b
Vinyl chloride
  and cancer, 112b
  metabolism, 70b
Violence
  intentional, 100
  political, 100
Viral disease
  foodborne, 251
  global warming and, 383b
  waterborne, 225t
Viruses
  carcinogenicity, 76b